ESSENTIALS FOR THE

EMERGENCY MEDICAL RESPONDER

ESSENTIALS FOR THE

EMERGENCY MEDICAL RESPONDER

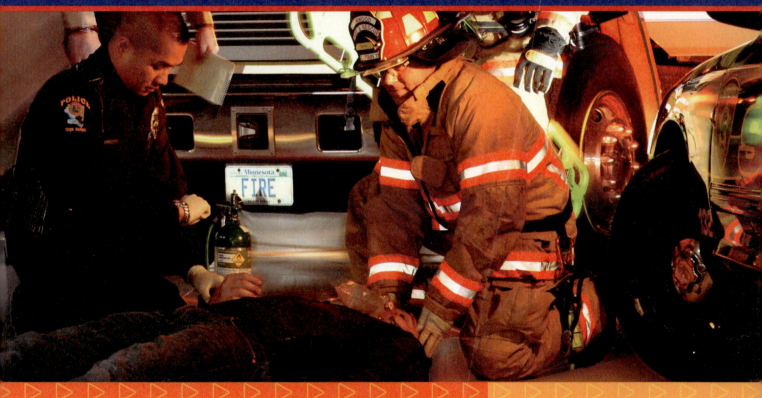

Joseph A. Grafft & Katherine Kuzma Grafft

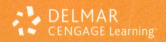

DELMAR
CENGAGE Learning®

Australia • Brazil • Japan • Korea • Mexico • Singapore • Spain • United Kingdom • United States

DELMAR
CENGAGE Learning™

Essentials for the Emergency Medical Responder
Joseph Allen Grafft and Katherine Kuzma Grafft

Vice President, Editorial: Dave Garza

Director of Learning Solutions: Sandy Clark

Senior Acquisitions Editor: Janet E. Maker

Managing Editor: Larry Main

Product Manager: Ramona J. Witcher

Editorial Assistant: Amy Wetsel

Vice President, Marketing: Jennifer Ann Baker

Marketing Director: Deborah Yarnell

Senior Marketing Manager: Erin Coffin

Senior Production Director: Wendy Troeger

Production Manager: Mark Bernard

Senior Content Project Manager: Jennifer Hanley

Senior Art Director: Casey Kirchmayer

For product information and technology assistance, contact us at
Cengage Learning Customer & Sales Support, 1-800-354-9706
For permission to use material from this text or product,
submit all requests online at **www.cengage.com/permissions**
Further permissions questions can be e-mailed to
permissionrequest@cengage.com

Library of Congress Control Number: 2011923723

ISBN-13: 978-1-4354-8784-0

ISBN-10: 1-4354-8784-2

Delmar
5 Maxwell Drive
Clifton Park, NY 12065-2919
USA

Cengage Learning is a leading provider of customized learning solutions with office locations around the globe, including Singapore, the United Kingdom, Australia, Mexico, Brazil, and Japan. Locate your local office at:
international.cengage.com/region

Cengage Learning products are represented in Canada by Nelson Education, Ltd.

To learn more about Delmar, visit **www.cengage.com/delmar**

Purchase any of our products at your local college store or at our preferred online store **www.cengagebrain.com**

Notice to the Reader

Publisher does not warrant or guarantee any of the products described herein or perform any independent analysis in connection with any of the product information contained herein. Publisher does not assume, and expressly disclaims, any obligation to obtain and include information other than that provided to it by the manufacturer. The reader is expressly warned to consider and adopt all safety precautions that might be indicated by the activities described herein and to avoid all potential hazards. By following the instructions contained herein, the reader willingly assumes all risks in connection with such instructions. The publisher makes no representations or warranties of any kind, including but not limited to, the warranties of fitness for particular purpose or merchantability, nor are any such representations implied with respect to the material set forth herein, and the publisher takes no responsibility with respect to such material. The publisher shall not be liable for any special, consequential, or exemplary damages resulting, in whole or part, from the readers' use of, or reliance upon, this material.

Printed in the United States of America
1 2 3 4 5 6 7 15 14 13 12 11

DEDICATION

My words cannot express my intense thanks to my wife Kathy, co-author of this text, for her dedication and sacrifice to making this project a success. She has been by my side as an encourager and helper and is the real reason this work is completed. With almost 40 years of health care experience, Kathy continues to be a wonderful, dedicated health care professional who is extremely competent and never stops caring for her patients.

To my dear friend Dr. Mike Wilcox, who has been my medical director for many years and is always there for me.

To all the hard working and dedicated career and volunteer EMRs serving their communities and providing a much needed safety net. They are an inspiration to present and future EMR providers, as well as to me.

J.A.G.

To my husband Joe who has spent countless hours in the field of EMS as a professional provider, educator, volunteer, and nationally recognized leader. He has inspired, encouraged, and mentored many EMS providers as well as myself. He has taught not only the importance of being a caring professional but has also consistently practiced it. Joe's impact on the EMS field has been called a legacy by his peers, and he deserves that honor because of his selflessness, contributions, and dedication.

To our children, Jason and Jessica, who spent many family outings in EMS-related activities and who have become competent and caring in the field of EMS.

K.K.G.

TABLE OF CONTENTS

FOREWORD

In 37 years as a medical director for several Emergency Medical Responder organizations, I have found the need for textbooks that properly prepare my crews for the work they will be doing in the field. The text must be up-to-date, easy to understand, and complemented with pictures and graphics. It must be concise to a point, where it can be easily used as a reference.

The text, *Essentials for the Emergency Medical Responder*, authored by Joe and Kathy Grafft, fulfills all of the requirements that I have mentioned. The book is easy to read. It is full of pictures and diagrams that beautifully complement the topics in each chapter. It has bullet point summaries that can be used as references as the Emergency Medical Responder moves from the role of student to the role of provider.

I believe you will agree with me that *Essentials for the Emergency Medical Responder*, written by seasoned EMS educators, will become a valuable tool for your EMS organizations. It may also become an increasingly important resource as Emergency Medical Responders assume a greater role in provision of patient care in underserved communities throughout our nation.

Michael R. Wilcox, MD,
FACEP, FAAFP

PREFACE

THE INTENT OF THIS BOOK

As a student taking this course, it is the authors' desire for you to become an excellent health care provider, advance in your technical skills and knowledge base, and be able to demonstrate a caring attitude to the patients you are called to serve. Because many times you are the first trained responder on the scene, safety and critical thinking skills will be necessary for both you and other emergency providers to properly manage and assess virtually any patient with whom you come in contact. This text will equip you with the necessary tools to provide excellent care, and above all else, through the practice of personal and scene safety, prepare you to *go home* after the call. Our vision is that through this text, an instructor with passion can facilitate the learning process and be awe inspiring to the student.

The current EMR has no comparison to the first responder of yesteryear. There is a rich history dating back to the 1970s with a course called "Crash Injury Management," which was offered primarily to firefighters and law enforcement. The next evolution came about in the 1980s, when the "First Responder" course opened the door to many different providers who not only cared for trauma and medical patients but also worked as athletic trainers, formed industry emergency response teams, or assisted at various community-sponsored events. New curriculum developed in the late 1990s did not include use of oxygen, suction, airway adjuncts, and AEDs. It became apparent that the scope of practice needed to evolve and provide additional tools for the initial responders to work effectively at trauma and medical scenes as the first link in the emergency response system. Hence the creation of the "Emergency Medical Responder" course.

Essentials for the Emergency Medical Responder is intended to bridge the gap and provide a stepping stone to allow the EMR to move up the provider level. This book meets and exceeds the 2009 National EMS Education Standards, which provide the essential breadth and depth of each provider level building on the skills and knowledge of the previous level. It prepares the EMR in all domains—cognitive, psychomotor, and affective. Of utmost importance is your willingness as an EMR to *dare to care* about the people who are sick or injured and temporarily entrusted to your care.

WHY WE WROTE THIS BOOK

We both have a deep burning desire and passion to educate the first trained person on the scene, which is often the EMR. We have taught thousands of students and hundreds of classes over the years, and the EMR classes have been the most enjoyable. The EMR is truly the individual who can make a tremendous difference in the outcome for the patient, whether a medical or trauma patient. Proper assessment and management of airway, breathing, and circulation; proper spinal stabilization; secondary or rapid survey issues; and a rapid transport decision can reduce death and disability.

We have used several different first responder texts and presently, emergency medical responder books in university, public, law enforcement, and firefighter classes, and none has measured up to what *Essentials for the Emergency Medical Responder* can provide. We had the desire, and frankly the vision, to move outside the box of the current educational and academic setting to create a useable, easily comprehensible, organized book that truly meets the needs of today's EMR.

This text includes expanded sections on patient assessment, patient communication techniques, emphasis on proper documentation, working with special populations, triaging patients, and scenarios for the EMR student to critically think through a medical, trauma, or environmental event. The incorporated scenarios reinforce learning and critical thinking as well as provide exercises to simulate during classroom time. We have placed Competency Skill Sheets in Appendix B, and a PCR documentation form in Appendix C. These are also available online at CengageBrain.com (see Note in Appendices) for your convenience, and will serve to reinforce the essential skills required of an Emergency Medical Responder.

You, the future EMR, hold the tools of your training to benefit the patients to whom you will come in contact. You can demonstrate care, concern, and empathy for both physically and emotionally hurting patients. You can effectively maintain safety standards and insist on safety as a primary goal so all EMRs can return home safely. Finally, you the EMR are entrusted with the awesome responsibility of lessening pain and suffering and being there with a comforting touch to those who desperately need you in their time of crisis—and as authors, we are privileged to be a part of that process.

SPECIAL FEATURES

Essentials for the Emergency Medical Responder has many features intended to motivate the student to read and learn the knowledge and skills presented in each chapter. Some of these include:

- The text follows the latest National EMS Education Standards, as well as the 2010 AHA CPR guidelines and the CDC Field Triage Scheme.
- The safety and wellness of the EMR and others on the scene are emphasized.
- Information the EMR will need for an organized systematic approach to assessment, interventions, and critical thinking in the field is included. Easy-to-follow patient assessment flow charts are included.
- Concise information of anatomy, physiology, and an emphasis on pathophysiology allows for enhanced understanding and application.
- There is heavy concentration on communication and patient documentation with scenarios and a sample PCR form for implementation.
- There are bullet point summaries that can be used as references as the emergency medical responder moves from the role of student to that of provider.
- Review questions at the end of each chapter are helpful for evaluating student knowledge of the concepts presented in the chapter. In addition to the review questions, Chapters 8, 10, and 11 have exercises that encourage the student to apply critical thinking skills and test the student on assessment, management, and documentation.

- There is an introduction to medical terminology. EMRs must know certain medical terms so they can understand human anatomy, physiology, and pathophysiology; properly assess trauma and medical patients; and communicate with hospital staff. *Essentials for the Emergency Medical Responder* attempts to introduce the medical terms at appropriate times in a manner that the EMR can understand and explain to the patient.
- Pictorial step-by-step skills use photos and descriptions to allow the student to see the proper methods used to perform the essential functions of your profession. Each skill is included at the end of the chapter to avoid interrupting the flow of learning and is referenced in the applicable discussion within the chapter. Use these as a guide to practice skills in a lab along with competency skill sheets found in the appendices.
- Amplification of special populations including obstetrics; pediatric; neonates; geriatric; and behavioral, physical, and cognitive challenges. The student is introduced to wheelchair considerations and various medical devices they may encounter while performing a secondary survey. Handling behavioral crises in patients experiencing substance abuse and psychological and emotional episodes is addressed. Specifics are provided in the awareness of assessment and management of the patient of abuse and neglect.

INSTRUCTOR RESOURCES (CD-ROM)

ISBN: 978-1-4354-8783-3

The *Instructor Resources CD to accompany Essentials for the Emergency Medical Responder* provides a variety of tools for instructors to enhance the learning experience and to assist students in learning the essential skills and information needed to prepare them for the field. Our Instructor Resources helps you, the educator, facilitate student learning within the guidelines of the National EMS Education Standards and the 2010 AHA guidelines. Assistance in planning and implementing your programs for the most efficient use of time and other resources is provided. Tools on the CD-ROM include:

- **Administration** section includes a description of the course materials included on the CD in addition to practical information and advice for conducting an EMR course.

- **Correlation to the National EMS Educational Standards and D.O.T. Paramedic Curriculum** maps out the EMR/First Responder content and provides instructors with the chapters and pages where the corresponding content is covered in the book.

- **Lesson Plans** include an outline of each chapter, with correlations to the accompanying Power-Point® presentations. A helpful guide for classroom instruction, they are provided in Word format so instructors may revise according to local practice variations and regional and state medical protocols.

- **Answers to Chapter Review Questions** at the end of each chapter are provided, as well as answers to assessment *Scenarios* and Glasgow Coma Scale *Exercises* at the end of Chapters 8, 10, and 11.

- **PowerPoint®Presentations** include a complete presentation for each chapter that combines key points with photos and graphics. Each presentation correlates directly to a corresponding Lesson Plan.

- **Computerized Test Bank** contains hundreds of questions and covers the content in each chapter. ExamView® format allows instructors to manage test administration in the classroom. Instructors may create or edit tests based on existing questions and add or delete questions to fit local practice variations and regional and state medical protocols—all in this user-friendly program.

- **Competency Skill Sheets** highlight skills necessary for Emergency Medical Responder practice and provide a baseline for skills learning and for testing. Each competency skill sheet provides a breakdown of the critical thinking steps involved in successfully completing a skill and is included in Word format to allow instructors to add specifics based on their local requirements and regional and state protocols and procedures.

- **Image Gallery** contains photos and graphics from the book and offers an additional resource for instructors to enhance classroom presentations.

ABOUT THE AUTHORS

For information on topics or to provide feedback on the textbook, please check out the authors' website at http://www.customizedsafetytraining.com.

JOSEPH ALLEN GRAFFT, MS, NREMT

Joe Grafft's interest and eventual career as an EMS provider began with his father Charlie Grafft, a police chief and later county sheriff. Despite having little and living in a boxcar without running water the first 12 years of Joe's life, his father modeled volunteerism. In 1959, at the age of 12, Joe began taking first aid and rescue classes from his father and became part of a junior rescue squad. Instilled in him was the importance of care and concern for the patient. His father's words of wisdom still resound after all these years, "Have a reason for what you do and treat everyone with respect and dignity!" How true these words are today!

In 1965, Mr. Grafft began working for an ambulance service while attending college. In 1968, he became a CPR instructor with the Minnesota Rescue and First Aid Association and a member of the Minnesota Para-rescue team. He became a Nationally Registered EMT in 1974 and shortly thereafter became a licensed EMS instructor and a Regional Faculty for the AHA. Receiving a bachelor's degree and later a master's degree in health education and EMS management, Joe began his professional teaching career in the high school setting while continuing to work in the ambulance service and as an athletic trainer. Joe's passion for the youth in EMS was demonstrated when he started a high school program in 1976, called Opportunities in Emergency Health Care (OEC). This program trained high school students to be EMTs and was the first such program in a high school in the nation. The high school had two ambulances staffed by paramedics and EMTs who mentored the students. The National Registry of EMTs awarded the OEC Program with the outstanding EMT training site. The ambulances made 5,000 runs per year. These same students won ten consecutive World Championships in EMS. The OEC program is still in existence 35 years later and has expanded to several other high schools in Minnesota. Joe has always realized the importance of working with youth as he continues to be a guest lecturer in high schools.

Mr. Grafft became the EMS director in 1988 for a hospital paramedic system. In 1990, he became the first EMS manager for the Minnesota State Board of Vocational Education—Fire Center, later becoming the Minnesota State Colleges and Universities, Fire/EMS/Safety Center, Chancellors Office. In this position as an EMS manager, he supervised and provided leadership for 53 campuses.

Grafft is past president of the National Association of EMS Educators (NAEMSE), International Rescue and Emergency Care Association, and Minnesota Ambulance Association; past chair of the AHA-ECC Committee in Minnesota; author of the *Issues in Spinal Care* course; secretary of Advocates of EMS; current treasurer of the National Association of EMS Educators; served on the NREMT Board of Directors for 13 years; and a conference presenter. He has written several articles for EMS journals and has authored a book titled *EMS in a Secured Facility*. Joe is a Nationally Certified Instructor for NAEMSE and is licensed by the Minnesota EMS Regulatory Board.

Currently, Mr. Grafft is a community faculty member at Metropolitan State University, School of Law Enforcement and Criminal Justice, a position he has held since 1995. He coordinates education and training and is the chief instructor for the Minnesota Department of Corrections, the Minnesota Department of Natural Resources, and the Civilian Corps (CCC). Grafft is a Safety Compliance Specialist for XCEL Energy and teaches the San Diego Border Patrol in basic and advanced wilderness medicine. Joe and Kathy provide EMS training through their company Customized Safety Training, LLC.

KATHERINE KUZMA GRAFFT, BS, RN, OCN

Kathy Grafft has been a health care professional since 1973, receiving a BS degree from the University of Minnesota. As a Registered Nurse, she has had extensive experience working as a CCRN (critical care RN) in a Level One Trauma Center and has expertise in working with special needs populations.

Ms. Grafft's career began in 1974 by teaching first aid for the American Red Cross. Soon after, she became a CPR instructor and an NREMT. Kathy and Joe have spent countless hours over the years volunteering their time teaching EMS to thousands of people from communities, churches, organizations, businesses, and schools. She has been blessed by serving internationally with medical missions in Guatemala, Ecuador, and India. She, along with Joe, had the privilege of teaching EMS courses in Tanzania and the Philippines.

Ms. Grafft's certifications include EMR instructor, BLS Training Center faculty instructor, ACLS, PALS, and OCN. Presently, she is an RN educator at North

Hennepin Community College as well as works as a perioperative and infusion/oncology nurse. Kathy continues instructing in EMS for Customized Safety Training.

ACKNOWLEDGMENTS FROM THE AUTHORS

Essentials for the Emergency Medical Responder would not have been possible without the support, guidance, and participation of the contributors and reviewers, and for this, we owe them our sincere thanks.

CONTRIBUTING AUTHORS

We are grateful to have the following contributors participate in the writing of *Essentials for the Emergency Medical Responder*.

Steven Collins, DOM, RN, EMT-P, was a paramedic in Las Vegas and Florida before becoming the director of Continuing Education for Emergency Medicine at Valencia College in Orlando. He then became an RN and held the position of education director for Highlands Hospital in North Carolina. After 20 years in Western medicine, Steve returned to Chinese medical school and practiced for ten years in Minnesota before returning to Florida. In addition to his practice, Dr. Collins continues to teach.

Christopher C. Miller, MS in clinical psychology, BA in business management, associate's degree in engineering, EMT-P, retired from a major metropolitan fire department and a small wild land urban interface fire department. Mr. Miller has more than 30 years of broad experience in the delivery of patient-centered, high-quality emergency medical services, fire suppression, technical rescue, and hazardous materials response and mitigation.

Chris Nollette, EdD, NREMTP- LP, has been involved in EMS since 1979. He has worked as a field paramedic for a large metropolitan service, a flight medic, and a SWAT medic and served on the special medical detail for the city when the current sitting president came to town. Dr. Nollette's degree is in curriculum and instruction with a minor in adult education. He has served as the president of the National Association of EMS educators, a board member for national accreditation, a founding member of the American Heart

Association's Scientific Sub-committee on Education, and many other EMS- and fire-related committees. Nollette is the current director of the EMS program for Moreno Valley College, part of the Riverside Community College District System in southern California.

David M. Schwartz, MA in educational leadership from the University of St. Thomas, had a 34-year career in law enforcement and more than 24 years as chief of police and director of public safety, Forest Lake Minnesota. Currently, Mr. Schwartz is a community facility member at Metropolitan State University and Compliance Training Specialist with XCEL Energy. Schwartz lives in Hugo, Minnesota.

CONTRIBUTING EDITOR

We are grateful to have the following contributor participate in the editing of *Essentials for the Emergency Medical Responder*: **Jason A. Grafft, M.Ac, NREMT**

REVIEWERS

To the reviewers, who provided an honest evaluation of the content in this book and guidance, we extend our appreciation. Their comments helped us keep our facts technically accurate and with the latest of standards. We, the authors, sincerely want to thank these reviewers for their time and effort.

John W. McBride, MD, FACC, FAHA, retired
Chair, MN ECC Regional Committee; Regional Faculty, BLS
Instructor, ACLS Instructor, First Responder Instructor
Saint Paul, MN

Tony Caliguire, associate's degree in science, NREMT-P
Instructor for Hudson Valley Community College Paramedic Program
Troy, NY
Lieutenant Paramedic for Village of Scotia Fire Department
Scotia, NY

Courtney Moreno, BS in biology, UC Berkeley, 2001; NREMT
CPR and Basic EMT Instructor (AHA certified)
Employed by UCSF

Basic EMT Clinical Instructor at UCLA (2009-2010) and CIEMT (2008-2010)
Field Training Officer, McCormick Ambulance (2008-2010)
San Francisco, California

Larry Torrey, RN, EMT-P
Tufts Medical Center
Department of Emergency Medicine
Boston, MA

Michael Wilcox, MD, FACEP, FAAFP
EMS Educator for Minnesota State Colleges/ University Systems
New Prague, MN

Bill Young
Lead Paramedic Instructor
Garden City Community College
Holcomb, KY

THANK YOU FROM THE AUTHORS

We want to single out the Linwood Township Fire Department, Linwood Township, Minnesota, who donated their time and expertise to demonstrate many of the skills presented in this text. We cannot thank them enough!

Also, many thanks go out to the STEP Program of Forest Lake Area Schools—District 831 of Forest Lake, Minnesota. We are grateful to the teachers and their students, severely challenged young adults, for sharing vital information and serving as models for the book.

Thanks to Tony Orrechia, MD, for sharing his expertise on special populations.

We would like to express our sincere thanks to Delmar, Cengage Learning for this opportunity and for their patience and guidance through the entire process. We especially want to thank Ramona Witcher, Janet Maker, Amy Wetsel, Casey Kirchmayer, Jennifer Starr, Jennifer Hanley, and the photographer Michael Gallitelli.

CLOSING THOUGHTS FROM JOE AND KATHY

We wish you well as you begin your new adventure and experience the rewards of becoming a skilled, dedicated, and caring Emergency Medical Responder.

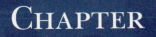

CHAPTER 1

EMERGENCY MEDICAL RESPONDER AND EMERGENCY MEDICAL SERVICES

LEARNING OBJECTIVES

By the end of this chapter, the reader should be able to:

- Name the components that make up Emergency Medical Services (EMS).
- Identify the purpose of the public safety answering points (PSAP).
- Define medical oversight.
- Explain the difference between quality improvement (QI) and quality assurance (QA).
- Describe the roles and responsibilities of an Emergency Medical Responder (EMR).
- Explain how ethics affect interactions with patients, health care professionals, and the public.
- Identify three types of medical errors.
- Explain the three types of consents.
- Differentiate between abandonment and negligence.
- Explain the Good Samaritan Law.
- Define culture of emergency services.

INTRODUCTION

An Emergency Medical Responder (EMR) is an individual who has special training in emergency medicine for prehospital care. The EMR is an essential part of the Emergency Medical Services (EMS) and is often the first trained provider to arrive on the scene. Training includes knowledge and skills in basic medical and trauma assessment and management, airway and oxygen management, bleeding control, cardiopulmonary resuscitation (CPR), and defibrillation. An EMR obtains training according to the United States Department of Transportation's (DOT) (governmental agency responsible for safe transportation on U.S. roadways) current guidelines. Along with being trained, the EMR needs to be professional, following the legal and ethical scope of practice for the EMR. As an EMR, you may be the patient's first contact with the medical system, and your actions will likely affect the outcome of the patient's condition. You may not only affect a patient's medical or trauma outcome but also—and more importantly—you may affect the patient's lasting opinion of the entire emergency medical services profession.

What Is EMS?

Emergency Medical Services (EMS) is a coordinated network of professionals whose function is to provide a variety of medical services, such as prehospital medical and trauma care and transportation for those in need of emergency care. The level of service dispatched to an emergency call will vary based on the need of the patient, the population and topography of the service area, and local standards of care. The level of EMS system varies widely in different cities, regions, and states. Typically, the EMS system is initiated with a call for service and ends with the delivery of the patient to a hospital (Figure 1-1). The level of care a patient receives en route depends on the training of the EMS service provider, available resources, the patient's condition, and local protocols.

Components of EMS

EMS is the gateway to the health care system and has components in the private and public sectors. EMS may be provided by a public service, private service, third service, or a combination.

Public EMS

Public EMS is EMS services provided by a city, county, or other political subdivision funded by a combination of user fees and taxes. These services may be provided as part of a local fire or police department, or third service. Considerations that guide the public services include the size of the service area, population, revenue available, and the community standards for delivery of the services. Available funding sources often dictate the level of services provided as well as what type of delivery service to be used.

The **fire-based EMS** is one in which EMS services are provided by fire departments. It has a strong history with EMS. From career fire departments to volunteer services, answering medical and trauma related calls is considered part of their duties. The fire service often has special units established for medical response.

Private EMS

For many areas, a **private EMS service** is in place to handle emergencies. These services are both for-profit and not-for-profit operations that may or may not work in conjunction with public services. Hospitals are commonly providers of such private services. These private services often offer more than emergency response. For some, medical transfers are a large part of their funding base.

Third Service

Third service is an EMS operation not integrated within other agencies such as fire or police, which may serve as the backup or primary responder. Large cities such as New York City and Boston have third service agencies that function as primary responders. In other locations, a fire-based service may arrive on the scene and discover the call is for a different level of service than they provide. The fire-based provider would then notify a third service to handle the call while providing patient care until they arrive.

Other EMS Response Positions

In addition to the previously described EMS providers, many EMRs work in industrial settings as part of an **Emergency Response Team (ERT)**. ERTs are trained to handle emergency responses specific to the industry with whom they are employed. Additionally, EMRs are used in wilderness medicine response and athletic training and as standby at community events.

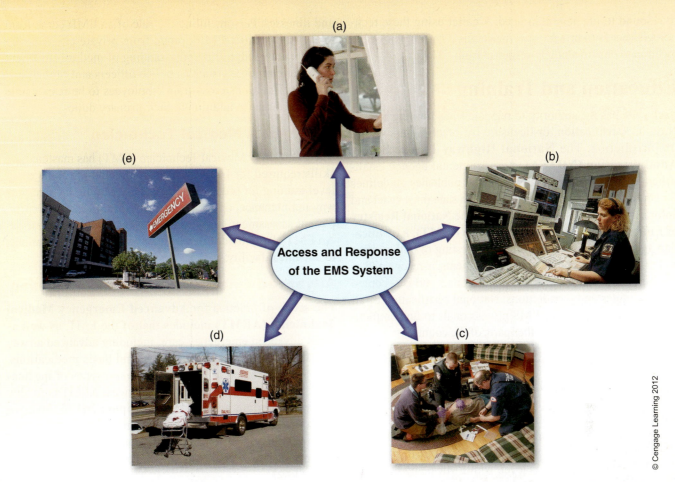

Figure 1-1 Access and response of the emergency medical services (EMS) system: (a) The EMS system is initiated when someone recognizes there is a problem or emergency and calls for help. (b) An emergency medical dispatcher answering a call. (c) The function of an EMS system is to provide a variety of medical services, such as out-of-hospital medical and trauma care. (d) Additional EMS resources continue the care and transport of the patient. (e) The EMS system ends with the delivery of the patient to a hospital or medical facility.

© Cengage Learning 2012

Public Safety Answering Points

Dispatch of EMS services is most often initiated with a 9-1-1 call to a **Public Safety Answering Point (PSAP)** call center. This center is a local dispatch office staffed with professionals employed to receive 9-1-1 calls from the public and dispatch the required service to the caller as soon as possible. PSAPs may be part of a sheriff's office, local fire or police department, an ambulance service, or a regional office covering all emergency services. Often PSAPs are part of county government, but large cities, state agencies, and governmental services may have their own call centers.

The 9-1-1 System

Most calls for medical assistance come via the **9-1-1 system**, the U.S. national emergency number. Not all telephone systems are configured to dial 9-1-1 directly. You will need to know if a prefix is required to reach an outside line in your service area before being able to connect to the 9-1-1 system. In some buildings, for example, the caller may need to dial a "9" first to get an outside phone line.

Enhanced 9-1-1

Hard-wired telephones have **enhanced 9-1-1**. With enhanced 9-1-1, the operator receiving the call immediately sees the name and address associated with the telephone number and what fire, police, and rescue agencies serve that address. This enhanced 9-1-1 system provides the dispatcher with useful information about the resident or address that is then relayed to the responding agency.

Technology and 9-1-1

Technologies such as cellular telephones and global positioning satellite (GPS) services, such as OnStar, have made it easier to contact a PSAP in an emergency. These systems, however, have ongoing problems. Calls from cellular telephones and GPS services are routed to the closet PSAP tower. At times, the tower routing the call may be in a different jurisdiction or even a different state from where the call originated. Without reliable data and directions, many factors such as large buildings, topography, rural areas, or unfamiliar cities make it difficult for emergency personnel to respond to the person in need. A caller using these technologies needs to provide specific details regarding his or her location to ensure a timely response from EMS.

Education and Training

Each state has the authority to regulate EMS training by registration, certification, or licensure for practitioners within its jurisdiction. The **National Highway Traffic Safety Administration (NHTSA)**, a governmental agency established to make national highways safer, publishes guidelines for education and training; however, each state must enact and enforce its own rules and regulations. The **National Registry of Emergency Medical Technicians (NREMT)**, a certification agency established to standardize testing of both written and practical skills competency requirements, is recognized as the national standard for EMS professionals and is accepted by most states and jurisdictions. National certification of all levels makes it easier for EMS professionals to find employment locally as well as in other parts of the country.

EMS Training Levels

Even with national certification, EMS employees should expect any jurisdiction in which they work to have their own **scope of practice**, which is the legal description of the limit of care that an EMS provider can give based on the provider's EMS training level and certification. Every EMS provider level builds on the previous level, with EMR being the entry level.

Educational requirements vary from state to state. Although NHTSA publishes minimum recommended educational guidelines for training, some states and agencies choose to exceed these recommendations; others do not. Typically, EMS professionals need to recertify every two years. It is largely up to the EMR providers to keep track of their continuing education hours and recertification deadlines. State EMS offices or local agencies may assist EMS providers with the process.

Emergency Medical Responder

EMR is recognized as the entry level for emergency medical service. The U.S. Department of Transportation recognized a need for responders trained to the EMR level, which is beyond first aid but not as high as the next established level, the **Emergency Medical Technician (EMT)**. The Department of Transportation (DOT) was designated by Congress as the lead agency after a "White Paper" written in 1966 established a need for national criteria for EMS. Because ambulances travel on the roadways, Congress thought it was logical to place EMS under the DOT. It was soon realized that ambulance providers did more than respond to emergencies on the roadways, so their role was expanded to consider emergencies in all environments. Agencies then began to employ personnel trained to recognize life threats, provide basic life support interventions, and mobilize necessary resources to appropriately assess and treat patients' injuries

and illnesses. Persons filling the role of an EMR come from every walk of life. EMRs range from private citizens who desire a knowledge and understanding of medical treatment to career employees, such as police officers and firefighters. Many jurisdictions cross-train employees to be responsible for EMR duties in addition to their primary duties.

Emergency Medical Technician

The Emergency Medical Technician (EMT) has mastered the skills required for EMR and has completed the basic entry level training for prehospital care. This training includes airway maintenance, oxygen administration, bleeding control, patient assessment, and limited medication administration. An EMT also provides rescue and transportation of patients to a medical facility.

Advanced Emergency Medical Technician

The scope of practice for **Advanced Emergency Medical Technician (AEMT)** includes that of the EMT, as well as some advanced emergency care, including advanced airway management, intravenous therapy, and basic medications. AEMTs are trained to administer several types of medications and place advanced airway devices. AEMTs are able to provide certain **advanced life support (ALS)**, invasive lifesaving procedures and interventions. AEMTs fill a valuable role in EMS systems that may not be financially able to support a large number of emergency responders trained to a higher level.

Paramedic

Paramedic is the highest level of training for prehospital providers. A paramedic must have ALS training in airway management, cardiac monitoring, and administration of medications. Paramedics have typically completed college-level courses covering comprehensive patient assessment, advanced airway management, intravenous access techniques, expanded medication administration, and cardiac arrest management. In the private sector, ALS ambulance services and fire departments are the largest employer of paramedics today.

Authorization to Practice

Each state independently regulates the practice of medicine within its borders. EMR professionals are certified to practice in a specific state, county, or region.

Medical Director

An EMR works on his or her own certification in conjunction with medical direction from a licensed physician. Each EMS agency has a **medical director**, a person of the highest medical authority, usually a physician licensed as a Doctor of Osteopathy (DO) or a Medical Doctor (MD), who provides direction of on-scene activities, establishes written protocols for EMS providers, and grants variances to individual providers that allow them to exceed their standard scope of practice. The medical director also provides advice and medical oversight, which includes written and verbal instructions for prehospital patient care.

Protocols

Protocols are medical guidelines established by an agency's medical director or by a regulatory authority that play an important role in the delivery of EMS. Based on a carefully developed set of procedures, protocols form a decision tree that an EMR can follow. Without protocols, the responder would have to determine alone what procedures to perform and what techniques to use. The medical director may be able to expand or restrict the scope of practice for EMR providers in their system. If statewide protocols allow expansion of the scope of practice locally and the medical director chooses to expand the scope, he or she is responsible for training and verifying that every provider is able to competently perform every skill (Figure 1-2).

Quality Management

Quality management ensures not only the quality of the service but also the means by which to achieve the highest quality of service. Quality management is imperative to ensure patient safety and the reduction of errors. Quality management includes two components: **quality assurance (QA) and quality improvement (QI)**. QA in the EMS field is the monitoring and evaluation of all aspects of EMS services to ensure or improve the quality care the EMS system provides. For EMS, QI is a formal review and analysis of performance and processes within the EMS agency with the goal of reducing medical errors and needless loss of life. Part of this process is to make sure the EMR has the knowledge, tools, and

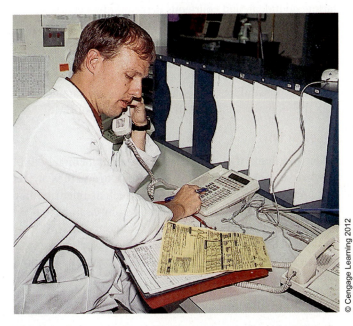

Figure 1-2 Medical directors are often involved in the training and scope of practice of emergency medical providers.

competencies to improve the quality of emergency medical care. With the assistance of the medical director and agency, it is the EMR's responsibility to stay up to date on training and advancements in technology and practice standards.

Policies and Procedures

For EMS staff to perform their duties, they must have a framework of written policies and procedures from which to work. **Policies** inform EMRs of what is expected and what is not allowed. Typically, EMS agencies have policies regarding personal conduct, driving emergency vehicles, drug and alcohol use, off-duty behavior, grooming, use of equipment, patient care practices, gratuities, and professional conduct. **Procedures** list the employer-required steps to follow when providing patient care. Common procedures for EMS agencies include proper use of specialized equipment; disposal of sharps and biohazards; and how to report exposures, medical errors, and omissions. Policies and procedures are to be routinely evaluated for QA to ensure they are meeting the needs of both the patients and the providers. Many organizations have a **sunset clause** that requires policies and procedures to be reviewed every three to five years or as they expire to keep them updated. Each agency writes, revises, and enacts its own set of policies and procedures to fit the conditions of the area it serves. It is imperative that EMRs ask a supervisor for clarification when unsure about a policy or procedure.

Roles and Responsibilities of the EMR

An EMR has many roles and responsibilities. EMRs must be ready, safe, caring, and professional.

Readiness

To meet the expected standards of both the EMS system and the public, EMRs must come to work ready to respond. Readiness is not just showing up to work on time. Readiness also involves being physically fit, being rested, and being alert to meet the demands of the position. The public expects EMRs to be fully trained and competent with each skill required in a medical emergency. That training includes classroom training and practical hands-on instruction, as shown in Figure 1-3. EMRs are responsible for keeping the provided equipment and supplies stocked and in working order and for being familiar with the operation of all equipment and supplies.

Safety

Safety is the responsibility of every EMR. To be part of the solution, EMS professionals must put their own personal safety first. Ignoring personal safety could make the provider become part of the problem rather than the solution. EMRs must realize that when faced with a dangerous situation, there will be both psychological and physiological changes

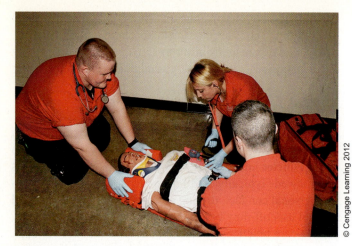

Figure 1-3 Emergency Medical Responders practicing in a skills lab.

that take place that can hamper both their thought processes and ability to react. Getting under control and keeping emotions intact will assist in performing the required duties. Without control, fine motor skills are decreased, field of vision narrows, and mistakes can be made that affect both the outcome for the patient and the EMR's own well-being. To be a part of the solution, the EMR must be able to safely enter the scene and keep the patient safe from further injury. After the EMR's safety is ensured, the next step is to provide for the safety of the patient and bystanders.

Caring for Patients

The initial treatment a patient receives has a strong influence on the outcome of the patient's condition. For many victims of medical and trauma emergencies, contact with emergency services is the first point of entry into the health care system. Most people have limited knowledge of what services EMS has to offer. Their only expectation is that they will receive care when they call for help.

Communication

Direct communication with the patient is a valuable resource for the EMR. Medical problems that may not be easily recognized are often verbally communicated to the EMR. Symptoms described by the patient can be indicators of an underlying condition that would not otherwise be perceived. EMR providers need to extend good verbal communication beyond just the patient to fellow responders, medical directors, and witnesses to the incident.

Patient Advocacy

The EMR must be a **patient advocate**, meaning a person who makes sure that the care a patient receives is in the patient's best interest. A victim of trauma or medical problems may be in a vulnerable position to accept care that he or she would not want under normal circumstances. On scene, this means ensuring that care provided to the patient is appropriate to his or her condition and sensitive to his or her requests.

The EMR must understand that the choices in caring for a patient should be made in the patient's best interest and not influenced or affected by the EMR's personal beliefs. Any personal biases that the EMR might have regarding race, religion, sexual orientation, or political views cannot be allowed to affect the care given to patients.

Continuous Care and Transfer

After you provide care for a patient, it is your responsibility to continue with that care until you are able to transfer their care to an equal or higher trained EMS provider. Transferring care is an important component of the service an EMR provides. Failure to do so is a criminal offense called patient abandonment. After you have started care for a patient, you must follow through with that care until your patient receives the higher level of care needed and expected.

Patient Confidentiality

While providing care, you will receive information about an individual that is private in nature. You have a legal responsibility to keep that information away from those who are not authorized to have it. Your must protect the patient's **confidentiality** or privacy and ensure that patient's medical information is given only to the patient's health care provider. Bystanders, friends, and even police officers and firefighters who are not involved are not entitled to the personal data of the patient. The only individuals who can receive personal data about the patient in your care are the EMS personnel or hospital staff to whom you turn over the patient's care.

Professionalism

EMR is considered a professional position. **Professionalism** is defined as the behavior, goals, or qualities such as a skilled, caring, confident, and courteous demeanor that characterize a medical professional. EMS demands and expects its members to act professionally on the job as well as in their personal lives. EMS professionals are held to higher standards than regular citizens. Understanding this expectation and accepting the responsibilities that go along with it are paramount for both the individual and organizational success of EMS.

Character

When you think of character, you should immediately think of what your personal core values are. **Core values** are the basic personal beliefs and behaviors, such as integrity, fairness, respect, honesty, courage, and compassion, that are considered important and necessary among the EMS profession. These values have a foundation based on personal integrity and should direct you in everything you say or do in your profession.

Ethical Behavior

This lifestyle is based on **ethical behavior**, doing what is right based on a set of moral principles and values. At times, it may be easier to claim to be ethical than to actually be ethical. The cost of doing what is right is often high, but the repercussions of being unethical greatly exceed that cost. EMRs need to rely on core values, especially in dealings with coworkers. Coworkers will form and maintain opinions of you based on how they perceive your behavior. You must conduct yourself on and off duty in a manner that is above reproach. The reckless use of chemicals, illegal acts, and lack of morals will not only ruin your credibility but also that of your agency.

Additional Responsibilities to Consider

In addition to the other responsibilities of the EMR, the interaction with bystanders and the use of on-scene bystander technology need to be taken into consideration.

Bystanders

Bystanders, both known and unknown by the patient, will be present at most scenes. It is likely that EMRs will interact with bystanders. Bystanders can potentially provide information as to their connection to the patient, whether they witnessed the incident, and if they know what happened to cause the injuries. All of these considerations will help the EMR more fully understand what information is available.

Technology

In today's electronic world, an EMR can be reasonably certain that pictures or video of the scene may be taken. Additionally, text messages may be sent describing what the sender perceives to be taking place. These bits of information can be used to give EMR providers an idea of what took place before EMS arrived, as well as during the incident response.

Medical Errors

Medical errors can be skill, knowledge, or rule based. **Skill-based errors** take place because the EMR failed to follow the correct procedures required to do the skill. This can be caused by the EMR's not knowing the correct methods required, failing to follow the correct procedures, or by taking shortcuts that may have saved time but resulted in a mistake being made. **Knowledge-based errors** occur when the EMR does not have the information needed to accomplish the skill. These mistakes occur when the EMR has not had the opportunity to receive the training or has failed to take advantage of new skills that are available. **Rule-based errors** occur when policies and procedures are not followed. If we allow ourselves to attempt skills that are outside of our scope of practice, we put the patient as well as our occupation in jeopardy. EMRs must understand the limitations to the procedures they are allowed to perform and stay within those limits.

After EMS professionals acknowledge that there will be failures, they must work to reduce the number of errors made. Reviewing run reports as well as encouraging the EMR to ask for assistance are important tools. Reducing errors takes a concentrated effort by both the EMR and the agency. The agency needs to have an environment that promotes education and training based on the best available technology to give EMRs the best chance for success.

Research Activities

In the performance of routine duties, an EMR collects data on the patient. **Research data** are essential and may consist of information such as the type of injuries or illnesses cared for, time and date of the occurrence, equipment used, treatment given, number of patients, conditions of patients, and delivery point of victims. **Data collection**, specific health care information collected and documented by the EMR, is used for consideration of future health care needs and practices. This information can lead to an expanded scope of practice, acquisition of new equipment, and additional training. These things all raise the quality of service delivered.

Legal Considerations

EMRs have legal standards to uphold in the performance of their duties. Consent, treatment of minors or emancipated minors, abandonment, negligence, assault and battery, and the Good Samaritan Law are all legal considerations that must be fully understood by EMRs.

Consent

After identifying themselves to the patient, the EMR should ask for permission or consent to provide care to the patient. **Consent** refers to voluntary agreement by a person to allow something to take place. The EMR should be familiar with informed consent, expressed consent, and implied consent.

Informed consent is consent given by a responsive patient after the EMR has provided an explanation of the risks and benefits of care or treatment that is to be given. **Expressed consent** is the act of a competent adult or emancipated minor verbally advising a medical provider to proceed with treatment. **Implied consent** is the legal presumption that a patient who is unable to verbally express agreement to treatment would agree to be treated in certain circumstances, such as potentially life-threatening injuries.

Treatment of Minors and Emancipated Minors

Generally, children younger than the age of 18 years, or age 21 years in some states, are considered minors and are not legally permitted to give consent for their medical treatment. Consent for treatment must be obtained from a parent or legal guardian. When a parent or legal guardian is not on the scene, an adult sibling, close relative, or school official can give permission under the doctrine of *in loco parentis*, which translates to "local parent." Parents often sign authorization forms giving other adults such as coaches or chaperones permission to provide consent for medical treatment for their child. If the child has a life-threatening or limb-threatening emergency situation and there is no parent or legal guardian available, implied consent allows the EMR to treat a minor.

If a minor is married, pregnant, in the military or financially independent, and no longer lives with a parent or guardian, he or she is considered to be an **emancipated minor** and is legally responsible for his or her own decisions and consequences of those decisions. It is important to know your state laws for the definition of a minor and emancipated minor in regard to age and situation.

Abandonment

In the prehospital setting, patient **abandonment** occurs when an EMR begins emergency medical assistance to a patient and then leaves that patient, still in need of care, unsupervised. If an EMR starts providing care to a patient, the EMR must continue to provide that care until services are no longer needed or until other adequate services have been secured to assume care for the patient. Failure to do so is a crime that may lead to suspension or loss of employment. Patient abandonment is considered a form of misconduct for the EMR, and the responder can be held responsible for any injuries that result. Patient treatment begun must also be continued even if the EMR becomes aware that the patient has no means to pay for the services rendered. Abandonment under these circumstances would be considered beyond the protection of the EMR's medical liability insurance.

Negligence

Negligence is the failure to provide care in a manner that upholds accepted medical practices and standards of care. Sometimes this failure results in the further injury of the patient. An EMR is negligent if he or she fails to treat a patient in a manner that is commonly accepted as the norm for his or her position. Negligence is the cause of most liability actions taken against EMRs and their agencies. Four common elements found in cases of negligence by an EMR include (1) the presence of a duty to act, (2) failure to act on that duty, (3) injuries or damages were received by the patient, and (4) actions or inactions of the EMR caused the injuries or damages to the patient. Successful suits against an EMR can result in both the loss of professional certifications as well as monetary penalties.

Assault and Battery

The EMR must remember that every patient who is legally and intellectually capable of making decisions has the right to refuse treatment. An EMR can be held liable if treatment is provided against a patient's will and without consent. Charges of assault and battery can be filed against the EMR. **Assault** refers to a case in which a patient is afraid that he or she may be touched without having given consent. **Battery** refers to actually unlawfully touching the patient against his or her wishes.

Good Samaritan Law

Some laws have been established to assist health care workers. The **Good Samaritan Law** is a law that is meant to provide legal protection for certain people who voluntarily administer emergency assistance to an injured or ill person in good faith and with reasonable care. In most states, a person is not obligated to render care unless such care is specified in a job description. However, some states consider it an act of negligence if a witness does not call for help.

The Good Samaritan Law helps a rescuer who is not expecting a reward and who provides reasonable care in good faith. An example of unreasonable care might be removing an injured person from a car without consent or necessity and in doing so aggravating the victim's injuries. Consent should be obtained from the victim if possible, but it is considered implied consent if the victim is unable to respond or, in the case of a minor, there is no parent or guardian present. The best ways to protect yourself from legal liability are to act on behalf of the victim, stay current in training, obtain professional help, and do not perform procedures that you are not trained to do. The Good Samaritan Law varies from jurisdiction to jurisdiction, so it is important to be familiar with your state's laws.

Culture of EMS

The **culture of emergency medical services** refers to the structure and history of an EMS agency. Each agency has a particular organizational structure and culture. The EMR must respect and understand this culture to become a part of it. For instance, whereas fire and law enforcement have a very structured system with specific hiring, training, and duty requirements, other private responders may be based at hospitals or other locations and develop their own culture. Additionally, industrial response teams have their distinct culture. No matter what culture you find yourself in, the most important component will always be the successful treatment of the patients. If you can keep that in mind, then the culture of your organization can be successful for both the patient and the responders.

SUMMARY

The EMR is an important part of the EMS system. Individuals who choose to enter this exciting field will find many challenges but will also receive many personal rewards for their duties performed. The standards to become an EMR are meant to establish minimum requirements for the position. A successful EMR must see this level is a starting point and must always strive to acquire the latest training and most up-to-date skills. Under the guidance of a medical director, an EMR will have the opportunity to compile the skills that best serve the community. EMRs must demonstrate ethical behavior and professionalism; keep up to date through continuing education; be aware of legal considerations regarding patient care; and above all, provide quality patient care within the individual's scope of practice.

REVIEW QUESTIONS

1. EMS units that are provided by a fire-based service are considered to be _____.
   a. Public units
   b. Third-party units
   c. Private units
   d. Community units

2. In EMS, what is the highest level of prehospital care?
   a. Paramedic
   b. Emergency medical responder
   c. Firefighter
   d. Emergency medical technician

3. What organization sets the standards for EMRs?
   a. National Association of Emergency Medical Technicians (NAEMT)
   b. National Highway Traffic Safety Administration (NHTSA)
   c. National Registry of Emergency Medical Technicians (NREMT)
   d. United States Association of Emergency Medical Services (USAEMS)

4. Typical recertification of training for an emergency medical responder is every _____.
   a. Two years
   b. Three years
   c. Eighteen months
   d. Four years

5. What position is in charge of the EMS system oversight?
   a. Paramedic supervisor
   b. Medical director
   c. Surgeon general
   d. Fire chief

6. What location answers 9-1-1 calls made from a cellular telephone?
   a. Local police department of the registered owner
   b. State highway patrol
   c. Nearest local Public Service Answering Point (PSAP)
   d. County sheriff of the registered owner

7. Before entering the scene of an unknown medical problem, what question should the EMR ask first?
   a. Is the scene safe?
   b. Is assistance on the way?
   c. Whose jurisdiction is this?
   d. Will my radio work at this location?

8. As an EMR, your *scope of practice* is established by the _____.
   a. Fire chief
   b. The agency that employs you
   c. The individual state and local community
   d. The training you have

9. The decision algorithm that an EMR follows is part of the _____.
   a. Agency rules
   b. Training standards
   c. National certifications
   d. Agency protocols

10. What kind of failure is caused by an EMR not understanding how to perform a medical procedure?
    a. Knowledge-based failure
    b. Skill-based failure
    c. Rules-based failure
    d. Scope of practice failure

11. Leaving a patient unattended in a life-threatening condition is an example of _____.

    a. Abandonment

    b. Triage

    c. Negligence

    d. Assessment

12. Allowing your personal biases to influence how you treat a patient is an example of _____.

    a. HIPPA standards

    b. Agency protocols

    c. Ethical standards

    d. Medical direction

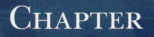
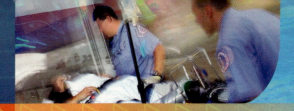

CHAPTER 2

SAFETY AND WELLNESS

LEARNING OBJECTIVES

By the end of this chapter, the reader should be able to:

- Name the three categories of health screenings.
- List methods for stress management.
- Explain routes of pathogen transmission.
- Define an exposure control plan.
- Explain types and uses of standard precautions.
- Describe safety recommendations for biohazards.
- Differentiate among cleaning, disinfection, and sterilization.
- Define hazardous materials.
- List steps for safely lifting and carrying patients.
- Name the methods for an emergency patient move and non-emergency patient move.

INTRODUCTION

Safety and wellness are defined as maintaining physical, emotional, and psychological health on the job. Safety and wellness are essential to a successful career in Emergency Medical Services (EMS) and should be considered as important as patient care. Emergency Medical Responders (EMRs) encounter, on a daily basis, critical and emotionally charged events that cause mental and physical stress to their bodies. EMRs should follow safety and wellness guidelines to protect themselves, their patients, and others involved in the incident.

EMRs should strive to provide quality care for every patient. However, quality patient care is dependent on EMRs taking care of themselves as well. This chapter discusses the principles of personal health, a safe working environment, and lifting and moving patients. EMRs must take personal responsibility to put into practice the principles of good health and safety.

Personal Health

Personal health is the state of your physical, medical, and psychological well-being. There are many ways to maintain a healthy body and a healthy mind. Before beginning any fitness program, contact your personal or departmental health care provider for a health screening. A health screening is a baseline measurement of common health indicators such as blood pressure, cholesterol, motor function, immunizations, physical agility, and psychological health. Subsequent periodic screenings may be required by your health care provider. Typically, health care providers recommend yearly health screenings.

Health Screenings

Health screenings fall into three categories: physical, medical, and psychological. After baseline measurements for physical, medical, and emotional health are determined, the EMR needs to consider how to stay healthy on the job.

Physical Screening

A physical screening includes a dexterity assessment that evaluates the function of your bones, joints, and muscles.

Medical Screening

A medical screening checks your immunization status, looks for the presence of disease processes, and assesses fundamental health indicators such as blood pressure and cholesterol level.

Psychological Screening

A psychological screening assesses your emotional health by measuring factors such as stress, depression, and coping mechanisms.

Immunizations

Immunizations increase a person's resistance to certain infectious diseases by exposing the person to weakened or dead pathogens of a particular disease. This exposure causes the body to create specific antibodies that protect the body against that disease. Certain immunizations are required by most emergency services agencies. Given the likelihood of exposure to infectious disease on the job, there is no excuse for exposing yourself and your loved ones to unnecessary risk. The following immunizations should be current before first patient contact.

- Tetanus
- Hepatitis B
- Measles, mumps, and rubella (German measles)
- Varicella (chicken pox)
- Influenza

You should also have a recent tuberculosis screening.

Stress

EMS is a high-stress job that could affect your career, as well as life outside of work. A career or voluntary work in emergency services will tax your body and mind, sometimes to unreasonable levels. For example, humans are not built to frequently lift a 350-pound body and easily cope with the death of a child or deal with the fears, anxiety, and pain experienced by the patient, friends and family (Figure 2-1). EMRs face stressful situations on a regular basis in the course of their duties. They may internalize the emotions and pain of emergency situations (Figure 2-2). An EMR will find it difficult to provide excellent care to victims if the EMR is sick, injured, angry, or depressed. You owe it to yourself, your family, your friends, and your patients to stay well and get help when you need it.

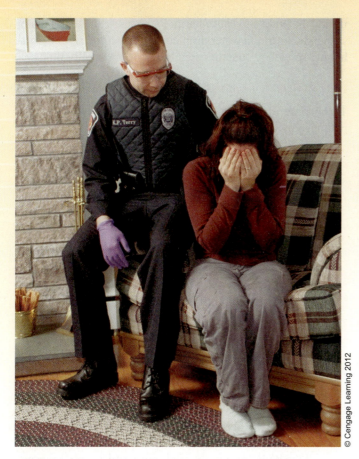

Figure 2-1 EMR's must learn to deal with the fears, anxiety, and pain experienced by the patient, friends, and family.

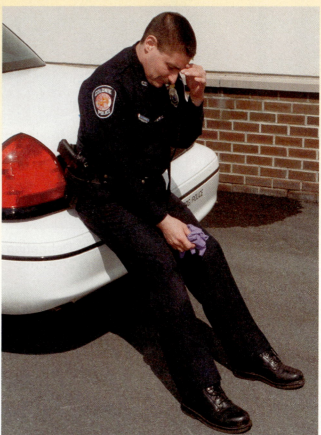

Figure 2-2 The Emergency Medical Responder may internalize the emotions and pain of stressful emergency situations.

Stress Management

Stress management is any method used to control the factors causing stress. Eating a healthy diet, getting enough exercise, enjoying hobbies, journal writing, spending time with loved ones or friends, and getting adequate sleep are proven ways of preparing the body to deal with stress of the job and controlling the effects of stress accumulated on the job. Making time for the things you enjoy will help you deal with the daily stressors of work.

Warning Signs of Stress

Knowing the common warning signs of stress are necessary in order to manage it (Figure 2-3), because the physical effects can continue to be felt for many weeks after the incident. Common warning signs of stress include:

- Irritability
- Feelings of anxiety, guilt, or sadness
- Difficulty with work or excessive absenteeism
- Lack of or an increase in appetite
- Increased alcohol or drug use
- Lack of interest in sex
- Isolation
- Insomnia or an increase in sleep

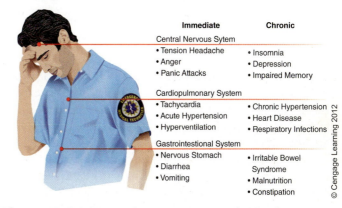

Immediate	Chronic
Central Nervous Sytem	
• Tension Headache	• Insomnia
• Anger	• Depression
• Panic Attacks	• Impaired Memory
Cardiopulmonary System	
• Tachycardia	• Chronic Hypertension
• Acute Hypertension	• Heart Disease
• Hyperventilation	• Respiratory Infections
Gastrointestional System	
• Nervous Stomach	• Irritable Bowel
• Diarrhea	Syndrome
• Vomiting	• Malnutrition
	• Constipation

Figure 2-3 Stress has numerous physical effects. Some reactions are immediate, but others are delayed.

Critical Incident Stress Debriefing

Sometimes emergency services personnel respond to traumatic incidents that may overload their coping mechanisms. These situations could include traumatic situations such as the death of a child, the death of a coworker, multiple casualties, or the death of a family member. Stress management in these situations is vital, and the responder may need to undergo

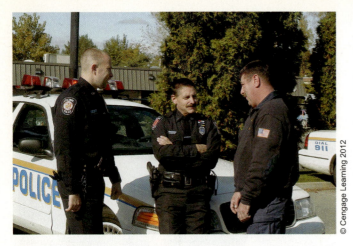

Figure 2-4 A Critical Incident Stress Debriefing can begin with a defusing a few hours after the incident.

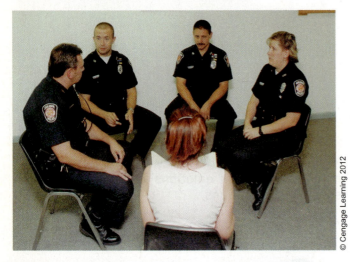

Figure 2-5 A more formal debriefing may be held one to three days after the critical incident.

a **Critical Incident Stress Debriefing (CISD)**. A CISD is a structured conversation between the individual who has experienced a traumatic event and a mental health professional, a peer trained in CISD, or a CISD team. This conversation may reduce the stress after an exceptionally difficult incident. CISD is confidential. EMRs cannot be disciplined or fired for what they say during a session. CISD typically begins with a defusing as soon as resources are available, typically within 24 hours of a critical incident, Figure 2-4. A more formal debriefing, led by a mental health professional or team, may be held one to three days after the incident (Figure 2-5) if needed. The CISD is designed to help the EMR make sense of his or her reactions and may be an important first step in preventing ongoing stress.

Infectious Disease

An **infectious disease** is any disease that can be transmitted from one person to another or from an animal to a person. Infectious diseases are caused by **pathogens**, microscopic organisms such as bacteria, viruses, or parasites that can

invade the body and cause harm. Pathogens can be **airborne**, suspended in air on water droplets or dust particles, or **bloodborne**, spread by contaminated blood or other body fluids.

Pathogen Transmission

To become infected, the body must first be exposed to a pathogen by one of the following routes of transmission:

- *Fomites:* Inanimate objects such as door knobs, metal surfaces, hand towels, bedding, or equipment in the responding unit
- *Vectors:* Living things such as mosquitoes, flies, fleas, and ticks
- *Direct contact:* Physical contact with an infected medium such as blood, secretions, or contaminated water
- *Inhalation:* Pathogens suspended in the air can enter through the lungs during respiration
- *Ingestion:* Eating, drinking, or swallowing an infected medium
- *Inoculation:* Direct entry into the body through a break in the skin, including open wounds, needle sticks, and animal bites

Healthy, intact skin can protect your circulatory system from the outside world and is the best defense against infectious disease transmission. An open wound will allow access to the body and is an easy place for pathogens to invade. Other areas of the body, such as the eyes, nose, and mouth, are especially vulnerable to pathogens. A medical responder may not know immediately whether he or she has been exposed to or infected by a pathogen. Depending on the type of exposure, strength of the pathogen, and the body's defenses, signs and symptoms of infection can take weeks, months, or (in rare cases) years to develop. Table 2-1 lists the common infectious diseases an EMR may encounter while providing patient care.

Exposure

Patients are not required to disclose if they carry an infectious disease. Some states and jurisdictions require hospitals to notify EMS personnel if they have transported a patient with a confirmed infectious disease. However, the practice varies substantially across the country.

The EMR has three responsibilities related to infectious disease exposure:

1. Know the laws and regulations on infectious disease reporting—federal, state, local, and agency.
2. Follow standard precautions and use appropriate protective gear at all times.
3. Document and report any suspected exposure as soon as possible.

Exposure Control Plan

Employers are responsible for developing and maintaining written policies and procedures called an **exposure control plan** to prevent and document on-the-job exposure incidents, such as exposure to blood- and airborne pathogens. Employers

Table 2-1 Common Disease-Causing Organisms and Infectious Illnesses

Organism and Illness	Signs and Symptoms	Mode of Transmission
Adenovirus (common cold)	Runny nose, cough, sore throat, congestion	Contact with droplets
Varicella virus (chickenpox and shingles)	Rash (itchy or painful)	Contact with open lesions, airborne
Mycobacterium tuberculosis (tuberculosis)	Cough, sweats, weight loss	Airborne
Hepatitis type A virus	Fever, nausea, vomiting, yellow skin color	Contaminated food or water
Hepatitis types B, C, and D viruses	Fever, nausea, vomiting, yellow skin color, abdominal pain	Direct contact with blood or other body fluid
Herpes simplex 1 virus (oral herpes)	Painful lesions, usually around the mouth	Contact with saliva or wound
Herpes simplex 2 virus (genital herpes)	Painful lesions, usually in genital area	Contact with lesions
Human immunodeficiency virus (cause of AIDS)	Multiple infections such as pneumonia, thrush, herpes	Contact with blood or body fluids
Influenza virus (causes the flu)	Cough, fever, headache, vomiting, diarrhea, general malaise	Airborne
Methicillin-resistant *Staphylococcus aureus* (MRSA)	None (a bacterium that can inhabit a wound or healthy skin) or infection of wound	Contact with contaminated area
Neisseria meningitidis (a bacterium, one cause of meningitis)	Fever, rash, headache, stiff neck	Airborne respiratory secretions
Plasmodium malariae (blood parasite causing malaria)	History of exposure; fever, chills, headache, weakness, vomiting, diarrhea	Bite from a malaria-infected female mosquito
Enterobius vermicularis (round or pinworms)	Mostly asymptomatic; perianal itching, especially at night, causing skin tears, which can lead to bacterial infections	Ingestion of eggs, can be airborne, environmental contact, hand to mouth, contaminated clothing or bedding

© Cengage Learning 2012

are also responsible for arranging follow-up screening and treatment. For their best interest, employees need to document and report an exposure as soon as possible.

If exposed to an infectious disease by needle stick or contact with blood or bodily fluids, EMRs must, at a minimum, document when, where, and what happened on a **First Report of Exposure Form**.

- When the exposure took place (date and time)
- Where the exposure took place (address and location)
- What happened that led to the exposure (e.g., patient vomited in my face or stuck by needle after withdrawing it from the patient's arm)

This is the *minimal* information needed for documenting an exposure incident. If you become infected, your initial report may be scrutinized by your company for workers' compensation purposes. Poor documentation will obscure the facts and may significantly impact the benefits you receive. If notified by a supervisor or hospital that you may have been exposed to a pathogen, follow up with your employer and medical professional immediately. The First Report of Exposure Form should be completed within 24 to 48 hours after the incident.

Safe Work Environment

Health care workers are a high-risk population for work-related injury and illness. Many of the occupational hazards of prehospital patient care are unavoidable. Because it is impossible to keep track of everything that happens during patient contact, maintaining a safe work environment requires the EMR to have systems in place that mitigate hazards and encourage proper handling of dangerous or infectious materials. When starting your routine, take a moment and think of a safe work environment. Are you healthy and ready to work? Do you wash your hands and clean your uniform regularly? Do you follow standard precautions and keep personal protective equipment easily accessible? Attentive personal safety habits will easily translate to a safe environment for you, other responders, and your patients.

The EMR must strive to maintain a safe work environment by following specific safety guidelines. Habits and equipment are important, but the techniques used to avoid work-related illness and injury must also be considered.

Habits

- Hand washing
- Cleanliness and disinfection
- Sharps disposal
- Biohazard disposal
- Reporting

Equipment

- Soap and water
- Hand cleaner
- Exam gloves
- Eye protection

- Surgical mask
- N95 respirator or High- Efficiency Particulate Air (HEPA) filter mask
- Disposable gown
- Sharps container
- Biohazard containers and red bags
- Exposure incident report

Techniques

- Hand washing
- Flushing skin after an exposure
- Glove removal
- Eye flush
- Sharps handling
- Biohazard disposal
- Cleaning of equipment

Standard Precautions

Standard precautions are designed to reduce the risk of transmission of microorganisms from both known and unknown sources of infection. Based on the definition by the **Centers for Disease Control and Prevention (CDC)**, a governmental agency dedicated to disease prevention and control, standard precautions synthesize the major features of **universal precautions,** designed to reduce the risk of transmission of blood-borne pathogens, and **body substance isolation (BSI)**, designed to reduce the risk of pathogens from moist body substances. Standard precautions apply to all patients in any setting where medical care is delivered. Standard precautions are based on the principle that all blood, bodily fluids, secretions, excretions (except sweat), non-intact skin, and mucous membranes may contain transmissible infectious agents (Table 2-2).

Table 2-2 Standard Precautions for Infection Control

	WASH HANDS (PLAIN SOAP) • Wash after touching blood, body fluids, secretions, excretions, and contaminated items. • Wash immediately *after gloves are removed* and *between patient contacts*. • Avoid transfer of microorganisms to other patients or environments.
	WEAR GLOVES • Wear when touching *blood, body fluids, secretions, excretions*, and *contaminated items*. • Put on *clean* gloves just *before touching mucous membranes* and *non-intact skin*. • Change gloves between tasks and procedures on the same patient after contact with material that may contain high concentrations of microorganisms. Remove gloves promptly after use, before touching noncontaminated items and environmental surfaces, and before going to another patient and wash hands immediately to avoid transfer of microorganisms to other patients or environments.
	WEAR MASK AND EYE PROTECTION OR FACE SHIELD • Protect mucous membranes of the eyes, nose, and mouth during procedures and patient care activities that are likely to generate *splashes* or *sprays* of *blood, body fluids, secretions*, or *excretions*.
	WEAR GOWN • Protect skin and prevent soiling of clothing during procedures that are likely to generate *splashes* or *sprays* of *blood, body fluids, secretions*, or *excretions*. • Remove a soiled gown as promptly as possible and wash hands to avoid transfer of microorganisms to other patients or environments.
	PATIENT CARE EQUIPMENT • Handle used patient care equipment soiled with *blood, body fluids, secretions*, or *excretions* in a manner that prevents skin and mucous membrane exposures, contamination of clothing, and transfer of microorganisms to other patients or environments. Ensure that reusable equipment is not used for the care of another patient until it has been appropriately cleaned and reprocessed and that single-use items are properly discarded.
	LINENS • Handle, transport, and process used linens soiled with *blood, body fluids, secretions*, or *excretions* in a manner that prevents exposures and contamination of clothing and avoids transfer of microorganisms to other patients or environments.
	• Use *resuscitation devices* as an alternative to mouth-to-mouth resuscitation.

Federal Requirements

Other governmental agencies are in line with the CDC's policies regarding infectious disease protection. The **Occupational Safety and Health Administration (OSHA)**, a governmental agency created to maintain a safe and healthy work environment, requires that employers provide the necessary equipment and training for its employees and that all employees follow standard precautions and use appropriate **personal protective equipment (PPE)**, specialized clothing or equipment worn by employees for protection against health and safety hazards, when caring for all patients.

Prevention Practices

Standard precautions include a group of infection prevention practices that apply to all patients, regardless of suspected or confirmed infection status, in any setting in which health care is delivered. These practices include hand hygiene; use of gloves, gown, mask, eye protection, or face shield, depending on the anticipated exposure; and safe injection practices. Also, equipment or items in the patient environment likely to have been contaminated with infectious body fluids must be handled in a manner to prevent transmission of infectious agents. For example, gloves are to be worn for direct patient contact, heavily soiled equipment is to be contained, and reusable equipment is to be properly cleaned and disinfected or sterilized before being used on another patient.

Hand Washing

Of all the health safety recommendations, hand washing is the *first and best defense against infectious disease.* Health care workers' hands frequently come in contact with blood and body fluids, so it is not enough to quickly rinse and dry. EMRs must thoroughly clean their hands before and after each patient contact. Many pathogens are resistant to the small doses of disinfectants that are safe for repeated human use. Good hand-washing technique is critical because soap and water do not disinfect. Soap and water work together to lubricate (soap) and flush (water) pathogens from the skin.

If access to soap and water is not available, alcohol-based hand cleansers are acceptable. However, in the case of certain body substances, such as fecal matter or emesis, soap and water must be used as soon as they become available. The steps for properly washing your hands on the job are illustrated in **Skill 2-1** at the end of this chapter.

Personal Protective Equipment

EMRs must use PPE, which is designed to minimize the risk of infection for medical responders and patients. Some of this equipment will be used for each patient contact; others are only required in specific situations. What is used and when depend on the treatment to be given and the responder's level of comfort. If the patient has a strong, productive cough, covering the eyes and mouth is appropriate. Delivering a baby in the field requires sterile gloves, a mask, gown, and eye protection for the safety of the EMR, the mother, and the newborn. Examination gloves may be all the EMR needs to splint a jogger's deformed ankle. Whatever the situation, the EMR is responsible for properly using and disposing of appropriate PPE.

When donning personal protective apparel, the EMR should first put on a mask and eye protection. The ties should be tight and the mask secure so it will not fall down. The EMR should then put on a gown, if necessary. Assistance may be needed to tie the back of the gown. Finally, gloves should be put on and pulled up over the sleeves of the gown.

The EMR uses a reverse process to take off PPE. First, the gloves are removed and then the gown, mask, and eye protection. If the PPE is grossly contaminated from body fluids, the EMR may need assistance to disrobe to prevent accidental self-contamination. Specific instructions for donning and removing personal protective equipment are provided in **Skill 2-2. Skill 2-3** demonstrates the process for application of nonsterile gloves and removing contaminated gloves.

The following PPE are commonly used by EMRs:

- Exam gloves (two pairs of gloves are recommended for calls that have potential for gross contamination; Figure 2-6)
- Protective safety glasses with side guards
- Filtered masks (Figure 2-7)
- Surgical mask (Figure 2-8)

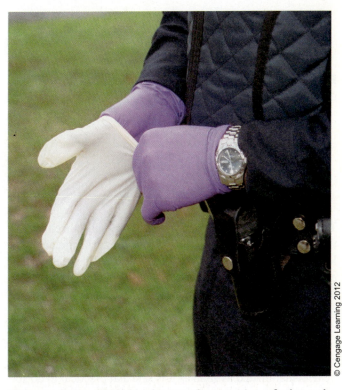

© Cengage Learning 2012

Figure 2-6 Double gloving (two pairs of gloves) is recommended for exposure to copious amounts of blood or body fluids.

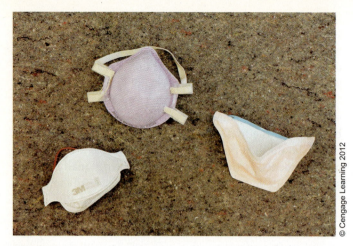

Figure 2-7 Typical filtered masks worn in Emergency Medical Services.

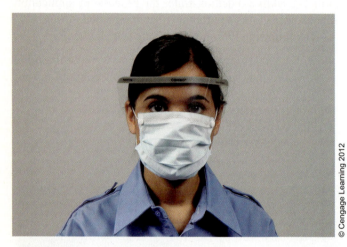

Figure 2-8 A combination surgical mask and eye shield.

- Disposable gown
- Uniform
- Boots

Biohazards

The EMR must be constantly aware of any substance that has the potential for spreading disease. **Biohazards** are any biological substance that may be infectious. EMRs are primarily concerned with blood and other bodily fluids, but anything that carries pathogens can be biohazardous. Contamination occurs after the EMR, his or her clothes, or a piece of equipment comes in contact with a biohazard. Contaminated people or equipment must not be allowed to come in contact with uncontaminated people or objects. A contaminated person must be decontaminated as soon as it is safe and practical to do so.

Disposal of Biohazards

In addition, contaminated equipment must be disposed of or cleaned as soon as is safe and practical. Disposable contaminated equipment such as gloves, masks, gowns, and respirators cannot be discarded with everyday items such as gum wrappers and soda receipts. They must be discarded in a biohazard bag, which is a heavy-duty red plastic bag with easily identified markings.

Cleaning, Disinfection, and Sterilization

After possible exposure to pathogens, nondisposable contaminated equipment such as backboards and the EMR's vehicle must be cleaned, disinfected, or sterilized before reuse. The EMR is responsible for any equipment used to treat patients. Cleaning, disinfection, and sterilization help keep equipment in good repair and minimize the risk of spreading an infectious disease.

Cleaning

Cleaning with soap and water removes particulate matter from clothing and equipment but does not kill pathogens and is not sufficient for removing blood or bodily fluids.

Disinfection

Disinfection uses hospital-grade cleaners that kill common pathogens present on the surface of an object. It is sufficient for cleaning the inside surfaces of vehicles, as well as some of the larger, nondisposable equipment that may have come in contact with the patient's skin or blood and bodily fluids. Disinfection, however, should not be used on contaminated laundry items, which must be washed separately. Always follow agency protocols for disinfection of equipment.

Sterilization

Sterilization requires chemical or physical (e.g., superheated steam, ozone) substances to eradicate pathogens on the surface of an object. Anything that comes in contact with nonintact skin, mucous membranes, or internal structures (e.g., muscles, bones, organs) should be sterilized before use and stored or disposed of in the proper container.

Sharps

The EMR must take special precautions when working with **sharps**, any items with corners, edges, or projections capable of piercing the skin. Contaminated or not, *all* sharps are dangerous and require special handling, OSHA recommends these steps when dealing with sharp objects.

1. Minimize contact by disposing of sharps immediately.
2. Do not recap, bend, or remove needles unless there is no alternative.
3. Never reach or stuff items into containers of sharps.
4. Keep sharps containers near the area of use.

All sharps must be disposed of in a specially designated, puncture-resistant, leakproof container, as shown in Figure 2-9. Typically, these containers are made of red plastic with a locking white or clear lid and quickly identified by label markings.

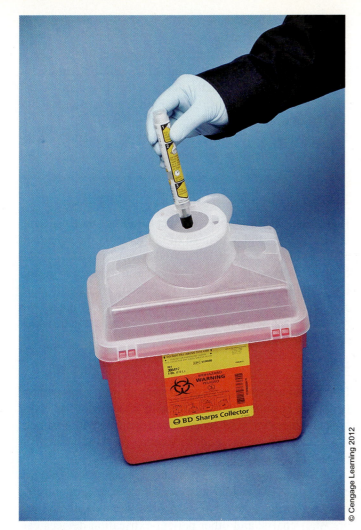

Figure 2-9 Needles must always be discarded safely in appropriate sharps containers.

Hazardous Materials (HAZMAT)

Hazardous materials (HAZMAT) are any items or agents (biological, chemical, or physical) that have the potential to cause harm, including sickness or death, to animals, the environment, or humans, either by themselves or through interaction with other items or agents after exposure. The list of hazardous materials is long and includes a surprising number of substances that EMRs come in contact with on a daily basis. Unless the EMR has special training in the use of decontamination equipment and handling of hazardous materials, he or she has no obligation to enter or manage a scene where hazardous materials pose a risk to responders or anyone else. Chapter 13 discusses hazardous materials and HAZMAT scenes in greater detail.

Most importantly, remember that the EMR's responsibilities are limited to recognition, notification, and assistance. After you recognize a HAZMAT incident, stay away. Notify dispatch and request specialized resources. Stay on scene in the **cold zone**, a designated safe area as established by the

HAZMAT response team, to assist other responders and provide patient care. In this zone, you will need minimum safety protection.

Lifting and Moving Patients

Lifting and moving is a fact of life for EMS personnel that accounts for a significant portion of sick days and workers' compensation claims. Patients are not typically found lying face up in an unobstructed area. Responders will need to move them from places where it is dangerous to walk; too small for more than one person; or difficult to apply appropriate **body mechanics**, the proper way to lift, push, or carry.

The main priority during a lift or carry is the safety of the responder as well as the patient. Proper body mechanics are a good start, but attentive planning does the rest. When going up or down stairs, make sure a spotter is used. If the ground is hard to walk on or slippery, make it as stable as possible and go slowly. Make sure that the route is clear before you make an emergency move and that additional personnel and equipment are available if needed.

Personal Preparation

The EMR's career and the patient's safety depend on exercising good judgment, being prepared for difficult situations, knowing when to request additional help, and using proper lifting techniques. The EMR must pay attention to the scene, plan the move, and have the equipment needed on hand. Most importantly, EMRs must prepare their bodies to do the job that is required.

Start each shift by warming up and stretching your back muscles. Figure 2-10 shows lower back exercises that can be done to improve back strength. Warming up and stretching help prevent injury and give you an idea of how your back feels before it is used. If the stretches or movements are uncomfortable or painful, consult your supervisor and health care provider immediately. The body compensates so well for small sprains and strains that many people do not notice a problem until it is far too late to resolve the issue. Do not be one of these people. Repetitive-stress injuries will permanently affect your ability to do an effective job because these injuries are aggravated by the actions you are expected to perform. Five minutes of stretching each shift and a visit to your supervisor or health care provider at the start of a problem may ensure good health until retirement.

Body Mechanics

Using good body mechanics during all aspects of the job is critical for EMRs to protect their bodies. Body mechanics, the proper way to lift, push, or carry, are essential to keeping responders safe on the job. Good body mechanics transfer the load to the large muscle groups in the thighs, abdomen, and back (commonly called the core). Engaging the core substantially reduces strain on the lower back and allows the responder to lift more weight more times without injury.

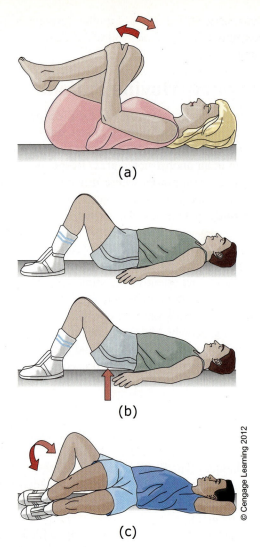

(a)

(b)

(c)

© Cengage Learning 2012

Figure 2-10 Back exercises reduce the risk of a back injury.

Guidelines for Safe Lifting

To get patients to the hospital, responders must first get them to the ambulance or air medical transport. If a patient is unable to walk, he or she will need to be carried. There are many techniques for safely lifting and moving a patient.

Simply memorizing safe-lifting guidelines will not keep you safe; it takes practice to apply these techniques properly. Proper lifting techniques as described next are demonstrated in **Skill 2-4** at the end of this chapter.

1. Position yourself as close to what you must lift as possible. Six inches or less is ideal.
2. Place your feet apart at a comfortable distance.
3. Turn your toes outward and shift the weight of your body toward your heels.
4. Keep your spine straight and eyes up.
5. Drop your hands to your sides and bend your knees until your hands are level with what is being lifted. It is okay to put one knee on the floor if it is safe to do so.
6. Grab the object with your palms facing up and hands a comfortable distance apart.

7. Make sure your arms and spine are straight and your head and eyes are up.
8. Initiate the lift with your thigh muscles and then engage your abdomen and back muscles. Your back muscles should feel tight from the pelvis to the shoulders.
9. Lift evenly and slowly enough for you to maintain control of what you are lifting.
10. Keep the weight close to your body as you move, making sure your arms and back are straight and your head and eyes are up.

Pushing and Pulling

If possible, push very heavy objects. Pulling strains specific muscle groups and puts most of the force on the shoulders and lower back. Pushing allows the body to stay close to the object. While pushing, keep your spine straight, eyes up, and hands in line with your shoulders. Pushing engages the core and keeps the body in a neutral position, which means the responder can work harder longer without as much risk of injury.

Know Personal and Equipment Limits

Patients do not come in standard sizes or weights. Some patients will be small enough for you to lift and move safely—typically these are your pediatric patients. You will need help lifting and moving most adults whether they are fit and trim or morbidly obese.

Anything used to move or secure a patient in the field has a load limit that must be heeded. There are no hard-and-fast numbers for the amount of weight that backboards, stretchers, stair chairs, and other patient-extrication devices can handle. It is the responsibility of the EMR to know the limits of the equipment used and to use it appropriately. Always follow the manufacturer recommendations for load limits on equipment used.

Before lifting anything, ask yourself two questions:

1. Is there enough help to safely execute this lift?
2. Is the right equipment available?

If the answer to either of these questions is "no," fix it before you lift.

Emergency Moves

An **emergency move** or rapid extrication is used when the risk of harm (fire, flood, unstable vehicle or gun fire) from the environment outweighs the risk of injury from the move. These moves are designed to be executed quickly by one or two people, making provisions if possible for cervical spine immobilization. Demonstrations of each emergency move listed can be found in **Skills 2-5** through **2-10** at the end of the chapter.

- Clothing drag, **Skill 2-5**
- Arm drag, **Skill 2-6**
- Blanket drag, **Skill 2-7**
- Rescuer assist, **Skill 2-8**

- Pack strap carry, **Skill 2-9**
- Firefighter's carry, **Skill 2-10**

Non-Emergency Moves

Non-emergency moves are used when there is enough time to plan and execute a patient transfer. These moves typically require two or more people and preserve the patient's spinal alignment better than emergency moves. Demonstrations of these non-emergency moves may be found in **Skills 2-11** through **2-18** at the end of the chapter.

- Chair carry, **Skill 2 -11**
- Extremity lift, **Skill 2-12**
- Carry transfer, **Skill 2-13**
- Draw sheet transfer, **Skill 2-14**
- Firefighter's drag, **Skill 2-15**
- Seat carry, **Skill 2-16**
- Use of the scoop stretcher, **Skill 2-17**
- Use of a stair chair, **Skill 2-18**

Skill 2-1 Hand Washing

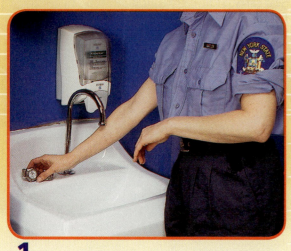

1 Remove any rings, your watch, or other jewelry that could trap contamination.

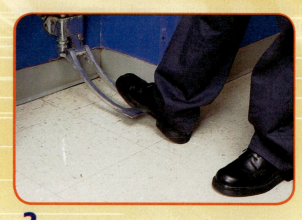

2 A deep basin sink and foot-pedal water faucets are preferable for washing hands. Adjust the hot and cold water to a comfortable lukewarm temperature.

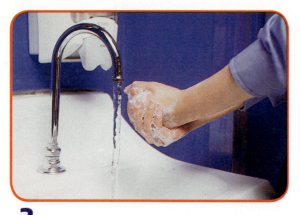

3 Wet the hands to the midforearm. After applying a liberal amount of soap, wash the hands carefully. The areas between the fingers deserve special attention. A hand brush may be used for contamination that is difficult to remove.

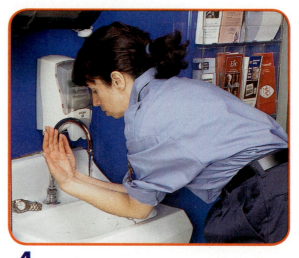

4 Thoroughly rinse the hands, allowing the contaminated water to run off the elbows.

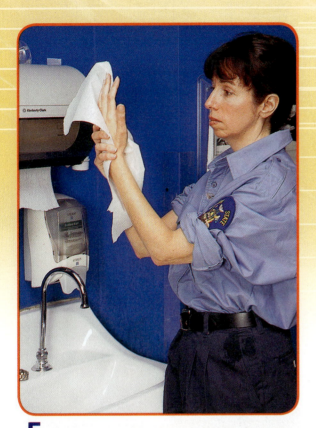

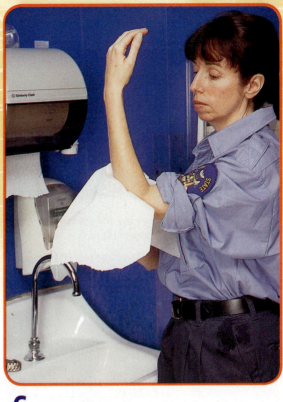

5 Turn off the water. Grasping a clean towel, turn off the faucet and discard the towel. Using a clean towel, dry the hands starting at the fingers. . .

6 . . . and working toward the elbow.

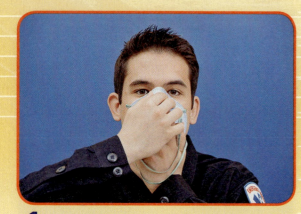

1 Grasp the top ties of the mask and position the metal strip in the mask over the bridge of the nose.

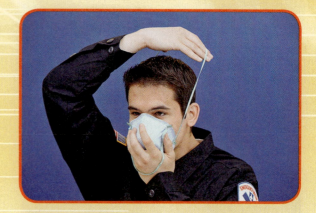

2 Pull the elastic straps over the head.

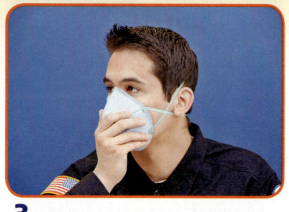

3 Grasp and pinch the metal strip around the bridge of the nose.

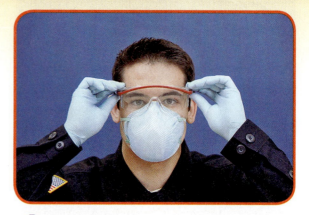

4 Pick up and put on the protective eyewear.

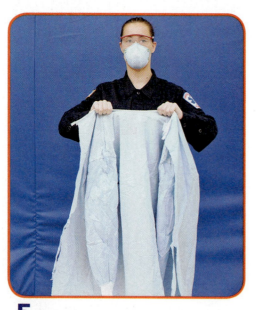

5 Grasp the gown by the collar and allow it to hang with the inside of the gown toward you.

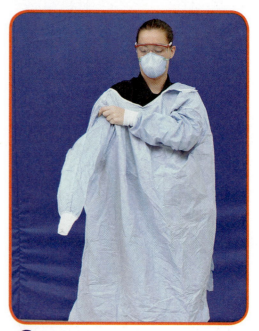

6 Place your arms in the sleeves.

© Cengage Learning 2012

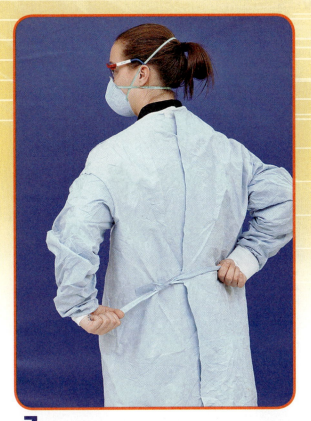

7 Tie the gown behind your back.

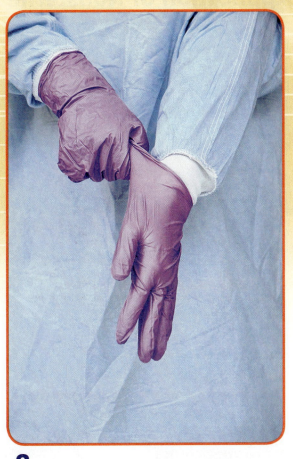

8 Pull on properly sized examination gloves. Each glove's collar should be over the sleeve of the gown.

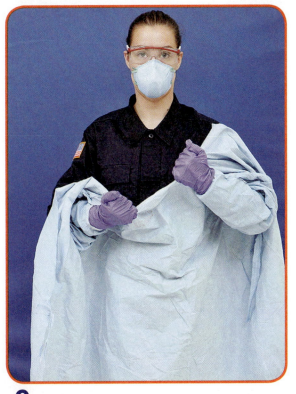

9 Remove the PPE by reversing the order and washing your hands afterward.

Skill 2-3 Donning and Removing Gloves

Application of Nonsterile Gloves

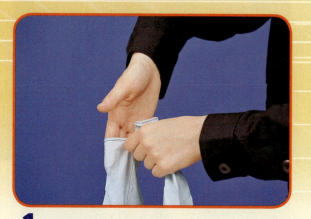

1 Select an appropriate size and type of glove for the job. Arrange one glove so the thumb is aligned with the thumb of the hand it is intended to go on.

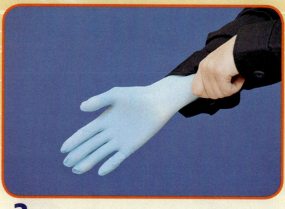

2 Grasp the front of the cuff with one hand while inserting the other hand into the glove. Be sure to place each finger within the appropriate finger section. Pull at the cuff to ensure that the glove is completely applied to the hand.

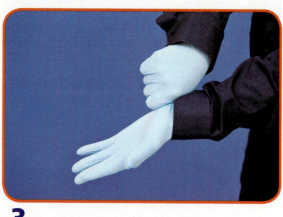

3 Repeat the process for the other hand.

Removal of Contaminated Gloves

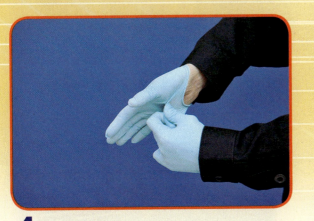

4 Grasp the palm or outside cuff of the left glove with the gloved right hand.

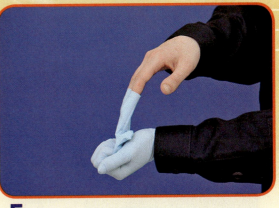

5 Pull the left glove toward the fingertips. The glove should turn inside out as it is removed.

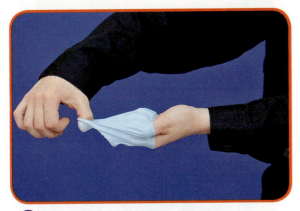

6 Hold the removed glove in the still-gloved right hand. Insert the thumb of the ungloved left hand under the cuff of the right glove, carefully avoiding any contaminated areas. Pull the right glove toward the fingertips, turning it inside out on itself as it is removed. The soiled left glove should remain rolled into a ball in the palm of the right glove after it is removed. The right glove should then be inverted over the left glove and the two gloves rolled together and disposed of properly in a red hazard bag. Gloves should never be left at the scene. Also, it is dangerous to snap or fling potentially contaminated gloves at any time.

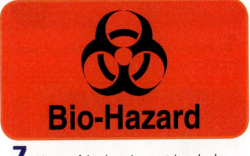

7 Dispose of the gloves in a container clearly marked with the biohazard label and wash your hands thoroughly.

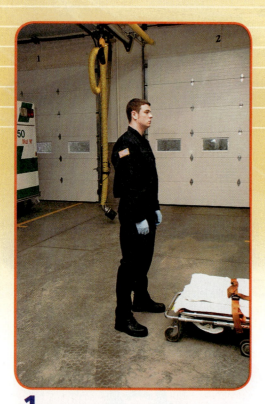

1 Position your feet about shoulder length apart, facing forward.

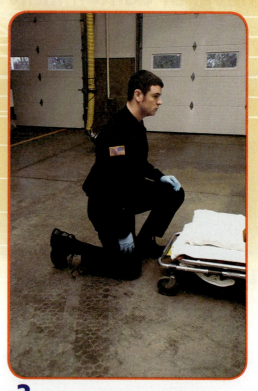

2 Lower your body by bending at the knees, one knee down, keeping your back straight.

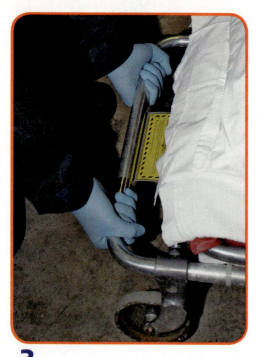

3 Grasp the object with both hands, palms upward, and then lift evenly and smoothly.

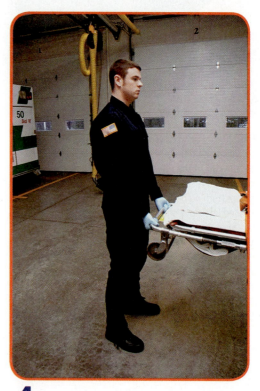

4 With your arms locked out straight, stands fully upright.

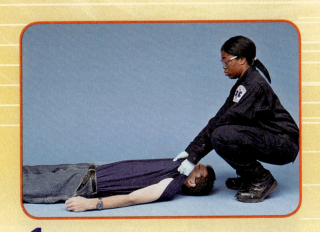

1 Grasp the patient's clothing at the collar while cradling the patient's head on your forearms.

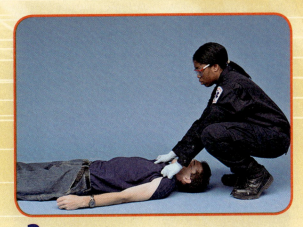

2 Crouching down with your back straight, walk backward.

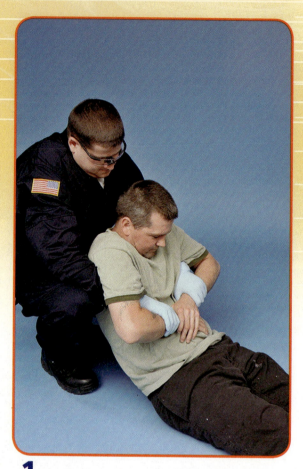

1 Kneeling down, slide your arms under the patient's arm and grasp the wrists across the chest.

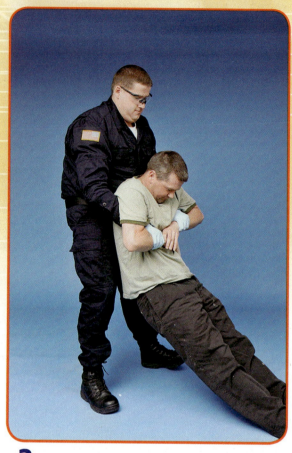

2 Standing up, walk backward.

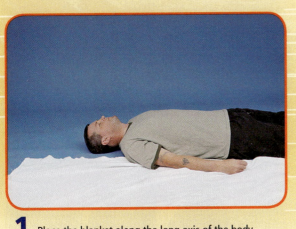

1 Place the blanket along the long axis of the body, leaving about one foot of material at the head.

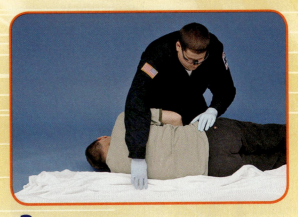

2 Logroll the patient onto the blanket, pulling the blanket underneath the patient.

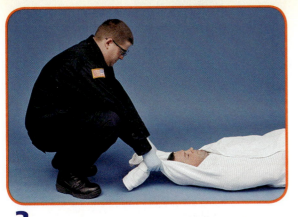

3 Wrap the patient with the blanket, protecting the patient.

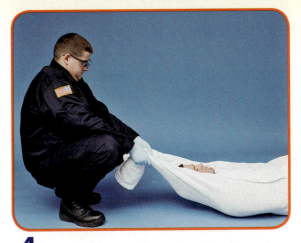

4 Roll up the excess material at the head and grasp the roll.

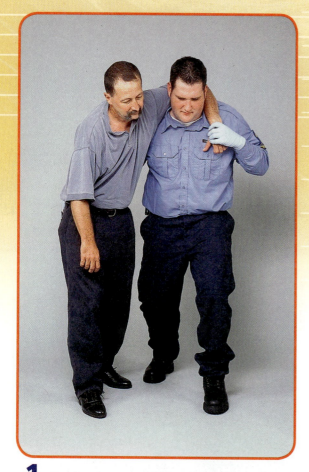

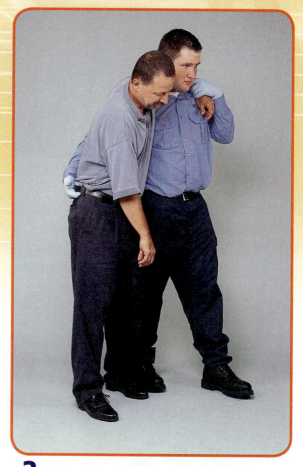

1 Crouch to the patient's level and swing one arm over your shoulders.

2 With one hand grasping the patient's beltline and another grasping the patient's wrist, stand and assist the patient with walking.

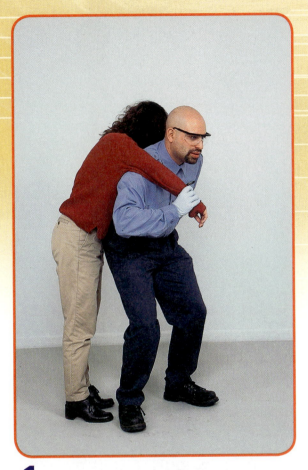

1 Crouching in front of the seated patient, grasp the patient's wrists and then pivot on your heels, draping the patient's arms over your shoulder in the process

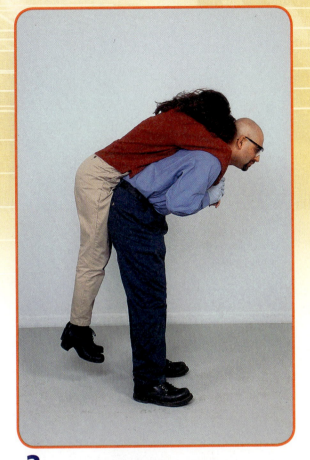

2 Stand, hoisting the patient onto your shoulders and off his or her feet. (This carry is useful if the patient who is being assisted suddenly tires and needs to be carried. Then you simply release the belt and step in front of the patient, grasping the free hand and placing it over his or her shoulders.)

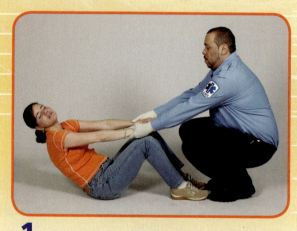

1 Stand toe to toe with the supine patient. Crouching down, grab the patient's wrists and roll the patient to a seated position.

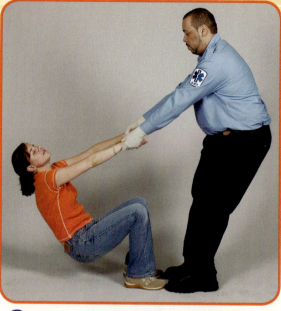

2 Without stopping, pull the patient as nearly erect as possible.

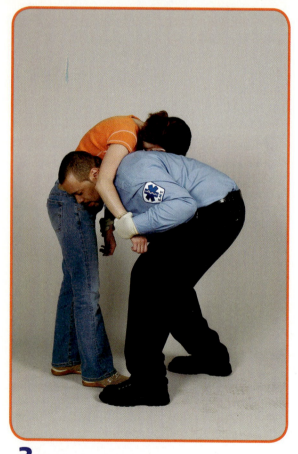

3 Quickly crouching again, place your shoulder into the patient's abdomen while simultaneously standing.

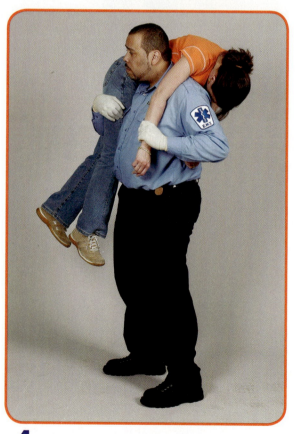

4 Put one arm through the patient's legs and grasp the patient's hand with your free hand. (Another EMR may help hoist the patient up onto your shoulders. The second EMR waits until the patient is up and your shoulders and then, grasping the patient's knee, helps hoist the patient.)

© Cengage Learning 2012

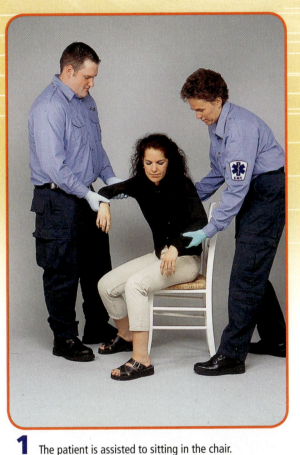

1 The patient is assisted to sitting in the chair.

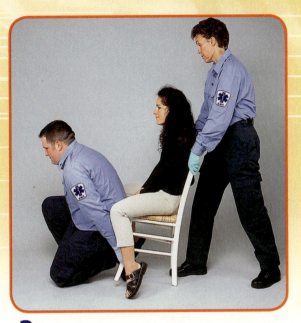

2 Kneel in front of the chair, facing forward and between the patient's legs. Reach back and grasp the legs of the chair.

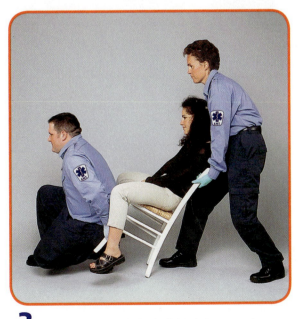

3 A second EMR, at the back of the chair, grasps the uprights of the chair and leans the chair backward.

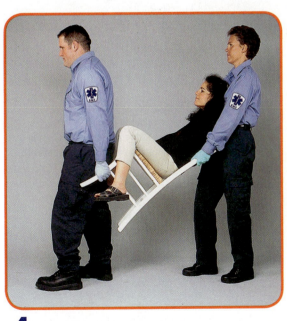

4 Simultaneously, the two EMRs lift the patient up and proceed to walk forward together.

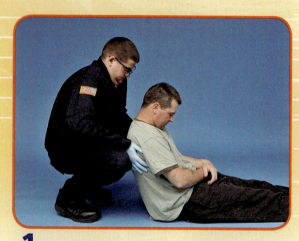

1 Kneel behind the patient and help the patient up to a sitting position. The patient can be rested against your knee for a moment.

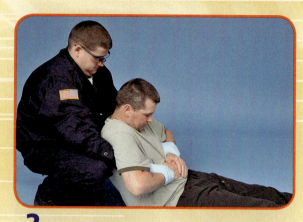

2 Reach under the patient's arms and grasp the patient's wrists, pulling them against the patient's chest tightly.

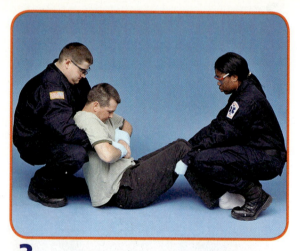

3 A second EMR then crouches. Reaching down on each side, the EMR grasps under the patient's knees. (In some cases, it may be more convenient to crouch beside the patient's knees and hook the arms under the patient's knees.)

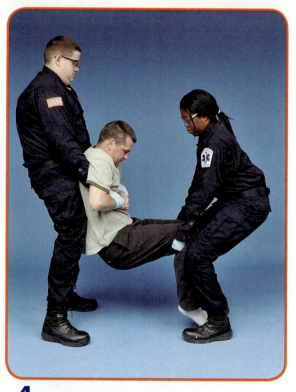

4 Simultaneously, the two EMRs stand with the patient and walk forward together.

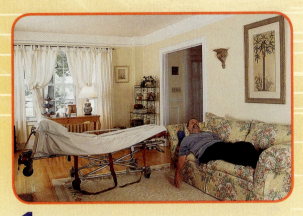

1 The first stretcher is placed with the patient's head at the foot of the other stretcher at a 90-degree angle.

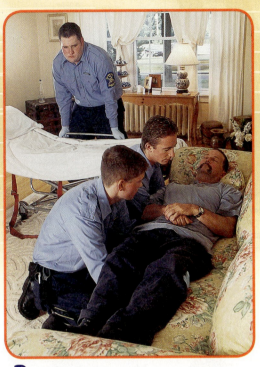

2 The two EMRs stand on the side of the patient, and the first EMR places one arm under the patient's head and neck and the other arm under the shoulders. The second EMR places his or her arms under the patient's lower back and buttocks.

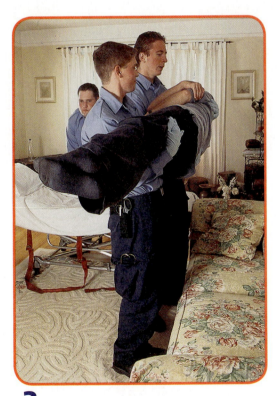

3 Simultaneously, the two EMRs hoist the patient to their chests. Shuffling sideways, the two EMRs move the patient to the awaiting stretcher.

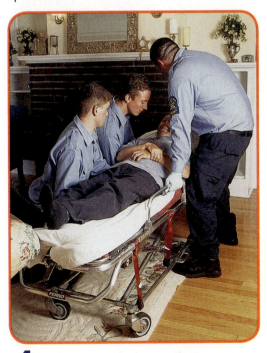

4 The patient is then gently laid onto the awaiting stretcher. Be sure that all stretcher straps are attached before moving the patient.

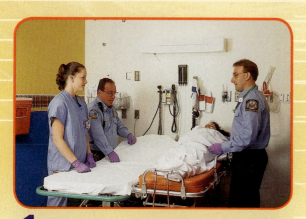

1 The two stretchers are placed side by side. Be sure that the stretcher brakes are engaged before moving the patient. Any side rails present will have to be lowered.

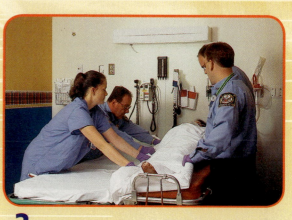

2 Two EMRs are on the one open side of both stretchers. Rolling the edge of the draw sheet or bed linen into a collar, the EMRs grab a firm purchase. (It is a good practice to have the two teams of EMRs pull vigorously against each other to test the strength of the sheet.)

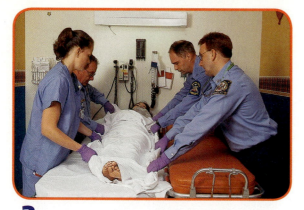

3 Simultaneously, the four EMRs slide the patient from one stretcher to the other in one fluid motion.

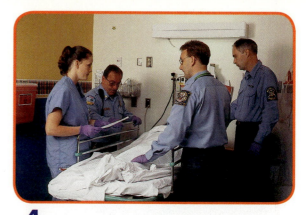

4 After the patient is on the new stretcher, replace the side rails.

© Cengage Learning 2012

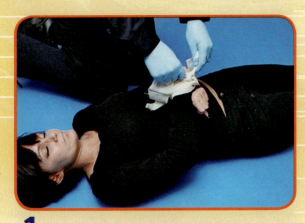

1 Using the triangular bandage folded into a cravat, secure the patient's wrists together.

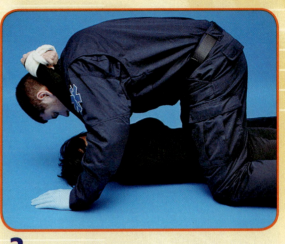

2 While on all fours, drape the tied hands over your shoulders and drag the patient.

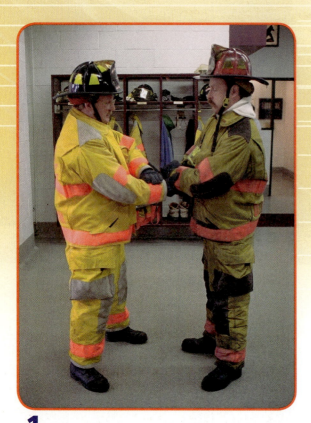

1 The two EMRs clasp arms. Each EMR grasps the other EMR at the elbow.

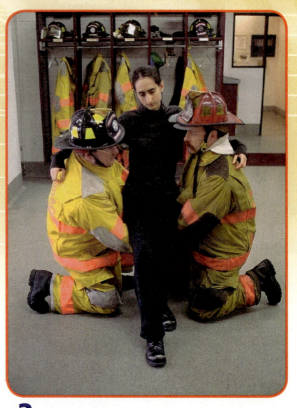

2 With one pair of arms high, the patient sits back into the seat that has been created. The EMRs then stand together at the same time.

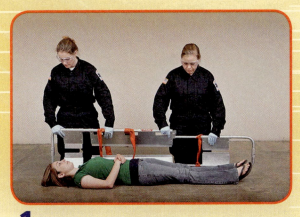

1 EMRs next to the patient estimate the need for equipment adjustment.

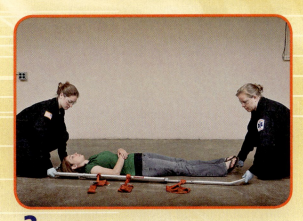

2 Place the two halves of the orthopedic stretcher on each side of the patient and adjust to the appropriate length for the patient.

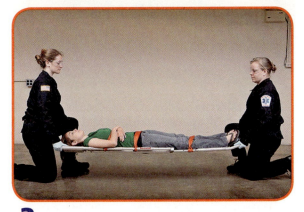

3 Logroll the patient onto the orthopedic stretcher and secure it with straps.

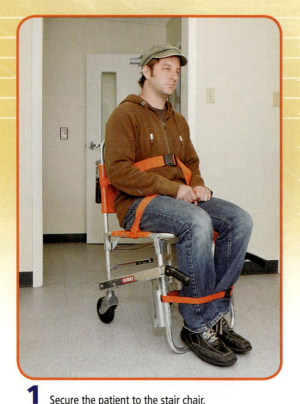

1 Secure the patient to the stair chair.

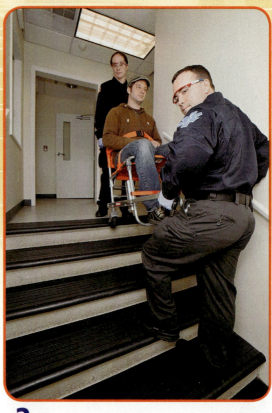

2 The EMRs take positions at the head and foot of the stair chair and lift the patient, extending hand rails as needed.

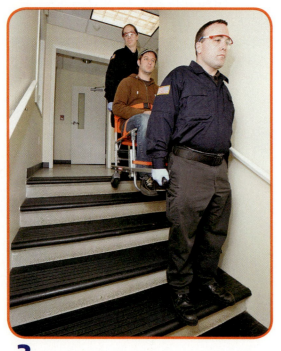

3 The EMR guiding the foot of the stair chair can face toward or away from the patient while carrying the patient down the stairs.

SUMMARY

To ensure a successful career, the EMR is responsible for practicing safety and wellness at home and on the job. EMRs must protect themselves, their patients, their coworkers, and their families from infectious diseases, stress, and physical injuries. To do this, EMRs must be knowledgeable of personal health practices, including health screenings, immunizations, and stress management. EMRs must also be aware of how diseases are transmitted and know the elements of a safe work environment. Furthermore, EMRs must be well versed in agency protocols and state and federal laws regarding standard precautions and know when and how these precautions are to be implemented. EMRs must use the proper PPE, use proper hand washing techniques, and use correct body mechanics to lift and move patients.

The EMR needs to understand that the potential for infection, stress, and injury is not entirely avoidable in emergency services and to draw upon basic knowledge of medical conditions and safe practices to make good decisions for a safe and healthy career.

▶ REVIEW QUESTIONS

1. Define *Critical Incident Stress Debriefing*.
2. Provide a brief description of three "routes of transmission" of exposure to a pathogen.
3. Define *standard precautions*.
4. What are biohazards?
5. What should you do if you think you have been exposed to an infectious disease?
6. Explain the differences among cleaning, disinfection, and sterilization.
7. What are your responsibilities if you find hazardous materials on scene?
8. List the guidelines for safe lifting.
9. Why should you push instead of pull?
10. Explain the difference between an emergency move and a non-emergency move.

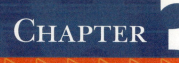

CHAPTER 3

THE HUMAN BODY

LEARNING OBJECTIVES

By the end of this chapter, the reader should be able to:

- Explain the differences among anatomy, physiology, and pathophysiology.
- Explain the meaning of common prefixes and suffixes and how they affect medical terms.
- Describe the common anatomical positions and their locations.
- List and describe the various systems of the body.

INTRODUCTION

As an Emergency Medical Responder (EMR), you must understand the body's structure and function. Basic knowledge is essential to understanding illness, injury, and the interventions you provide. As an EMR, you are not expected to have detailed knowledge of medical terminology, *anatomy* (study of the structure of an organism), *physiology* (study of the functions and activities of life or living matter), and *pathophysiology* (study of functional changes associated with or resulting from injury or disease). You are, however, expected to know enough to understand and communicate with other healthcare workers accurately and professionally. This understanding will also assist with reporting findings in a professional manner. Compare the two following reports:

1. His foot hurts, and it looks black and blue.
2. The patient's foot is deformed at the distal tibia/fibula, and the patient states a pain level of 9 at site of the injury. There is a hematoma approximately 2 cm x 2 cm in this area.

Both statements describe the injury. However, the second example reflects a more clear understanding of the injury and is a more technical communication.

Medical Terms

Medical terms combine standard prefixes and suffixes to create words and phrases that are precise and difficult to confuse with nonmedical terms. The EMR should be familiar with the basic forms that are used on the job every day.

Common Prefixes Used in Medical Terms

Some common prefixes and words that can be created from them are:

- **a-, an-:** an absence (aphasic—unable to speak; anuria—unable to urinate)
- **arterio-:** the arteries (arteriogram—a diagnostic study of the arteries)
- **brady-:** decreased speed (bradycardia—slow heartbeat)
- **cardio-:** the heart or cardiac function (cardiologist—a specialist of the heart)
- **dys-:** something different from the norm (dysrhythmia—an abnormal heart rhythm)
- **hemo-:** the blood (hemodynamic—circulation of the blood and forces involved with the movement of blood)
- **hyper-:** above normal limits or excessive (hyperactive—activity greater than expected)
- **hypo-:** below normal limits or less than (hypovolemic—below normal amount of volume)
- **naso-:** the nose and nasal passage (nasopharynx—the passage from the opening of the nostrils to the back of the throat)

- **neuro-:** of the nervous system (neurosurgery—surgery involving the nervous system)
- **oro-:** the mouth (oropharyngeal airway—a device that fits inside the mouth to open the airway)
- **tachy-:** increased speed (tachycardia—fast heartbeat)
- **vaso-:** the blood vessels in general, including arteries, veins, and capillaries (vasoconstricted—when blood vessels reduce in diameter or tighten up)
- **pneumo-:** air, lung (pneumothorax—air in the thorax, the space between the rib cage and lungs)

Common Suffixes Used in Medical Terms

Some common words that can be created from suffixes are:

- **-pnea:** breathing (apnea—the absence of breathing)
- **-therm:** temperature (hyperthermic—temperature greater than normal)
- **-plegia:** paralysis (hemiplegia, half paralyzed)
- **-itis:** inflamed (pharyngitis—inflammation of the throat)
- **-stomy:** opening (tracheostomy—opening in the throat)
- **-ist:** a specialist (cardiologist—heart doctor)

Anatomical Position

Health care providers use standard terminology to describe the different areas of the body. The **standard anatomical position** is the term for referring to the body's features. It is always the same, and all descriptions of the body, internal

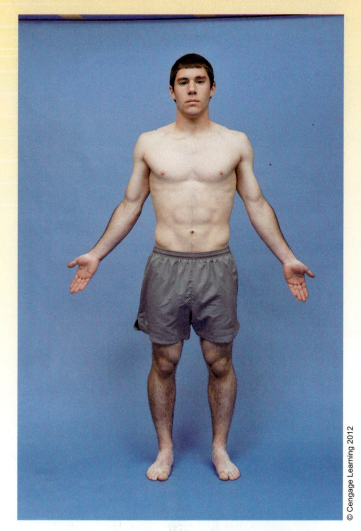

Figure 3-1 Standard anatomical position.

position), and the nose is medial to the ears. There is also a very important marker that runs from the middle of the **axilla** (armpit) to the center of the waist called the **midaxillary line**. The midclavicular line starts in the middle of each clavicle or collarbone and runs parallel to the midline.

When discussing any body part, **superior** means above, and **inferior** means below. The head is superior to the chest, and the chin is on the inferior part of the head. Closer to the center of the body is **proximal**, and farther away is **distal.** The elbow is proximal to the wrist but distal to the shoulder. Injuries or conditions that are noted to be farther away from the core of the body are designated as being **peripheral**, such as the condition called peripheral edema (swelling of the feet and legs). Examples of these standard planes of reference and directional terms are illustrated in Figure 3-2 (a, b).

Recumbent Positions

When a person is lying face down, he or she is **prone** (Figure 3-3a). If the person is lying face-up, he or she is **supine** (Figure 3-3b). Lying on one's side is a **lateral**

or external, are based on the natural position of the body. As shown in Figure 3-1, this position is assumed to be standing face forward with the legs slightly apart with feet pointing forward and the arms held at the sides slightly away from the body with the palms facing out.

Body Aspects

Invisible lines and planes are used to create points of reference on the body that may be used to describe the location of an injury. The front of the body is the **anterior aspect**, and the back of the body is the **posterior aspect**. The inside of the body follows this same rule. For example, a blow to the chest might cause an injury to the anterior aspect of the lungs.

Anatomical Locations or Directions

The **midline** of the body is the line that runs directly through the center of the body vertically and divides the body into left and right. Closer to the midline or middle of the body is **medial**, and closer to the left or right is **lateral**. The thumb is on the lateral aspect of the hand (when viewed in the anatomical

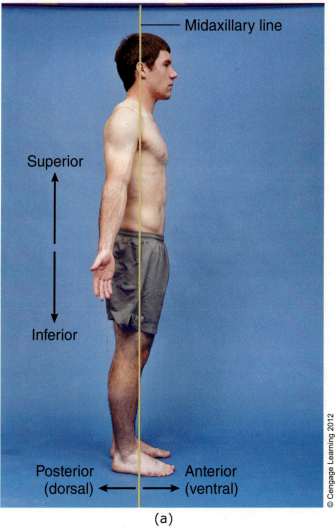

(a)

Figure 3-2 The standard planes of reference and directional terms.

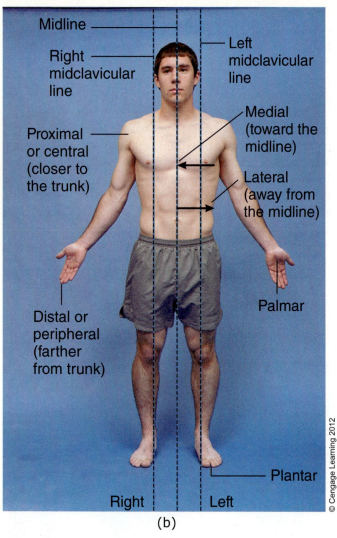

Midline

Right midclavicular line

Left midclavicular line

Medial (toward the midline)

Proximal or central (closer to the trunk)

Lateral (away from the midline)

Palmar

Distal or peripheral (farther from trunk)

Plantar

Right

Left

(b)

Figure 3-2 (*continued*)

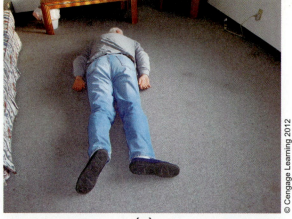

(a)

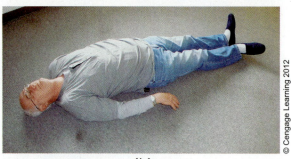

(b)

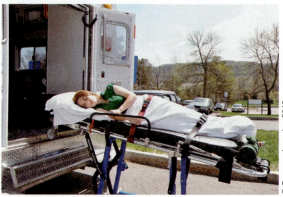

(c)

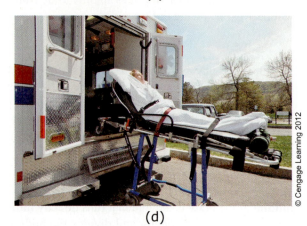

(d)

recumbent position (Figure 3-3c). A person sitting in a semi-sitting position with the head and chest elevated between 45 and 60 degrees is in a **Fowler's position** (Figure 3-3d). Sitting upright at 90 degrees is the **high Fowler's position** (Figure 3-3e). Sometimes patients in shock may be placed in a **modified Trendelenburg**, or shock, position, which is a supine position with the legs elevated 12 to 16 inches (Figure 3-3f).

Body Function

The human body is a fully functional unit made up of interdependent systems. Each of these is distinct and relies on each other to correctly regulate the body. For example, the skeletal system can be studied independently as the human skeleton. In the living, dynamic body, bones are fed by the circulatory system, and signals from the nervous system regulate muscle movement.

Changes to Body Function

Trauma and medical conditions can cause profound changes to occur within the body. If not identified or if left untreated,

Figure 3-3 (a) Prone position. (b) Supine position. (c) Left lateral recumbent position. (d) Fowler's position. (e) High Fowler's position. (f) Modified Trendelenburg position.

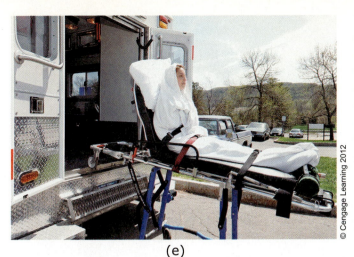

(e)

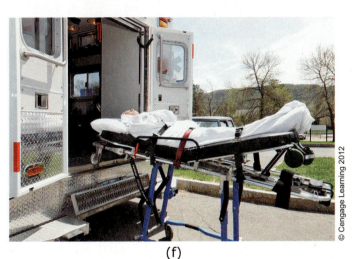

(f)

Figure 3-3 (*continued*)

these changes could lead to death or disability. An EMR must know when the body is working as it should, and more importantly, when it is not.

Compensatory Mechanisms

The human body uses many **compensatory mechanisms** to correct distinct deficits that come with illness or injury. These compensatory mechanisms are the reason we have fevers, our pupils dilate and constrict, our heart beats faster or slower, or we shiver. These are all examples of compensatory mechanisms our bodies use to remain as close to normal as it can. We measure and document these changes and collectively call the heart rate, respirations, blood pressure, and temperature the **vital signs**.

Overview of the Body

The human body includes a central structure called the **thoracic cavity** or chest cavity. The thoracic cavity is the space enclosed within the rib cage and is bordered inferiorly by a fibrous structure called the **diaphragm**. The **abdominal cavity** and its many organs of digestion and elimination lie below the diaphragm and above the pelvis. Superior to the thoracic cavity is the head, connected to the body by the neck. Also attached to the body are four limbs, two arms, and two legs. Externally, the body is covered by the skin and hair. Internally, the muscular and skeletal systems give structure and support as well as protect the internal organs. Many organs make up the remaining systems that perform the body's functions such as digestion, respiration, consciousness, **perfusion** (supply of oxygenated blood to organs or tissues throughout the body), waste management, and movement.

Although our bodies can withstand a fair amount of trauma or disease, we will see that the body is a rather delicate organism that can be seriously injured with little difficulty. Even so, one of the most profound and wonderful features of our bodies is that they have the capacity in many cases to adjust to injury or illness through compensatory mechanisms.

The Respiratory System

The respiratory system delivers **oxygen (O₂)**, a colorless, odorless gas required by the body to function normally, and removes **carbon dioxide (CO₂)**, a colorless, odorless gas naturally formed in the tissues of the lungs. CO_2 is toxic in large amounts but is essential to life in proper amounts. The respiratory system is the first part of the life-support chain and the focus of many basic life support interventions. EMRs are expected to understand the respiratory system well and be able to competently apply that knowledge in practice.

Respiration

Respiration is the act of breathing. Respiration begins with **inhalation**, air being taken in through the nose or mouth, past the pharynx into the **trachea** (windpipe) and then into the lungs. As the diaphragm moves down, negative pressure is created inside the lungs, pulling in air and causing the chest to expand. At the end of this cycle respiration ends with **exhalation**, the act of expelling air from the lungs. When the diaphragm moves up, positive pressure is created in the lungs, forcing air out. Figure 3-4 illustrates the process of inhalation and exhalation.

Respiration, which is ultimately controlled in the brain, regulates the amount of oxygen and carbon dioxide in the lungs. Normal breathing is regulated by the amount of carbon dioxide in the blood. Because the blood bathes the brain, the brain is constantly aware of the body's carbon dioxide level and adjusts respiration in an attempt to maintain the proper balance of oxygen and carbon dioxide (Figure 3-5).

Upper Airway Structures

Air passes into the body through the nasal passage or through the mouth or oropharynx. The **epiglottis**, a small flap that closes over the trachea when swallowing is initiated, prevents food from going down the wrong pipe, the trachea. If something solid accidentally does go down the trachea,

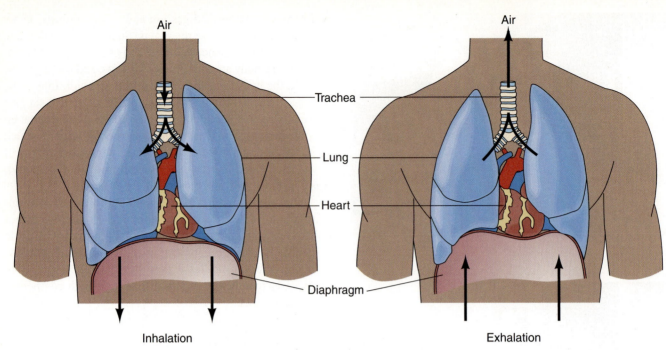

Figure 3-4 The diaphragm separates the thoracic cavity from the abdominal cavity and moves upward or down during the process of ventilation.

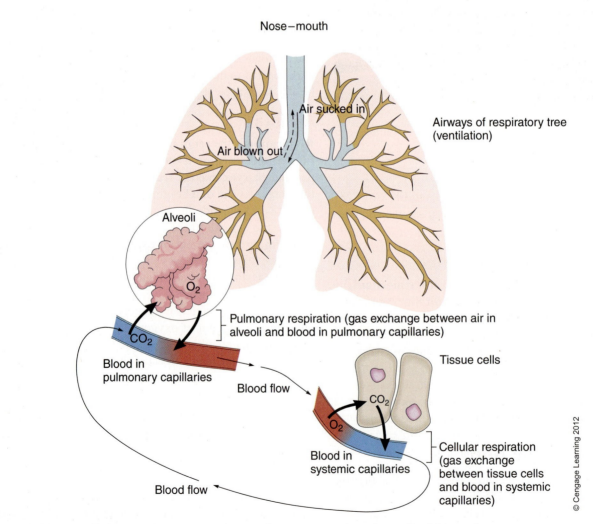

Figure 3-5 Cellular respiration consists of oxygen and carbon dioxide exchange.

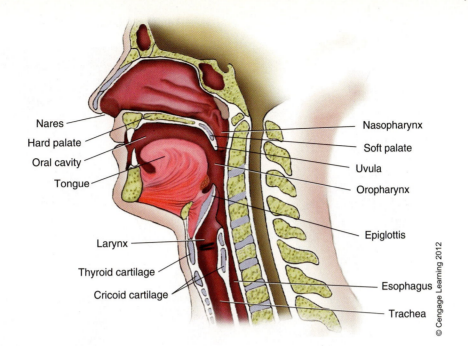

Nares
Hard palate
Oral cavity
Tongue
Larynx
Thyroid cartilage
Cricoid cartilage

Nasopharynx
Soft palate
Uvula
Oropharynx
Epiglottis
Esophagus
Trachea

© Cengage Learning 2012

Figure 3-6 The structures of the upper airway.

we normally, involuntarily cough it up. If we are unable to cough it out, our airway is said to be obstructed. Liquids also are expelled through coughing. Liquids are more likely than solids to be absorbed into the respiratory system or to be retained and create a breeding ground for disease. The larynx or voice box is located below the epiglottis. Structures of the upper airway are shown in Figure 3-6.

Lower Airway Structures

The trachea bifurcates, or splits, into the right and left **bronchi** (large air tubes leading from the trachea to the lungs) at the carina (ridge-like structure, which projects from the lowest tracheal cartilage) so air can enter the right and left lobes of the lungs. The bronchi branch into smaller, more numerous pathways called **bronchioles**, much like a tree branch. The bronchioles terminate in small sacs called **alveoli.** The alveoli are in direct contact with the lungs and are covered with blood vessels. There, oxygen binds with hemoglobin, and carbon dioxide is released from the blood into bronchioles and exhaled. Structures of the lower airway are shown in Figure 3-7.

EMR Applications for the Respiratory System

Respiration can be impaired by obstruction, depression of the respiratory center, swelling, or trauma. Obstruction of the airway can occur in an unconscious patient if the tongue falls back and blocks the airway. This blockage can be cleared by simply tilting the head back and lifting the chin to move the tongue out of the way or inserting a device to reestablish an open route. Another cause of obstruction is a foreign object lodged in the trachea (food, toy). Swelling or trauma to the area directly surrounding the trachea as well as injury to the

lung itself also can obstruct the airway and impair respirations. A decrease in function of the respiratory center of the brain may be caused by drugs, trauma, or medications.

When a patient is unable to breathe adequately because of tumors, injuries, muscular or neurologic disease, neck surgery, or coma, a **tracheostomy** (an opening made in the anterior neck and windpipe) can be surgically created. This opening may be temporary or permanent depending on the patient's condition. A curved, rigid plastic tube called a **tracheostomy tube**, or "trach," is inserted into the stoma opening to keep it from collapsing (Figure 3-8).

The Circulatory System

The human circulatory system is made up of three major parts: the heart, which is the pump; the veins and arteries, which make up the pipes; and the blood, which is the fluid. The heart, blood vessels, and blood of the circulatory system are illustrated in Figure 3-9.

The heart is a marvelous pump-like organ and one of the first organs to form in an embryo. It sits in the center of the chest, is about the size of your fist, and is partially covered by the lungs. The heart is composed of **cardiac muscle**, a special type of muscle that is able to generate its own electrical impulse. It has four chambers, two upper **atria** and two lower **ventricles**, which are the primary pump chambers of the heart. The right and left sides are divided by the septum, a thick muscular wall. Blood is held in each chamber until it is pumped through another chamber, vein, or artery. A cross-section of the heart showing the four chambers is shown in Figure 3-10.

Blood enters the heart through the vena cava into the right atrium and passes into the right ventricle through the tricuspid valve. From there it goes through the pulmonary

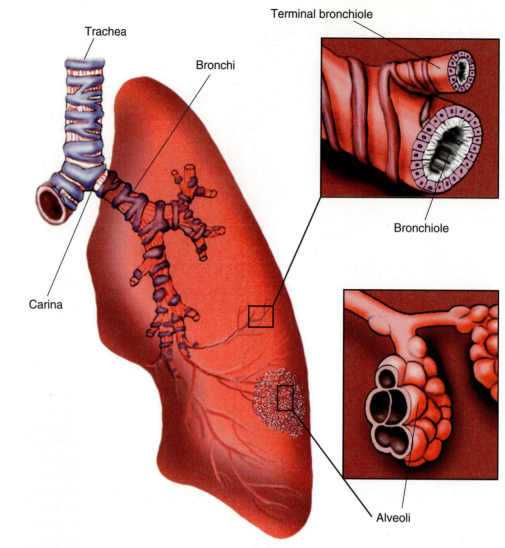

Figure 3-7 The lower airway structures.

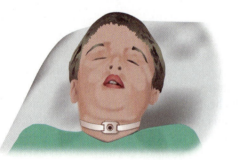

Figure 3-8 A patient with a tracheostomy breathes through a surgically created opening in the anterior neck.

valve into the pulmonary artery and enters the lungs. This is known as pulmonary circulation (Figure 3-11). There, it picks up oxygen and releases carbon dioxide. Blood then enters the left atrium and travels to the left ventricle, which pumps out oxygenated blood into the aorta and then out to the arteries. This circulation is known as systemic circulation (Figure 3-11).

Blood Pressure

When blood exits the heart, it does so under incredible force. This event can be heard as the heartbeat, felt as the pulse, seen as a rhythm on a monitor or **electrocardiogram (ECG or EKG)** and measured as blood pressure. **Blood pressure (BP)** is the amount of pressure placed on the vessels leading from the heart. The blood pressure is composed of two numbers written as a fraction (for example 132/84 mm Hg). The top number, or **systolic blood pressure**, represents the amount of force on the vessels pushing the blood out of the heart into the system. When this occurs, blood with oxygen and nutrients is able to reach the body cells. The bottom number, or **diastolic blood pressure,** is the pressure of the blood in the vessels at rest between heartbeats when there is no force.

EMR Applications for Blood Pressure

Hypertension is diagnosed when multiple blood pressure readings are higher than the normal value (usually greater than 140/90 mm Hg for an adult; prehypertension is 120/80

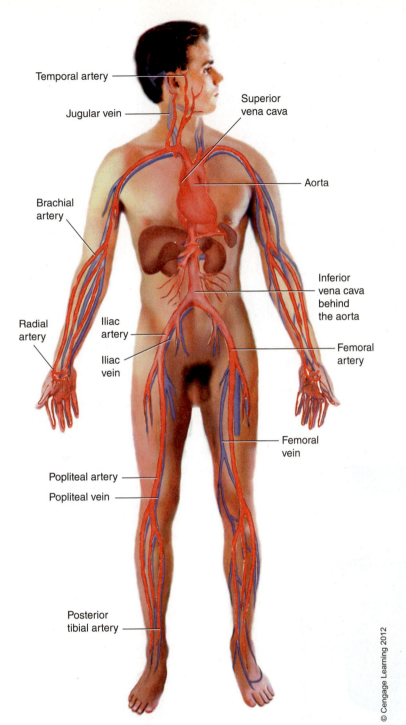

Figure 3-9 The circulatory system is made up of the heart, veins, arteries, and blood.

© Cengage Learning 2012

to 140/90). With hypertension, vessels can become scarred, hardened, or less elastic overtime. Because of this, blockage or rupture may occur and lead to a heart attack, stroke, or organ damage.

Hypotension is a blood pressure that is lower than normal value (approximately below 90 mm Hg systolic for an adult, with some exceptions). Hypotension may cause lightheadedness, loss of consciousness, or cells to die if severe and prolonged.

Heartbeat

The heartbeat is an electrochemical phenomenon. Starting at the sino-atrial (SA) node high on the right atrium, it follows a pathway to the atrioventricular (AV) node, which is located above the border of the right ventricle. This signal stimulates the atria to contract as it travels to the AV node.

The AV node is the gatekeeper of sorts. It allows clean signals to pass through to the ventricles. The signal then

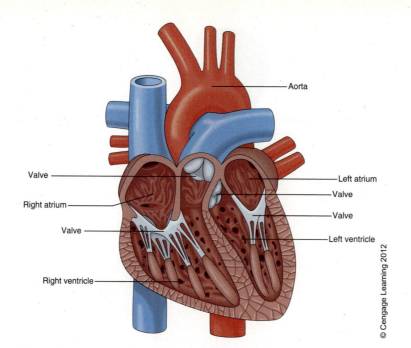

Figure 3-10   Cross-section of the heart showing the four chambers.

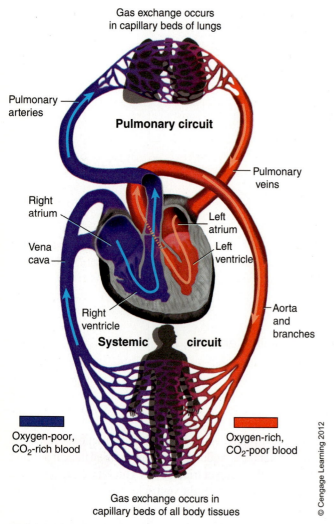

Figure 3-11   Blood flow through the heart and the body.

splits down the heart through the bundle branches and stimulates the ventricles to contract through the pathway of the Purkinje fibers (Figure 3-12). Besides this automatic electrical response, the heart can respond to signals from the body such as increased oxygen demand, hormones such as epinephrine, or medications that cause it to speed up or slow down. The average adult heartbeat is 60 to 100 times per minute. If the SA node does not function, the AV node will stimulate the heart to beat at 40 beats/min, just enough to sustain life.

EMR Applications for the Heartbeat

In cases of cardiac arrest, the heart will stop beating completely, creating a lack of rhythm known as **asystole**, which appears as a flat line on an ECG. When electrical signals in the ventricles become completely disorganized, causing the heart to quiver, it is called **ventricular fibrillation (VF)**. Rapid **ventricular tachycardia (VT)** happens when electrical signals to the ventricles fire too fast and do not allow the heart to fill adequately with blood. In all three cases, the heart does not create enough blood flow to sustain life.

When the heart's electrical system does not work or the heartbeat is too slow to adequately pump blood a device such as a pacemaker, automatic implantable cardioverter-defibrillator (AICD), or combination can be implanted into the person's chest wall (Figure 3-13).

Blood Vessels

The **blood vessels** are a complex set of tubes that carry the blood to and from the heart and lungs. Blood vessels that lead away from the heart and carry oxygenated blood are called **arteries**, and vessels that lead to the heart carrying deoxygenated blood are **veins**. Arteries branch out into **arterioles**

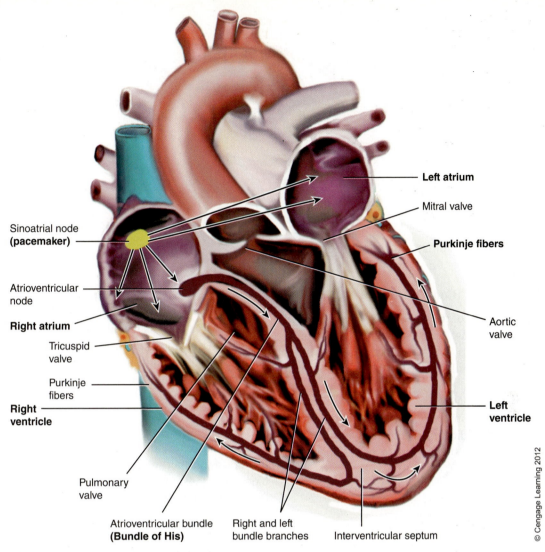

Figure 3-12 Conduction system of the heart.

Labels on the figure:
- Sinoatrial node (pacemaker)
- Atrioventricular node
- **Right atrium**
- Tricuspid valve
- Purkinje fibers
- **Right ventricle**
- Pulmonary valve
- Atrioventricular bundle (Bundle of His)
- Right and left bundle branches
- Interventricular septum
- **Left atrium**
- Mitral valve
- **Purkinje fibers**
- Aortic valve
- **Left ventricle**

© Cengage Learning 2012

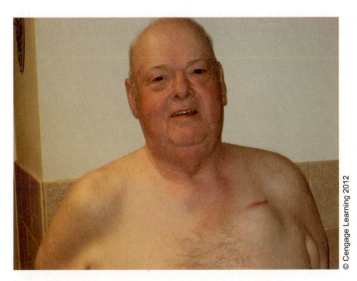

Figure 3-13 An implantable device for regulation and continuation of a heartbeat lies below the surgical incision.

© Cengage Learning 2012

(small blood vessels that branch from the arteries) and then into **capillaries**, tiny blood vessels that connect to **venuoles**, vessels that drain the deoxygenated blood from the capillaries and take it to the veins. The relationship among arteries, veins, and capillaries is shown in Figure 3-14.

There are significant anatomical differences between arteries and veins. Because arteries carry blood to the body and away from the heart, they are under greater pressure than veins. Arteries are wrapped in a layer of muscle and innervated by nerves. These muscles and nerves give the arteries more control over the flow of oxygenated blood. For example, arteries with a clean cut will spasm in an attempt to restrict blood loss and will constrict (narrow) if the body becomes **hypothermic** (body temperature below 95 degrees Fahrenheit) in an effort to maximize the blood supply to the head and thorax.

Although veins have one-way valves, they do not have muscles or nerves. Therefore, veins rely on the pressure of the heart and arteries to circulate the blood back to the heart.

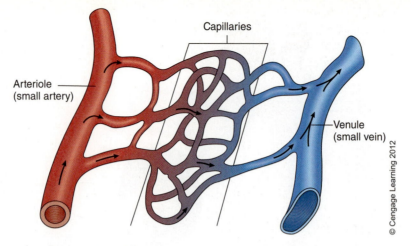

Figure 3-14 Arteries, veins, and capillaries.

EMR Applications for Blood Vessels

Depending on the pressure of the blood vessel, the EMR will see differences with bleeding. An artery with its intense pressure will spurt out blood, a vein with less pressure allows blood to flow out, and a capillary bleed with the least amount of pressure will ooze blood.

Upon assessment, an EMR may find that a patient's vein is accessed with a type of intravenous (IV) tubing. Patients receiving long-term IV medication therapy may have IV tubing secured in an arm or chest area (Figure 3-15). Patients on kidney dialysis may have a permanent dialysis access created by a fistula or graft. This allows the artery and vein to be connected to a dialysis machine to clean the blood. A fistula and a graft are illustrated in Figure 3-16. The EMR should not take blood pressures in an arm with IV tubing or a dialysis access and should avoid interfering with any area where an IV line is inserted.

Blood

Blood is a mixture of liquid and solid parts. The liquid is **plasma**, a transport medium for the other components in the blood. The most prominent solids are red blood cells, white blood cells, and platelets.

Red Blood Cells

Red blood cells (RBCs) are flat, round, and concave on each side. They have no nucleus and cannot reproduce by themselves. They are manufactured in the marrow of long bones such as the sternum and femur. Oxygen attaches to RBCs (like iron to a magnet) and is carried through the blood. The higher the concentration of oxygen, the brighter red the blood

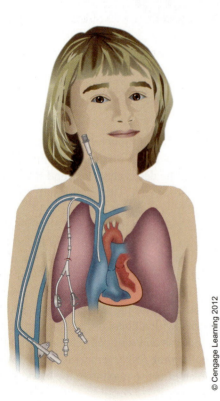

Figure 3-15 Central venous catheters are used to administer intravenous medication and to withdraw blood samples from the venous system.

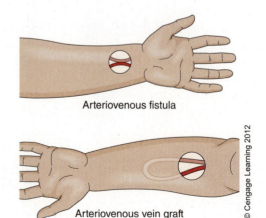

Arteriovenous fistula

Arteriovenous vein graft

Figure 3-16 A fistula or graft is a surgically created access to a vein and artery for dialysis. Formation can also be in the upper arm.

appears. Carbon dioxide is a free gas that is unattached and flows in the plasma. Gas exchange occurs as the blood washes through the lungs where, in the alveoli, the lungs deposit oxygen into the RBCs and pick up carbon dioxide to exhale.

EMR Applications for Red Blood Cells and Oxygenation

There are many reasons why the body might not absorb oxygen or obtain adequate amounts of oxygen from the blood. Oxygen can be displaced from the hemoglobin by things such as cyanide or carbon monoxide (CO). Oxygen can be impaired by diseases, such as sickle cell anemia, that affect the shape of the RBCs. An inadequate amount of hemoglobin caused by a major bleed or insufficient respirations will also cause a decrease in oxygen. The EMR will notice initial signs of lightheadedness, fatigue, and pale skin color in these patients that can progress to loss of consciousness or death.

White Blood Cells

The primary role of the **white blood cells (WBCs)** is to fight infection. They are formed in the bone marrow but differ from RBCs because they have a nucleus and tend to be aggressive. WBCs attack, attempt to neutralize, and remove anything that is a threat to the body. Usually they attack foreign objects such as bacteria. Although immune response is complicated, the aggregation and release of huge numbers of WBCs is a hallmark of infection, usually bacterial.

EMR Applications for White Blood Cells and Infection

A surge of WBCs is often accompanied by a fever. The body can handle a temporary state of being several degrees either warmer or cooler with little difficulty, but when the temperature rises excessively, organs such as the brain and the kidneys may experience permanent damage.

When WBCs are decreased, the patient's immune system is compromised. There can be many causes for a low immune system, including infancy (immune system not fully developed), advanced age, disease, medications such as chemotherapy, and radiation therapy.

EMRs will provide care to patients with compromised immune systems. Precautions must be taken to avoid introducing infection to the patient or EMR. If you have a cough or the patient is coughing, wear a mask to protect the patient and yourself. As is appropriate for all contact, proper hand washing and use of gloves are of vital importance.

Platelets

One of the wonders of blood is its ability to form clots by a component of the blood called platelets. Clot formation is a complex process that begins when the integrity of the circulatory system is disrupted. When the circulatory system has a leak, as in a cut, or when a change occurs in the inside wall of a blood vessel, platelets release chemicals that stimulate a **thrombus** (a clot), to assist in controlling a bleed.

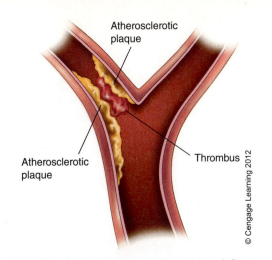

Figure 3-17 © Cengage Learning 2012

Figure 3-17 Platelets and other blood factors can adhere to the irregular surface of a plaque, resulting in a thrombus.

EMR Applications for Platelets as a Clotting Mechanism

A thrombus or an **embolism** (a thrombus that moves) is a common cause of heart attack (myocardial infarction), cardiac arrest (the heart stops beating), stroke, or extremity pain. Sometimes a thrombus can be the cause of a **pulmonary embolism**, where the clot travels to the lung and blocks an artery in the lung, often resulting in sudden, severe shortness of breath. Figure 3-17 illustrates how clots are formed.

A deficiency of platelets causes an inability of the blood to clot effectively. Clotting disorders are often the result of genetic disease, cancer, or a disease process, but many medications such as Coumadin and aspirin can interfere with the clotting mechanism of blood. Over-the-counter (OTC) supplements, such as herbs, may also interact with prescription medications to inhibit the clotting process. A patient with this condition may bruise easily, have prolonged bleeding, or bleed from body cavities such as the nose.

Remember that the skin does not have to be broken for blood loss to occur. When a bruise or **hematoma** occurs, blood pools under the skin until the clotting mechanism can stop the bleed. Some parts of the body, such as the upper leg and abdomen, can hold a large amount of blood internally. Medical and trauma events can cause internal bleeding when the body is unable to clot the area involved. It is possible to "bleed out" internally without ever having an open wound.

The Integumentary System

The skin is the body's largest organ. It is comprised of several layers, each with specific functions. The epidermis is the thinnest outermost layer. It protects the other layers of the skin from the environment and is constantly being reformed. Below the epidermis is the dermis. This layer is richly fed by blood and is made up of connective tissue and serves as the foundation for structures such as hair follicles, sweat glands, sebaceous glands (oil glands), and blood.

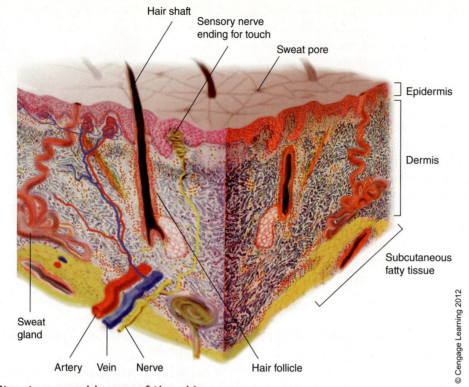

Hair shaft

Sensory nerve
ending for touch

Sweat pore

Epidermis

Dermis

Subcutaneous
fatty tissue

Sweat
gland

Artery   Vein   Nerve

Hair follicle

© Cengage Learning 2012

Figure 3-18   Structures and layers of the skin.

The lowermost layer is the subcutaneous or hypodermis. It is composed of adipose (fat) and collagen (responsible for skin elasticity and structure). The purpose of the hypodermis is twofold: it supplies the upper layers of the dermis with blood, and it attaches the skin to the muscles and bones. Figure 3-18 shows the layers and important structures of the skin.

Skin Functions

The skin performs several functions for the body:

- Protection of the internal organs and the body in general; protects the body from the environment, bacteria and other organisms
- Regulation of temperature through vasodilation or vasoconstriction of the vessels, such as perspiration (which tends to cool the skin) and shivering (tends to warm the skin)
- Prevention of dehydration by keeping the fluids of the body inside
- Absorption of chemicals or topical medications (those applied on top of the skin)
- Sensation of touch, heat, cold, pressure, and injury, which is accomplished by the nerve endings
- Excretion of waste through perspiration

EMR Applications for the Integumentary System

Generally, skin is a uniform color determined by pigmentation in the dermis. Variations in skin color are normal for people of different ethnic and racial backgrounds.

However, several skin colors should alert an emergency responder. **Shock** is a medical emergency in which organs and tissues of the body are not receiving an adequate flow of blood, resulting in inadequate oxygenation of cells, tissues and organs. When there is insufficient oxygen to tissues, the skin may turn cold, pale, ashen, blue (cyanotic), or mottled (blotchy). In a person with dark skin, the EMR may need to look under the lower eyelid and inside the lips to determine a change in skin color. It is important for an EMR to observe the skin for temperature, color, and moisture because these may indicate poor oxygenation or shock, which are serious conditions that require immediate treatment (discussed further in Chapter 8).

Regulation of temperature (thermal regulation) and moisture is controlled by the opening and closing of pores in the skin. When this regulatory mechanism is affected by conditions such as extreme temperature, shock, anxiety, or any stress on the body, the skin can become hot and dry or cool and clammy.

The Digestive System

Most of the digestive system organs are contained in the abdominal cavity, which is broken down into four quadrants, using the umbilicus as the center point. Each quadrant is named either left or right and upper or lower. The four quadrants and their organs are pictured in Figure 3-19. It is important for the EMR to know which organs are contained in each quadrant.

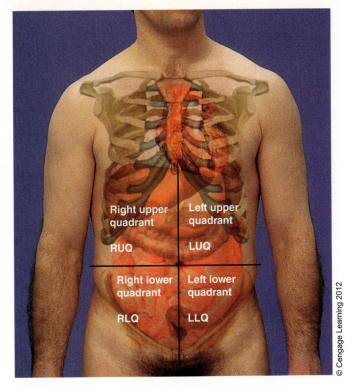

Figure 3-19 The four quadrants of the abdomen.

Digestion is the process by which we ingest products, turn those products into usable energy by the body, and then remove the waste. This process occurs in one long tube called the alimentary canal, which is formed by the mouth, esophagus, stomach, small intestine, large intestine, and rectum.

Food's Journey: Beginning to End

When solids or liquids are introduced into the mouth, it secretes salivary enzymes that start breaking down foods. As food is chewed, it mixes with salivary enzymes so the food slides down the esophagus easier. Food travels down it in a bolus, a clump of chewed and partially digested food called chyme. Food enters the stomach, a hollow muscular organ with many folds or rugae, which allow for expansion when large amounts of food are introduced. Digestive enzymes secreted by the pancreas and hydrochloric acid help break down food and other matter present in the stomach.

When the food is sufficiently churned, it is propelled from the stomach by a series of rhythmic contractions called **peristalsis** into the small intestine, where most of the digestive and absorption occurs. The gallbladder releases bile produced by the liver and helps break up fats. The liver additionally cleanses toxins from the body and changes food into energy. Nutrients are extracted from the chyme as it passes through the small intestine, the longest part of the digestive tract.

When the bulk of the nutrients are removed, the remainder passes into the large intestine and are deposited into the rectal vault before being released through the anus. The entire process of digestion may vary depending on the body's need for nutrients or the health of the digestive tract. The process of digestion and elimination is illustrated in Figure 3-20.

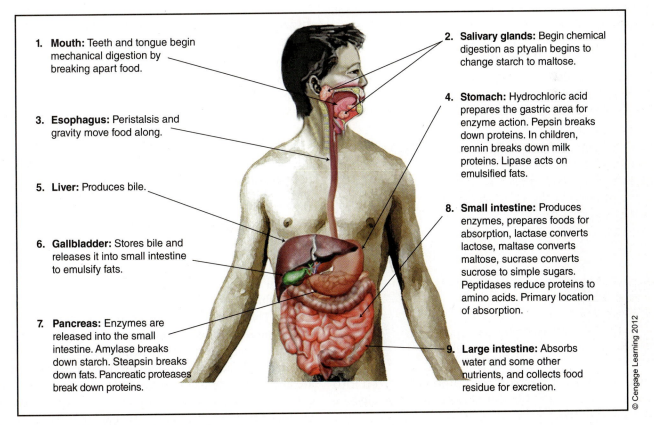

1. **Mouth:** Teeth and tongue begin mechanical digestion by breaking apart food.

2. **Salivary glands:** Begin chemical digestion as ptyalin begins to change starch to maltose.

3. **Esophagus:** Peristalsis and gravity move food along.

4. **Stomach:** Hydrochloric acid prepares the gastric area for enzyme action. Pepsin breaks down proteins. In children, rennin breaks down milk proteins. Lipase acts on emulsified fats.

5. **Liver:** Produces bile.

6. **Gallbladder:** Stores bile and releases it into small intestine to emulsify fats.

7. **Pancreas:** Enzymes are released into the small intestine. Amylase breaks down starch. Steapsin breaks down fats. Pancreatic proteases break down proteins.

8. **Small intestine:** Produces enzymes, prepares foods for absorption, lactase converts lactose, maltase converts maltose, sucrase converts sucrose to simple sugars. Peptidases reduce proteins to amino acids. Primary location of absorption.

9. **Large intestine:** Absorbs water and some other nutrients, and collects food residue for excretion.

Figure 3-20 The gastrointestinal system.

EMR Applications for the Digestive System

EMRs may encounter digestive system emergencies ranging from trauma to disease. Trauma to the abdominal cavity or disease processes in the abdominal structures or organs can result in symptoms or physical changes that the EMR should recognize.

Abdominal Cavity Trauma

The digestive tract in the abdomen is susceptible to injury or trauma because it is not protected by the ribs. Solid organs, such as the liver and pancreas, in the abdominal cavity can bleed in traumatic situations and are impossible to control in the prehospital setting. Hollow organs such as the stomach and intestines can spill their contents into the abdominal cavity as a result of injury. Such a spill can be life threatening.

Appendix

Attached to the large intestine in the lower right quadrant is a small piece of tissue called the appendix. It has no known function but can become inflamed (appendicitis) by trapped material. When inflammation occurs, the appendix may need to be removed. If it ruptures, it can spill bacteria into the abdominal cavity, leading to pain and a severe infection.

Emesis

Many conditions or illnesses may cause a patient to expel **emesis** (vomit) from the stomach. Emesis has a repugnant odor because it is composed of partially digested food combined with digestive enzymes. Emesis may potentially contain pathogens, so the EMR should wear proper personal protective equipment.

Openings in the Abdominal Wall

Interruption of the digestive process caused by disease, dysfunction, or removal may result in the need of a patient to have a feeding tube such as a gastrostomy tube (GT) inserted into the

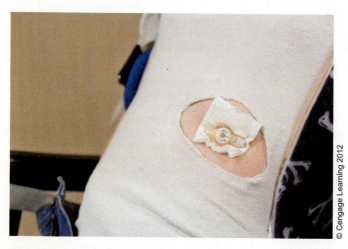

Figure 3-21 A gastrostomy tube is inserted into the abdominal wall for the purpose of receiving liquid feedings.

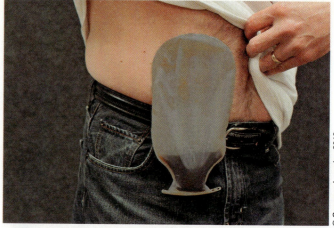

Figure 3-22 A patient may have a colostomy for elimination.

wall of the abdomen for the purpose of receiving liquid feedings (Figure 3-21). Patients with these conditions may also have a colostomy or a surgical stoma (an opening in the lower abdominal wall) to divert feces into an external bag, Figure 3-22.

The Endocrine System

The endocrine system is composed of organs called glands, which produce hormones. **Hormones** are chemical messengers that travel in the bloodstream to tissues or organs. Hormones can change the way an organ or cell functions. Figure 3-23 shows the glands that produce hormones and describes the effect of each hormone.

EMR Applications for the Endocrine System

The EMR must be aware that the pancreas produces the hormone **insulin** (Figure 3-24), which assists in the body's utilization of glucose. Glucose is vital for cell function. If the pancreas does not produce insulin, it is impossible for glucose to be transported to the body's cells. When a person has insulin-dependent diabetes mellitus, the pancreas may produce no insulin, not enough insulin, or there may be an ineffective use of insulin, and the patient must take injections of insulin on a daily basis. A patient may also receive insulin delivered by an insulin pump (Figure 3-25).

The Urinary System

The urinary system consists of the kidneys, ureter, bladder, and urethra. These and other associated structures are illustrated in Figure 3-26. As food and liquids are digested, the excess fluid passes from the digestive tract into the bloodstream. This fluid is either absorbed by the body or excreted by the kidneys. When blood passes through the kidneys, it is washed of excess waste by nephrons, the primary structure of the kidneys responsible for urine production. There are approximately one million nephrons in each kidney to collect and process urine. Urine passes down ureters into the **bladder,** a large muscular sac that holds the urine until

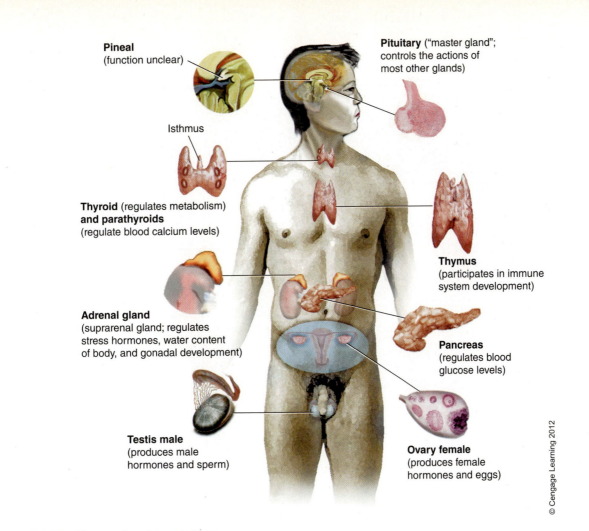

Pineal
(function unclear)

Pituitary ("master gland";
controls the actions of
most other glands)

Isthmus

Thyroid (regulates metabolism)
and parathyroids
(regulate blood calcium levels)

Thymus
(participates in immune
system development)

Adrenal gland
(suprarenal gland; regulates
stress hormones, water content
of body, and gonadal development)

Pancreas
(regulates blood
glucose levels)

Testis male
(produces male
hormones and sperm)

Ovary female
(produces female
hormones and eggs)

© Cengage Learning 2012

Figure 3-23 The endocrine system.

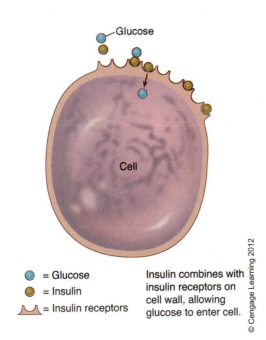

Glucose

Cell

= Glucose

= Insulin

= Insulin receptors

Insulin combines with
insulin receptors on
cell wall, allowing
glucose to enter cell.

© Cengage Learning 2012

Figure 3-24 Insulin is the carrier of glucose
from the blood into the cells.

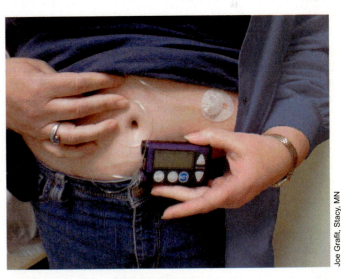

Joe Grafit, Stacy, MN

Figure 3-25 A person who must receive insulin
may receive his or her insulin delivered by an
insulin pump.

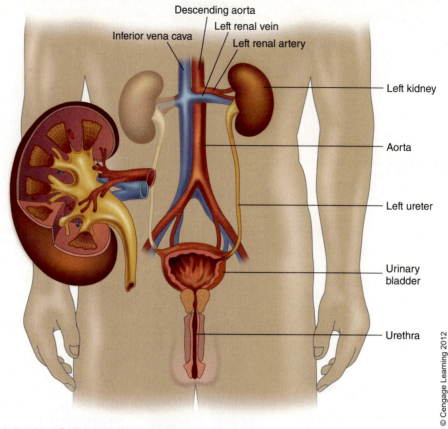

Figure 3-26 Structures of the urinary system.

Descending aorta
Left renal vein
Left renal artery
Inferior vena cava
Left kidney
Aorta
Left ureter
Urinary bladder
Urethra

© Cengage Learning 2012

elimination. Urine exits the body through a tube called the **urethra**. Urine is composed mostly of water and is normally a sterile fluid when it exits the body.

EMR Applications for the Urinary System

Many illnesses have indicators that can be found in the urine. A person with diabetes may release glucose, protein, and ketones through the urine. Some infectious processes cause either WBCs or RBCs to show up in the urine. Certain diseases and medications can cause chemicals to be released in the urine, which can be tested for a specific diagnosis. Pregnancy can also be determined through analysis of the urine.

A patient with a dysfunction of the urinary system may have a urinary catheter connected to a drainage bag for urine collection. This catheter is a long flexible tube that runs through the urethra and is anchored in the bladder by a water-filled balloon. If a patient's bladder has been removed, there will be a surgical stoma created called a urostomy in the abdominal wall to divert urine into a bag. A suprapubic tube placed directly into the bladder and drains urine into a bag may also be visible with your assessments.

The Reproductive System

The reproductive organs differentiate male and female anatomy. The organs make reproduction and continuation of the human species possible. These reproductive organs also produce hormones. Hormones play a role in characteristics and function.

The Male Reproductive System

The penis is normally flaccid. It serves two functions: (1) the exit pathway of urine through the urethra and (2) the male sexual organ. During sexual excitement, the penis fills with blood, causing an erection. At this time, the bladder is shut out, making it almost impossible to void. The prostate gland blocks urine flow while it assists with the expulsion of semen, called ejaculation. The testes are located in the scrotum, a sack that hangs directly behind and beneath the penis. The testes are responsible for the production and storage of semen. The scrotum allows thermal regulation of the testes by contracting and relaxing. Figure 3-27 illustrates the structures associated with the male genital system.

EMR Applications for the Male Reproductive System

The penis and testicles, because of their relatively unprotected location, are subject to serious injury from trauma.

Priapism, a prolonged erection of the penis without sexual stimulation, may be caused by certain medications, illicit drug use, carbon monoxide poisoning, or a spinal cord injury.

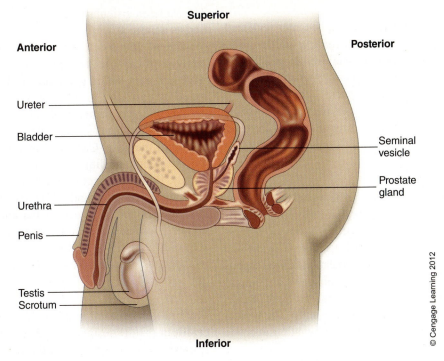

Figure 3-27 The male reproductive system.

The Female Reproductive System

The female reproductive organs, consisting of the ovaries, fallopian tubes, uterus, and vagina, are located in the pelvic cavity (Figure 3-28). Guided by a complex set of hormonal signals, each month one of the ovaries (alternating every other month) releases an egg into the fallopian tube, which then travels into the uterus. Each ovary has a finite number of eggs. If an egg is not fertilized, another set of hormones causes menstruation, the shedding of the egg and uterine lining through the vagina. If the egg becomes fertilized, the woman's body immediately begins releasing hormones that guide the embryonic development all the way to and through birth. The entire gestational period lasts approximately 36 to 40 weeks. When a woman reaches puberty, her body begins the process of menstruation. When a woman's body stops menstruation, she enters menopause.

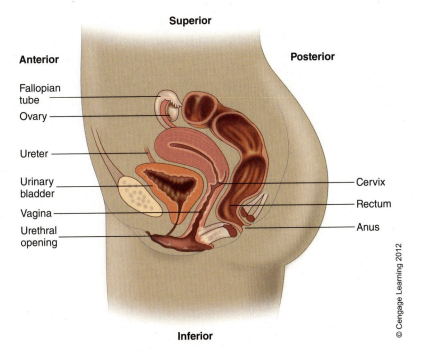

Figure 3-28 The female reproductive system.

EMR Applications for the Female Reproductive System

If an egg lodges in the fallopian tube and becomes fertilized, it is considered a tubal or ectopic pregnancy, which can be life threatening. The body can spontaneously abort a fetus at any time during the first few months of pregnancy. Vaginal bleeding can signal an impending emergency. It is the responsibility of the EMR to assess the safety and well-being of the mother and the unborn baby. Any deviations from the norm must be treated with urgency.

The Skeletal System

The axial skeleton includes the skull, the spinal column, and the bony ribs that are attached. The axial skeleton is illustrated in Figure 3-29. These bones form the axis or support that gives our bodies a basic form and structure. The skeletal system functions as a framework for protection of vital organs such as the brain, spinal cord, and thoracic and abdominal organs. The skeleton allows movement and produces RBCs in the long bones (femur, humerus, and sternum). The typical human body has 206 bones. Our bones are living tissue made mostly of calcium.

Joints

The skeleton articulates through joints. Joints can be classified as a point at which two or more bones meet to allow for movement. Joints define the body's range of motion. Within many joint capsules is a cushion, called bursa, a sac filled with lubricant called **synovial fluid.** Other joints are cushioned by cartilage. **Cartilage** is a substance that is not as hard as bone yet firmer than muscles. It connects and cushions bones in places such as the rib cage, the vertebrae, and the tip of the nose. Cartilage, tendons, and ligaments, have a difficult time healing due to a decrease of or lack of blood supply. Bones connect to other bones via **ligaments***, which are tough, fibrous strands of connective tissue. Internal organs are connected to each other and the skeleton by ligaments. Muscles connect to bones through **tendons,** which are connective tissue on the end of a muscle. The muscle is wrapped in a sheath called the fascia.

Cranium

The brain is encased in a group of fused bones called the **cranium** (skull) designed to protect it from external trauma (Figure 3-30). The bones of the face attach to the skull to

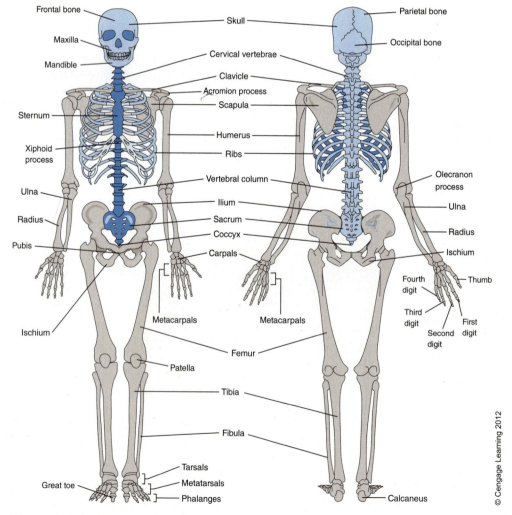

Figure 3-29 The axial skeleton (in *blue*) and the appendicular skeleton.

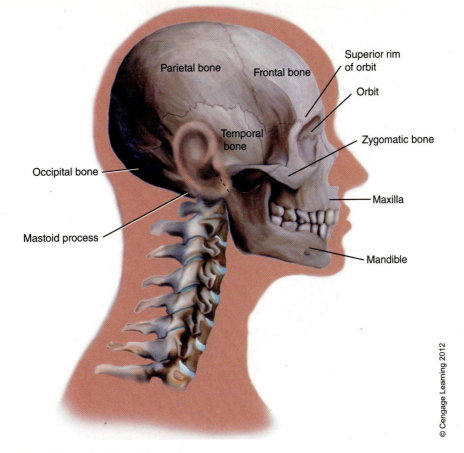

Figure 3-30 Bones of the skull and face.

protect the eyes and the upper airway structures. If the brain swells or fills with fluid, the cranium is unable to expand, and the brain can become injured.

Spine

The spine is a collection of 33 bones, or **vertebrae**. The vertebrae surround the spinal cord (the collection of nerves that run from the brain through the spinal column and branch out as peripheral nerves to body organs and tissues) and are separated from each other by cushions of cartilage, called discs.

The vertebrae are grouped by location. The top seven are the **cervical vertebrae,** which includes primarily the neck. Below the cervical vertebrae are the 12 **thoracic vertebrae** followed by the five **lumbar vertebrae**. The remaining vertebrae, the five **sacral** and four **coccyx,** are actually fused together. These sections of vertebrae and spinal cord can be seen in Figure 3-31.

Rib Cage and Sternum

The **thorax,** the part of the body between the neck and the abdomen, where the heart and lungs lie, is protected by the costal region, better known as the rib cage. There are 12 sets of ribs. Each rib originates from the spine and is connected to the sternum either directly or by a piece of cartilage with the exception of the two bottom pairs. These are the floating ribs, so named because they do not attach to the front and are only anchored to the spine.

The **sternum** itself is composed of three bones: the manubrium, which forms the top of the sternum; the sternal body, the longer center portion of the sternum; and the **xiphoid process**, which is a narrow cartilage tip at the bottom of the sternum. The anatomy of the rib cage and sternum can be seen at Figure 3-32.

EMR Applications for the Skeletal System

EMRs should avoid pressure on the xiphoid process while performing lifesaving measures with cardiopulmonary resuscitation (CPR) and while providing obstructed airway techniques.

A bone can be broken (fractured) with either indirect or direct force. EMRs should assume that a fracture will cause damage to associated nerves, muscles, vasculature, or soft tissue. Fractures are painful and potentially life or limb threatening.

Dislocations, although not usually life threatening, can be extremely painful, Dislocations are caused by extreme force resulting in two bone ends of a joint separating. Function is limited in the joint but may not be limited distal to the dislocation. An example of this is a patient who is unable to move a dislocated shoulder but is able to move his or her hand.

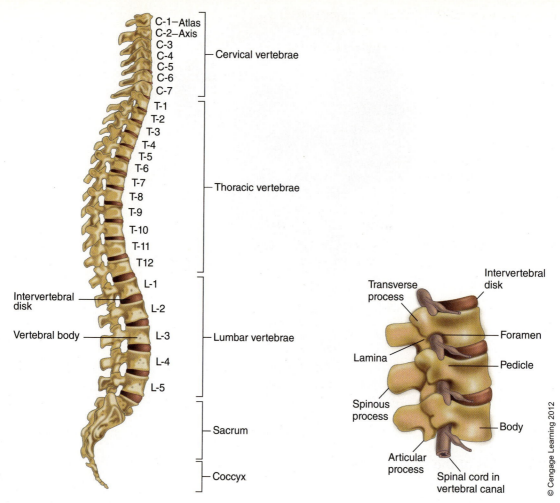

Figure 3-31 Anatomy of the spinal column.

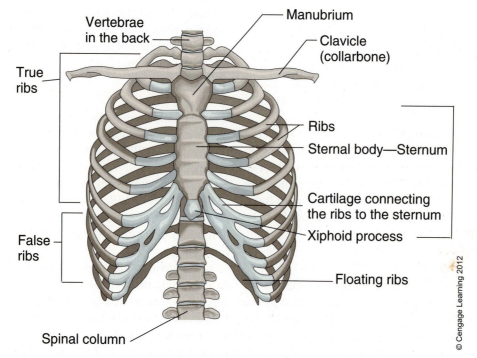

Figure 3-32 Anatomy of the rib cage and sternum.

Because the cranium is an immovable joint, injury to the brain can result in swelling and can cause traumatic brain injury (TBI) from pressure. This pressure within the skull is referred to as **intracranial pressure (ICP)**.

The Muscular System

The muscular system is designed to allow movement of the bones and assist the skeletal system in giving the body its shape. With more than 600 muscles adding mass to the body, the muscles assist in protecting the internal organs and other systems. Muscles are classified as cardiac, smooth, or skeletal. The heart is composed of cardiac muscle. Smooth muscles are found in the internal organs and allow for the bodily functions that do not require direct control and are said to be involuntary. It is generally only the skeletal muscles that are controlled voluntarily, directly and consciously.

Cardiac Muscle

As previously mentioned, cardiac muscle (the myocardium) is unique because it has the ability to self-contract and expand. Several places in the myocardium act as generators that create an electrochemical pulse. The rate of the heart beat or pulse changes with the oxygen demands on it. During situations, such as anxiety or exercise, there is a higher oxygen demand on the heart, causing it to speed up to provide more oxygen to the cells and organs. After the heart is formed in utero and begins beating, it does not stop until death. The heart, similar to any other muscle, can become weak if not exercised.

EMR Applications for Cardiac Muscle

Patients who experience heart failure have weak contractions of the heart that fail to move enough blood through their bodies. The left side of the heart is not strong enough to pump the blood out of the pulmonary circulation as quickly as it enters. This results in swelling (**edema**) of the extremities or fluid in the lungs heard as crackles. Figure 3-33 illustrates this process.

Smooth Muscles

Smooth muscles generally perform regulatory functions and are mostly involuntary. For example, the bladder is a smooth muscular sac that forces urine down the urethra as it empties. The colon is a smooth muscle organ that uses peristaltic waves to force feces through the intestines. Shivering or goose bumps are involuntary responses caused by pilo muscles below the skin. Involuntary responses from smooth muscle are automatically governed by the nervous system. When involuntary functions cease, danger follows.

Skeletal Muscle

Skeletal muscles provide for voluntary movements. Anatomically, the location of a skeletal muscle is the best indicator of its function. For example, the biceps and triceps

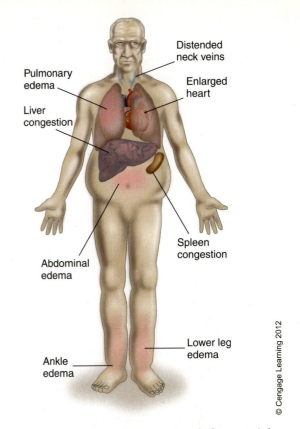

Figure 3-33 A poorly functioning left ventricle will result in a backup of fluid pressure in the pulmonary circulation, as well as other areas of the body. This backup of fluid is called edema.

dictate the action of the arm in relation to the forearm. This can be determined by noting where the muscles attach to the humerus, radius, and ulna.

When skeletal muscles are used, they produce lactic acid as a byproduct. Lactic acid causes the burning sensation during exercise. Lactic acid is flushed away by the bloodstream and excreted by the kidneys.

EMR Applications for the Skeletal Muscle

Muscular injuries occur when a muscle or muscles are stretched, torn, bruised, or cut. They commonly occur with bone fractures but can also occur from overexertion of the muscle. Muscle cramping can be a result of overuse of muscles or from dehydration.

The Neurological System

The nervous system controls voluntary and involuntary activities. The nervous system can be divided several ways. The **central nervous system** is made up of the brain and the spinal cord. The **peripheral nervous system** is composed of the nerves that come off the spinal cord and continue to the rest or the body. The **autonomic nervous system**, made up of the sympathetic and parasympathetic systems, controls the automatic functions of the body.

The Brain

The brain, encased in the cranium, is composed of the cerebrum, cerebellum, and brainstem. Each of these areas has subdivisions with special functions as shown in Figure 3-34.

- The largest part of the brain is the **cerebrum**. The cerebrum is composed of four lobes and divided bilaterally into the right and left hemispheres connected by the corpus callosum, a thick membrane that allows the two hemispheres to communicate with each other.
  - At the rear of the brain is the occipital lobe. Its primary function is related to vision. It translates signals received by the eyes into visual images. In addition, it may play a part in creating mental images.
  - On the sides of the brain are the temporal lobes. They are responsible mainly for auditory and speech processing.
  - Above the temporal lobes sit the parietal lobes. These separate the occipital lobes from the frontal lobes. The parietal lobes are responsible for integration of sensory information. They act as a sort of gatekeeper and central processor for our senses.
  - The frontal lobes sit at the most anterior aspect of the cerebrum. The frontal lobes are responsible for higher thought processes. Everything from cognition to abstract thinking and mathematical computation to emotional response is generated in the frontal lobes.
- The **cerebellum** sits on top of and slightly behind the medulla. Its primary function is motor control and balance. It may also play a role in emotional responses.
- The **brainstem**, which is the lower part of the brain, extends into the spinal cord. Survival functions are regulated here, which include breathing, digestion, alertness, heart rate, and blood pressure.

The brain is suspended in **cerebrospinal fluid (CSF),** which serves as a support or cushion within the skull. CSF is held in place by a series of membranes called the **meninges.** These membranes consist of three thin layers that encase the brain, brainstem, and spinal cord, keeping the CSF from spilling out.

EMR Applications for the Brain

CSF is normally a clear fluid. CSF from the ears or nose indicates a serious closed head trauma and can appear clear or pink tinged in color. The EMR should not stop the flow of CSF because it could increase pressure in the brain.

The brain essentially requires two things to function: oxygen and glucose. A lack of these from injury or disease can result in a severe decrease in consciousness that, if not corrected, will eventually lead to death.

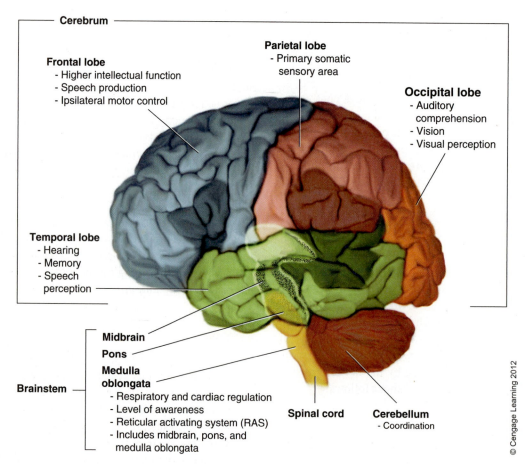

Figure 3-34 The brain and its subdivisions.

The Spinal Cord

The spinal cord extends through a hole in the base of the spine and runs along the back. It is encased in vertebrae, which are cushioned from one another by discs made of cartilage, which allows for limited movement. Nerves extend off the spinal cord and form longer nerve pathways that extend throughout the body. These nerves connect all of the muscles and organs of the body (Figure 3-35).

EMR Applications for the Spinal Cord

Injuries involving the spinal cord may cause total or some degree of paralysis or weakness. Injury can also cause a decrease or loss of sensation. The higher the injury or lesion is on the spinal cord, the higher on the body the involvement begins.

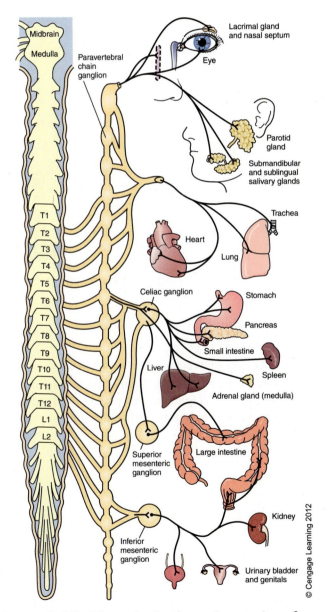

Figure 3-35 The spinal column is a series of vertebrae that house the spinal cord.

As an EMR, you can help prevent spinal cord injury by proper stabilization of the entire spine. If moving a patient causes a spinal cord injury, the injury is called a **secondary cord injury.**

Peripheral Nervous System

Peripheral nerves transmit information to and from the brain and spinal cord by electrochemical conduction. This is the same conduction used in the brain. Impulses travel electrically along the body of the nerve (the axon) to the tip (dendrite), where the impulse stimulates certain chemicals (neurotransmitters) to travel across the gap (synapse) that is present between all nerve cells. Depending on the stimulating impulse, specific neurotransmitters are released that cause a given response. For example, adrenaline causes the heart to speed up and the arteries to dilate. Figure 3-36 illustrates the actions of the peripheral nervous system.

Not all nervous impulses travel to the brain. Certain reflexes only travel to and from the spinal cord. Touching a hot surface, for example, stimulates heat receptors that cause an impulse to race to the cord from which the reflexive jerk is sent. The spinal cord reflexes roughly correspond to the level of the body that they innervate. The higher up the spinal cord, the higher on the body is the response.

EMR Applications for the Peripheral Nervous System

When an EMR checks circulation, movement, and sensation (CMS), the peripheral nervous system provides valuable information regarding movement and sensation. (This topic is discussed in Chapter 5.)

Autonomic Nervous System

The autonomic nervous system controls the automatic functions of the body. The cardiac muscle and the smooth muscles of the body are able to function automatically because of this system. The autonomic nervous system is divided into the sympathetic and parasympathetic nervous systems.

Sympathetic Nervous System

The **sympathetic nervous system** governs the fight-or-flight response. One way to think of the sympathetic response is how you would respond if you were walking through the woods and were suddenly approached by a large bear. It is an involuntary reaction to acute stress or alarm. It is controlled by the neurotransmitter adrenaline and is an instinctual response.

Parasympathetic Nervous System

The opposite response of the sympathetic nervous system is the **parasympathetic nervous system** response that governs rest and repose. This response calms or slows the body by balancing against the sympathetic nervous system to maintain a moderation in those responses. Relaxation techniques cause a parasympathetic response. The mediating hormone for the parasympathetic system is acetylcholine.

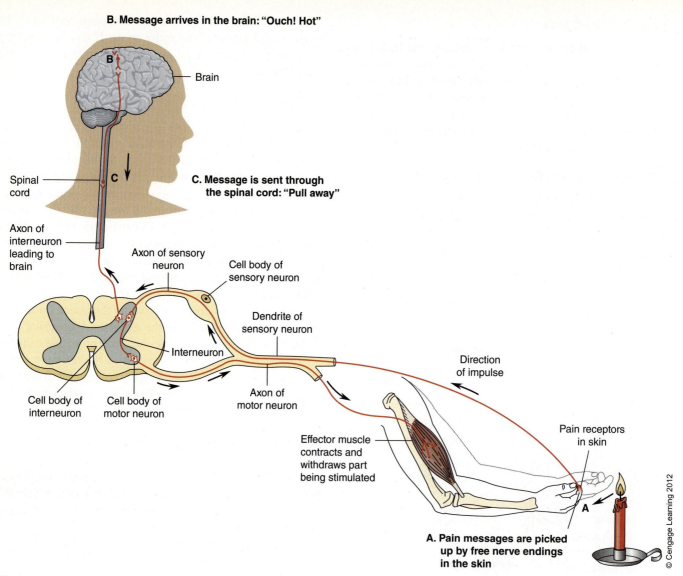

B. Message arrives in the brain: "Ouch! Hot"

Brain

Spinal cord

C. Message is sent through the spinal cord: "Pull away"

Axon of interneuron leading to brain

Axon of sensory neuron

Cell body of sensory neuron

Dendrite of sensory neuron

Interneuron

Cell body of interneuron

Cell body of motor neuron

Axon of motor neuron

Direction of impulse

Effector muscle contracts and withdraws part being stimulated

Pain receptors in skin

A. Pain messages are picked up by free nerve endings in the skin

© Cengage Learning 2012

Figure 3-36 The nerves in the peripheral nervous system take messages about the environment back to the brain.

EMR Applications for the Autonomic Nervous System

With a sympathetic nervous system response, the EMR will notice increased readings in the patient's pulse, respirations, blood pressure, and temperature, as well as increased sweating. Anxiety will be evident. The EMR must take time to assess the scene because the fight or flight response may impair the patient's judgment. This patient needs to be approached in a calm, reassuring, and nonthreatening manner.

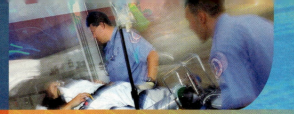

CHAPTER 4

INTERACTING WITH PATIENTS

LEARNING OBJECTIVES

By the end of this chapter, the reader should be able to:

- Define emotional intelligence.
- List the steps that bring about emotional intelligence.
- Define social intelligence.
- List steps for gaining rapport with patients.
- Explain the communication elements of good rapport.
- Explain the impact of dealing with death and dying.
- Define health care directive and explain the Emergency Medical Responder's role.

INTRODUCTION

Interacting with patients can be one of the most rewarding elements of working in the field of Emergency Medical Services (EMS). Emergency Medical Responder (EMR) personnel see a wide array of emotional responses and must respond with competence and compassion. Patient behavior can make initial care difficult. An EMR must come into this profession with more than just the required medical knowledge. They must also understand that patients are more than a diagnosis or a textbook example of a traumatic injury. Being competent in medicine is important; however, people skills are also a critical component of patient care. EMR providers must master emotional and social intelligence and learn the skills of good rapport and active listening to effectively provide the best care for their patients and for themselves.

Emotional Intelligence

Emotional intelligence[1] is the process of improving our strengths and weaknesses as we work through our inner conflicts. There are four steps to bringing about emotional intelligence, which are:

Step 1: Know Yourself

EMRs cannot interact with patients in a purposeful manner without first assessing their own strengths and weaknesses. In other words, you must know yourself before you can reach out and help someone else. Many communication problems stem from clouding the communication process with our own emotional struggles.

Step 2: Manage Your Emotions

To interact effectively with patients, we must begin by managing our own emotions to create a more predictable and better response to stressful situations. You must recognize what emotional factors affect you and then make a conscious effort to manage these emotions to provide the most effective care to the patient. EMRs must understand what inner emotions cause them to react negatively. Some examples might be:

- Difficulty working with someone who is drunk and has injured another person
- No tolerance for domestic abuse and called to a residence where abuse has occurred
- Must work on a child who has been beaten by a caregiver

In these examples, the EMR must rely on training and suppress personal emotions that might hinder patient care. If the emotional stress of the situation is too much, the EMR should turn over care to someone else.

Step 3: Motivate Yourself

The third step to emotional intelligence is self-motivation. You must motivate yourself from within. Although others may inspire us, motivation must be something that we do for ourselves.

Step 4: Have Empathy

Empathy is the identification with and understanding of the patient's situation, feelings, and emotions. Empathy is the cornerstone of becoming truly compassionate and effective as a caregiver when used appropriately. Kindness and compassion must be practiced every day so it becomes habit.

Social Intelligence

Social intelligence is defined as being intelligent not just about relationships but also in them.[2] In short, social intelligence is acting with wisdom when dealing with others in all social situations. Keep in mind that an unresponsive patient may hear everything you say.

Emotions are contagious. Start interactions with a smile, which is understood in any culture and language. A smile opens up communication in a nonthreatening manner. Although our best medicine comes from our compassion, maybe we could say that a smile is the way we deliver that powerful medicine.

Establishing Rapport

If EMRs establish **rapport**, a relationship with the patient based on trust, good communication is possible. Creating a connection is critical to helping a patient. Starting a conversation with the patient can be difficult for EMS professionals. What do we say? How do we say it? When do we say something? The first critical minutes will either break or create trust with the patient. It takes great skill to establish trust and a relationship with a stranger, particularly one who is frightened. EMRs only have a few minutes, sometimes only a few seconds, to establish rapport with the patient.

The first step in establishing this vital rapport with our patient includes getting centered, establishing an alliance, and gaining a contract.[3]

Step 1: Get Centered

Getting centered has little to do with the patient and everything to do with the EMR. The EMR must use empathy to put the patient first and gain his or her trust. What is said or done in the first few seconds may help or hurt the patient, so the EMR's focus must be on the patient's emotional, as well as physical, well-being.

Often the EMR will appear on the scene and immediately focus on the injuries. A better tactic is to make eye contact, introduce yourself, and act within seconds. An EMR must consciously ask one question at a time and give the patient time to answer. The EMR must focus on the answers and write down important information to avoid needing to ask the same question again, except when the patient's condition changes or when the answer given does not fit the signs and symptoms. Patients may feel helpless and may need to have the EMR's full focus centered on them.

Step 2: Establish an Alliance

After focus is centered on the patient, you must establish an alliance so the patient knows that you are working together. Tell the patient, "I am here to help you." Present yourself with confidence, compassion, and good character. Be honest and show respect. Explain what you are doing and why you are doing it with every intervention. This type of interaction will allow the patient to work with you and take some attention away from the circumstances, thus reducing the discomfort and instilling the patient with hope.

Step 3: Get a Contract

At this point, an EMR is in a position to create a contract with the patient. Get the patient involved and let him or her work with you. Statements such as: "Help me help you" or "We are in this together" encourage this behavior and help decrease the patient's stress, fear, and feeling of helplessness. Make sure the patient knows that he can make choices. Questions starting with, "Can you," "Will you," or "Would you like" facilitate the creation of the contract. When other emergency responders arrive, include the patient as you relay patient information to the next caregiver by verifying with the patient, at intervals, the accuracy of that information.

Communication Elements of Good Rapport

As an EMR works to gain and maintain rapport with a patient, some communication elements can be used to facilitate this process. These elements include active listening, body language, tone of voice, and touch. Additionally, understanding cultural differences in communication is essential in establishing rapport with patients.

Active Listening

EMRs see patients during extreme stress. Giving patients comfort and decreasing their stress can affect how they deal with their illness or injury. An EMR can help comfort and

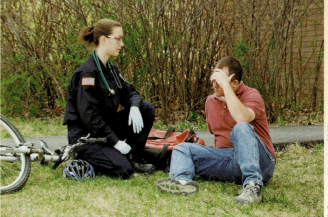

Figure 4-1 Active listening involves giving the patient your undivided attention and processing the information before responding.

© Cengage Learning 2012

decrease stress through a technique called **active listening**, which requires the listener to understand, interpret, and evaluate what is heard. Using this technique, an EMR listens carefully to the patient by giving the patient her undivided attention and processes the information before responding (Figure 4-1). The EMR can rephrase what the patient has said to ensure the information given was understood correctly. When EMRs listen to patients, they provide better medical care. When professionals fail to listen carefully, they could miss useful information. Patients may become frustrated or angry if they must repeatedly answer the same questions because the EMR did not listen the first time. In such situations, a patient may lose confidence in the EMR.

Body Language

EMRs must be careful about the body language used with patients and the patient's family members. Because more than 90 percent of communication is nonverbal, we must be aware of all nonverbal signals sent to patients and others on the scene. Simple moves can be misinterpreted and send powerful, negative messages. EMRs must not roll their eyes, sigh heavily, or stand over patients while speaking (which gives the illusion of talking down to the person). Some posturing, such as folding the arms, checking the time, or writing while only occasionally looking at the patient may send the wrong message. Some body language may indicate disgust or inconvenience with having to respond to the patient's needs.

Based on documented patient complaints, body language can make patients feel that a responder did not listen or did not respect them. When patients feel judged or that the EMR is uncaring, they may not cooperate and may look for reasons to complain or find fault with the care they received. To convey a positive message through body language, the EMR should kneel directly in front of the patient at eye level and show genuine concern through her facial expressions as shown in Figure 4-2.

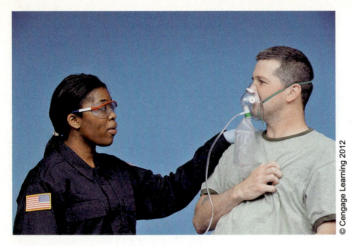

Figure 4-2 Kneeling in front of the patient at eye level conveys a positive message to the patient.

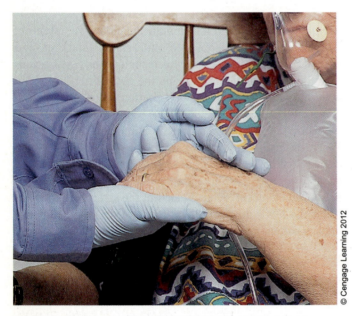

Figure 4-3 A simple touch can comfort and decrease a patient's stress.

Tone

Tone of voice or tone of questions can indicate to a patient whether a responder cares. Tone is critical in establishing trust and rapport with a patient. We must practice slow, clear, and even-toned speech when speaking with patients. The tone must be calm and supportive. Explain what you are doing as you care for the patient in a calm and reassuring manner.

Touch

Appropriate touch is a critical step in establishing rapport with a patient. Touch can be therapeutic and reassuring to a patient if the patient is comfortable with being touched (Figure 4-3). To assess a patient's comfort level, ask the patient if you can touch him or her on the shoulder before doing so. Be sensitive and watch for nonverbal cues from the patient such as facial expressions or pulling away from your touch.

Cultural Considerations

During the process of establishing rapport with a patient or the family, cultural differences must be taken into consideration. Some cultural considerations are personal space, direct eye contact, desire to communicate through another person, and refusal of care. Even though touch is comforting to most people you will encounter, others may find it unacceptable. Some patients may be reluctant to ask questions or reveal personal information. Be sensitive to cultural differences.

Negative versus Therapeutic Communication

As previously mentioned, a smile is important in establishing rapport, so be sure to smile when approaching a patient. Say, "Hello" and state your name, credentials, and agency. Ask the patient if she can tell you her name and ask why the patient called 9-1-1 or what help is needed. If a patient cannot respond, look for a family member or caregiver to provide that information.

Beyond the initial conversation, knowing what to say, can be difficult at times. An EMR may not know what is appropriate for some situations. Examples of what to say and what not to say are listed below. These are only suggestions, and you will need to find your own style as you encounter every new situation.

Negative Communication

Some statements should never be used with a patient. See the following for some examples:

- You shouldn't have done that.
- Why did you do that?
- You shouldn't feel that way.
- If I were you, I would. . . .
- You'll get over this.
- Everything will be alright.

Do not give false hope or say that the patient will get better. This is a critical error many EMRs inadvertently make, and it can be difficult for everyone if the patient's status of illness or injury later worsens.

Therapeutic Communication

Therapeutic statements can always be used with patients. The following are some examples:

- What can I do to help you?
- Can we work together?
- I will stay with you until EMS arrives.
- I will take care of you the best I can.
- Is there someone you would like me to call?
- What can I do to make you more comfortable?
- It's okay to cry.

Death and Dying

EMS professionals face death and dying during the performance of their duties, often in violent and unpredictable settings. Whether a patient with a terminal illness chooses to die at home or whether a death has been caused by a traumatic event, EMRs must treat all involved with compassion when responding to the scene.

Because critical patients cannot always be saved, EMRs must understand death and dying as well as the effect it can have on health care providers, patients, and patients' loved ones. If EMRs avoid dealing with death, the experience can be overwhelming. An EMR might become calloused and develop an indifferent attitude when faced with such patients and their families, which can then lead to numerous physical, emotional, and psychological problems long after the event. These effects can result in ongoing problems for the EMR, the EMR's family, and patients.

EMRs may try to cope with death and dying in unhealthy ways. They may use inappropriate coping strategies such as suppression of emotions; dehumanizing patients; labeling an episode as unavoidable; finding humor; failing to talk with peers, family, or friends about their experiences; or failing to address the problems. For some situations, an EMR may require a critical incident stress debriefing to ease the stress of the experience.

Caring for a Dying Patient

Death, or the fear of death, is an extremely stressful event that affects not only the health care provider but the patient and family as well. The EMR will observe that people express their grief in a variety of ways, often determined by whether the death is a sudden, unexpected loss or caused by a long-term illness during which the patient or family have had time to prepare.

Stages of Grief

Patients and family members may or may not experience all of the stages of grief. The duration of the stages varies with different people. The following is only a guideline.

- Denial: The patient denies that he or she is ill or dying. The patient is not convinced that it will happen to him or her, believing that this type of thing happens to others. In this case, allow the patient her denial and try to gather information from a loved one or friend.
- Anger: The patient may question, "Why me?" The patient is angry at his situation, himself, or those around him. Be understanding and sympathetic. Be a good listener and get permission to treat. Communicate what you will be doing. The patient may direct his anger at the EMR. Do not react in anger. Stay calm and speak calmly.
- Bargaining: A patient may turn to her faith, family, or herself to try to make a deal. She feels that she must have some control over her present condition and hopes to change it. Listening may be helpful at this point.
- Depression: The patient comes to the realization that the injury or illness is real. Sadness and a feeling of loss may overcome him. Ask if he would like you to call someone to be with him or tell him that you will stay with him

until others arrive. Ask if he would like something to make him more comfortable.
- Acceptance: The patient accepts her illness or injury. Although she may accept her fate, those close to her may not have reached the acceptance stage and may be angry with the patient for giving up. Do not give them false hope. Be an advocate for the patient, but at the same time, understand the feelings of the loved ones dealing with the loss. Keep extremely emotional individuals at a distance, giving them something to do, assigning someone to comfort them, and then asking the patient if it is alright to have them back on the scene.

Strategies for EMRs

The EMR must deal with these stages with great empathy. In other words, health care professionals must put themselves in the patient's and the family's place and feel their incredible sense of loss. EMRs can help their patients by following some common and effective strategies that can help make a very personal and powerfully painful experience a little more humanizing and bearable.

Active Listening

EMS professionals always wonder what to say. Many people do not care what you say and may not remember what you do say. They will, however, remember how you made them feel and how you cared to spend a moment to listen. Remember that people know that you cannot solve their problems. They really just want you to listen and show that you care. Additionally, the patient may want to express her last wishes to you.

Patience

Understand that patients may say or do things out of fear or anger because they have lost control of the situation. They usually are not angry with you, but they may vent to you. They feel lost and helpless. It may be the first time in their lives that they realize they are not really in control of life. Power is taken away from them, and their lives are out of order. Be patient. Be kind and understand that the situation is the focus of their grief.

Compassion

An appropriate touch on the shoulder or a kind gesture, such as getting a glass of water or helping with a pet, can be extremely powerful medicine. Take a moment to allow the patient to call family members. These acts show the patient that you are there to help and not in a hurry to leave.

Remaining Focused

It is critical to be honest with the patient and the family. Keep your conversation focused on the patient during these critical moments. Limit the number of professionals around the patient, so the patient and family are not overwhelmed, unless the illness or injury requires additional assistance. Remember to watch what you say to other responders around the patient and family. Keep your conversations low in volume and appropriate.

Consider Cultural Differences

You will observe a wide range of responses to death from various cultures. These may include open expressions of grief with calling out to the deceased, collapsing, wanting to wash the body and shroud it, a stoic acceptance, or a request to have someone from their faith present. Be respectful of patients and family members and their wishes.

Signs of Obvious Death

Most states have general guidelines stating that resuscitation efforts are not to be started if there are unambiguous (clear or precise) signs of death. The signs of obvious death include, but are not limited to, the following:

- Injuries not compatible with life such as decapitation: removal of head
- Postmortem lividity: reddish purple discoloration of dependent body parts, usually the areas on which patient is lying, if the person is unresponsive with no pulse or respirations
- Putrefaction: decomposition of the body
- Rigor mortis: generalized stiffening of all muscles of the body in an unresponsive, pulseless, breathless person

An EMR *cannot* declare someone dead. If there is any doubt in the EMR's mind whether a patient is dead, give CPR until relieved by another EMS person with the same or more training.

Health Care Directives

Patients have the right to make their own medical decisions. However, in a medical crisis, the EMR is obligated to begin lifesaving measures unless a **health care directive**, a legal document establishing the patient's written wishes for medical care, is presented for that patient. These documents vary from state to state and are usually initiated by patients, family, or guardians. These documents can be changed or cancelled by the patient at any time.

A health care directive outlines what medical care should be given in the event that the patient is incapacitated and unable to make medical decisions. A directive is ideally written by patients while they are able to make their own decisions. This directive also designates individuals to make decisions if the patient cannot speak. A good health care directive describes the kind of treatment or medical interventions, including resuscitation measures the patient wants to receive depending on the degree and type of illness. Directives usually list the types of treatment the patient does not want to receive. However, these documents can also specify that the patient wants a certain treatment no matter the degree or type of illness. When presented with an advance directive, EMRs should be aware of state laws; identify all parties listed in the directive; check for a signature; and if anything is uncertain, perform lifesaving measures.

Do Not Resuscitate (DNR)

A **Do Not Resuscitate (DNR)** is an order refusing cardiopulmonary resuscitation (CPR) if the patient's heart stops or if the patient stops breathing (Figure 4-4). DNR orders are accepted by doctors and hospitals in all states. An EMR must read the DNR order, identify the correct name and correct document for his state, and determine that the order is clear. If there is any doubt, care must be rendered. When documents cannot be provided or treatment instructions are not given by someone with authority, lifesaving measures should be started immediately while contact with the EMS professional's medical director is established for further instructions. Many EMS agencies may have a standing policy to provide patients with resuscitative measures until they are brought into a hospital setting where the DNR order can be addressed. EMRs must know the laws and policies for their service area before encountering these issues.

DNR DOCUMENTATION FORM #1

CONSENT FOR DNR ORDER
BY ADULT PATIENT WITH CAPACITY

PATIENT IDENTIFICATION PLATE

The patient's consent to a DNR order must be obtained at or about the time the order is issued. The patient's consent may be **either** oral or written.

ORAL CONSENT must be given in the presence of a physician and another witness.

Physician's Statement
I have provided the patient with information about his/her diagnosis and prognosis, the reasonably foreseeable risks and benefits of CPR, the range of available resuscitation measures, and the consequences of a DNR order. The patient has expressed the decision to consent to a DNR order orally in my presence.

_____   _____
Physician Signature   Date

Witness' Statement
The patient has expressed the decision to consent to a DNR order orally in my presence.

_____   _____
Witness Signature   Date

_____
Print name

ALTERNATIVELY, WRITTEN CONSENT may be given, and signed by the patient and two adult witnesses. If written consent is obtained, a copy must be placed in the chart.

After consent is obtained, the DNR order is to be issued by the attending physician, and entered on the Physician's Order Sheet.

    If the attending physician objects to a DNR order, he/she must either:
        — transfer the patient to another attending physician, or
        — notify the Medical Director that dispute mediation is required

REMINDER: The DNR order must be reviewed by the attending physician at least **every three days,** to determine if the order is still appropriate in light of the patient's condition. A notation must be made in the chart to reflect that review. It is **not** necessary to repeat the consent process when the order is reviewed.

Figure 4-4 An example of a Do Not Resuscitate (DNR) form.

SUMMARY

An EMR can prepare to communicate with patients by understanding the concepts of emotional intelligence and social intelligence. EMRs can communicate with and understand patients more effectively if they understand themselves. This chapter presented communication tools such as establishing rapport and listening actively to help EMRs quickly develop a relationship with the patient during a stressful and critical time. This special relationship will foster effective communication between the patient and health care provider so useful patient information can be obtained. Because not all EMS calls result in positive outcomes, it is critical for the EMR to have knowledge of the basics of death and dying. The EMR must be prepared to handle stressful calls, including ones during which health care directives call upon the EMR to respect the legal wishes of the patient.

REVIEW QUESTIONS

1. Emotional intelligence refers to:
   a. How the EMR handles inner conflicts
   b. How the EMR handles the patient
   c. How the EMR handles bystanders
   d. How the EMR handles EMS
2. Social intelligence refers to:
   a. How the EMR handles the patient
   b. How the EMR handles EMS
   c. How the EMR handles relationships
   d. How the EMR handles bystanders
3. How does the EMR accomplish the important task of establishing rapport with the patient?
   a. Establish an emotional tie to the patient.
   b. Establish an environment of safety.
   c. Establish a relationship with the patient.
   d. Establish a network with the patient.
4. What is the most important part of active listening for the EMR?
   a. To obtain key information from the patient.
   b. To obtain assistance from the bystanders.
   c. To perform your skills.
   d. To obtain additional resources.
5. Active listening does not consist of
   a. Explaining what you are doing to the patient
   b. Using eye contact
   c. Rephrasing what the patient says
   d. Being nonjudgmental
6. Which of the following is not an example of body language?
   a. Nonverbal communication
   b. Rolling your eyes
   c. Standing over a patient
   d. Verbal communication

7. In posturing, the EMR must be aware of
   a. The position the patient is placed in
   b. Checking the time
   c. Vital sign changes
   d. Any patient cues given
8. What should the EMR project in her tone with the patient?
   a. The EMR needs to speak in a slow, clear, and concise voice.
   b. The EMR needs to be factual.
   c. The EMR needs to check vital signs again.
   d. The EMR needs to be punctual.
9. The acronym DNR stands for
   a. Department of Natural Resources
   b. Do not resuscitate
   c. Deliver normal resuscitation
   d. Do not remediate
10. Role playing drills: What would you say or do in the following situations?
    a. Your patient that is unstable medically asks "Am I going to die?"
    b. Your patient asks "Why me? Why do things always happen to me?"
    c. You are performing lifesaving measures on a patient and a person identifies themselves as a relative stating "My uncle doesn't want heroic measures."
    d. Your patient starts screaming for their parent.

REFERENCES

1. Goleman D: *Emotional Intelligence*. Bantam Dell, 1995.
2. Goleman D: *Social Intelligence*. Bantam Dell, 1996.
3. Acosta J, Simon Prager J: *The Worst is Over*. Jodere Group, 2002.

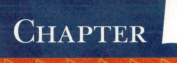

CHAPTER 5

PATIENT ASSESSMENT

LEARNING OBJECTIVES

By the end of this chapter, the reader should be able to:

- Describe the difference between a medical patient and a trauma patient.
- Describe how to manage unresponsive and responsive patients.
- Explain medical acronyms used to assess patients.
- Define critical thinking and how it pertains to Emergency Medical Responders.

INTRODUCTION

An Emergency Medical Responder (EMR) is often the first trained responder on the scene and is vital in the initiation of patient assessment. Patients may have both medical and trauma issues, and assessment protocols may differ depending on the condition of the patient and his level of consciousness. A **medical patient** is one who verbalizes or appears to have a disease, illness, or reaction. A **trauma patient** is one who has an injury that may or may not be visible to the EMR.

An EMR must assess the overall patient presentation to see the complete medical picture. Being familiar with systematic assessment guidelines and having critical thinking skills help EMRs obtain pertinent information to make appropriate treatment decisions. The patient assessment flow chart, as shown in Figure 5-1, is a visual representation of the patient assessment guidelines and tools used for unresponsive and responsive patients. Each major division in the chapter is represented by a section of the patient assessment flow chart.

Assessment

Whether a victim is considered a trauma or a medical patient, the initial assessment begins the same way with PENMAN, spinal stabilization if the mechanism of injury indicates, and establishing level of consciousness.

PENMAN

Prior to making contact with a victim begin with **PENMAN**, an acronym for personal and personnel safety, environmental hazards, number of victims, mechanism of injury, additional resources needed from your agency, and need for resources outside of your agency (Figure 5-2). PENMAN is used for the initial size-up of an incident. Following PENMAN allows the EMR on scene to assess the incident in a safe, methodical, and organized manner.

P—Personal and Personnel Safety

Assessing personal and personnel safety are the primary considerations when responding to and arriving on the scene of an incident. Make certain that you have the personal protective equipment (PPE) needed to be physically safe.

Additionally, the fire service apparatus (transport vehicle for personnel and equipment), the law enforcement squad (vehicle), and other specialized response vehicles need to be in safe operating condition. An EMR must know what equipment is available on the apparatus, squad, or specialized response vehicle as well as how to safely operate the equipment or safely assist in its use. Therefore, an EMR should be certain that the vehicle and equipment on it are safe and ready to respond.

E—Environmental Hazards

Environmental hazards are anything on scene than can harm the EMR. You will need a 360-degree perspective to identify environmental hazards. These hazards include vehicle traffic, leaking fuel at a traffic collision, the possibility of a shooter still on scene at a reported shooting, lightning and other weather hazards, down power lines, vicious dogs, and airborne contaminants, just to name a few. Some hazards can be mitigated to render the scene safe. If the scene cannot be made safe, an EMR should not be there. Rather, the EMR waits, or stages, until other responders can make the scene safe enough for the EMR to perform her duties.

N—Number of Victims

Victims are people on scene directly or indirectly affected by the event in one way or another. Victims have not been assessed or treated by the EMR. All people on scene are classified as victims. People cease being victims and become patients as soon as an EMR assesses and begins treating them. The EMR should determine the number of victims at a scene. If the victims are too numerous to count or cannot all be seen, the responder may have to estimate the number of victims. When estimation is required, it is better to estimate high rather than low.

M—Mechanism of Injury or Nature of Illness

The **mechanism of injury (MOI)** or **nature of illness (NOI)** involves an evaluation of the forces that caused the injury or the illness that has resulted in the patient's presenting medical condition.

MOI describes the event that causes the patient's injury or trauma, what happened at a scene, or what caused the

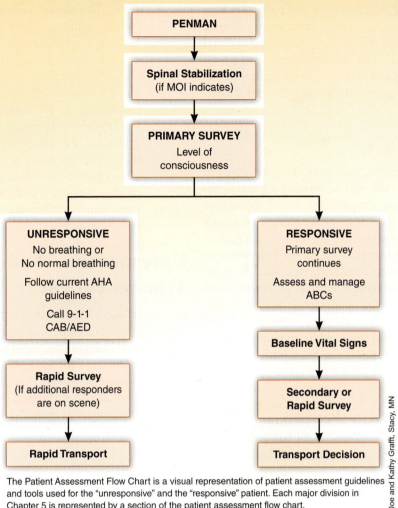

The Patient Assessment Flow Chart is a visual representation of patient assessment guidelines and tools used for the "unresponsive" and the "responsive" patient. Each major division in Chapter 5 is represented by a section of the patient assessment flow chart.

Joe and Kathy Grafft, Stacy, MN

Figure 5-1 Patient assessment flow chart.

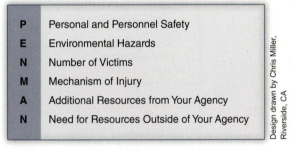

Design drawn by Chris Miller, Riverside, CA

Figure 5-2 PENMAN is used for initial scene size-up.

incident. Investigating how the victim or victims were injured will provide clues to the victims' injuries or illnesses. Upon arriving on scene, an EMR must determine the cause of the incident. If the incident was caused by hazardous materials, the site itself may continue creating more victims. As an adjunct to MOI, NOI is to be considered in any situation involving illness or medical emergencies. The EMR should note any potential contributing factors to the patient's condition

such as unusual odors in the home; medication bottles lying around; or an animal, reptile, or insects on site. For both MOI and NOI, the EMR should scan the area for clues.

A—Additional Resources Needed from Your Agency

An EMR must determine if additional resources are required from his agency and if those resources are immediately available. Examples might be additional EMRs, traffic control, and investigative personnel to secure the incident perimeter and initiate an investigation. These available resources should be requested as quickly as possible. Remember, it is always better to have too many resources than too few. Extra resources can be released or cancelled when it is determined that they are not needed.

N—Need for Resources Outside Your Agency

An EMR must ascertain the need for resources from outside the EMR's own agency or team as well. Outside resources should be requested as soon as the need is identified. These resources should provide the equipment and personnel necessary to complete the tactics and tasks necessary to mitigate the event. Common outside resources are hazardous material teams, search and rescue (SAR), Salvation Army, Red Cross, a medical examiner, and a chaplain. As with requesting resources from the EMR's agency, too many resources are better than not enough.

Spinal Stabilization

Upon approaching the patient, state your name, agency, and credentials. At this time, you will be forming a general impression or quick visual assessment of the overall appearance to determine priority of care. If there is evidence of a neck or back injury. your first physical contact with the patient is spinal stabilization. However if the patient is unstable or unresponsive and there is no assistance, continue lifesaving measures. If there is assistance, direct that person to maintain spinal stabilization as you continue to assess and manage the patient.

To stabilize the cervical spine, position yourself at the head of the patient and support the head with one hand on each side of the head, as shown in Figure 5-3. Try not to cover the ears so the patient can hear and answer questions. Avoid "yes" and "no" questions to keep patients from nodding or shaking their heads to answer. For example, instead of asking a patient if he has pain, ask a specific question about the pain, such as "Where is your pain located?"

Primary Survey

The primary survey, also called the primary assessment, begins with assessing the level of responsiveness or **level of consciousness (LOC)**. LOC is the measure of a person's response to stimuli determined by verbal communication with the patient or making physical contact to get a response. Responsiveness is initially assessed using the acronym **AVPU**.

A   Alert: The patient is alert and responds to verbal communication.
V   Verbally responsive: The patient alerts to your voice or loud sounds. He may follow simple verbal commands to open his eyes or squeeze your hand.
P   Painful stimuli response: The patient does not acknowledge the EMR and responds only to painful stimuli by withdrawing, uttering sounds, or facial grimacing. Painful stimuli may include a squeeze of the muscle extending from the neck to the shoulder, a firm gentle pinch to the ear lobe, or pressure applied to the cuticle of the thumb with a pen.
U   Unresponsive: The patient does not respond to any type of stimulus.

Unresponsive Medical or Trauma Patient

An unresponsive medical or trauma patient who exhibits no signs of life-sustaining perfusion (oxygenation and circulation) needs critical interventions, rapid survey, and immediate transportation. The steps for the EMR to follow in responding to the unresponsive patient are illustrated in Figure 5-4.

No signs of life sustaining perfusion include a patient who is unresponsive (Figure 5-5) and has any of the below characteristics.

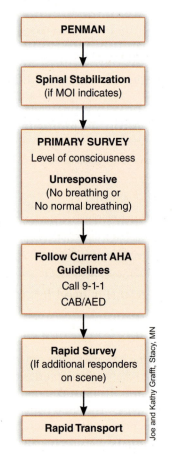

Figure 5-4   Responding to an unresponsive patient.

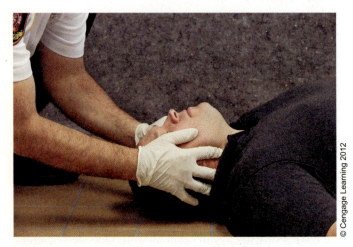

© Cengage Learning 2012

Figure 5-3   Manual spinal stabilization.

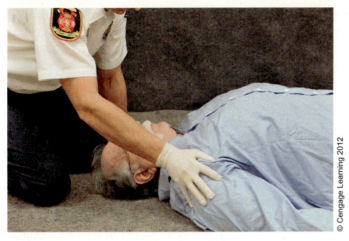

Figure 5-5 To establish unresponsiveness: shake and shout.

- No normal breathing, such as **agonal breathing** (slow breathing at a rate of approximately 3 to 4 breaths/min with shallow, irregular, or gasping breaths that often lead to apnea)
- Apnea (no breathing)
- No palpable pulse or a pulse less than 30 per minute for an adult and less than 60 per minute for a child or infant (per American Heart Association [AHA] guidelines)
- Skin that is cyanotic (blue), mottled or ashen and cool to touch

CAB for an Unresponsive Patient

After completing PENMAN, spinal stabilization, and AVPU, call 9-1-1, unless Emergency Medical Services (EMS) has been dispatched. Immediately check for unresponsiveness while simultaneously observing the patient's breathing. If the patient is unresponsive and not breathing or is not breathing normally such as gasping breaths, seek assistance in having an **automated external defibrillator (AED)** brought to the scene. An AED is a machine that can read the ECG and prompt the EMR to **defibrillate** by shocking the heart or prompt to not deliver a shock. A shock is delivered if the AED senses the dysrythmia of ventricular fibrillation (VF) or pulseless ventricular tachycardia (VT). VF is when the natural electrical impulse of the heart produces uncoordinated contractions of the ventricles. Pulseless VT is when the ventricles are beating too fast to provide an effective pulse, approximately greater than 180 beats per minute. Both of these dysrhythmias result in an inability of the heart muscle to provide adequate oxygenated blood supply to the body.

C—Circulation

After checking for unresponsiveness and breathing, circulation is assessed next by checking a pulse. To check a pulse in adults and children one year old or older, tip the patient's head back with the head tilt and then **palpate** (feel) for a central pulse, which is the **carotid pulse**. Place two to three fingers, not the thumb, at the patient's Adam's apple

(a)

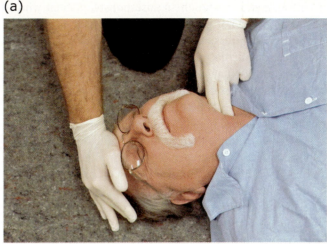

(b)

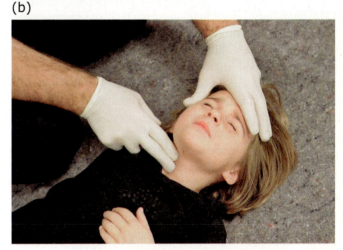

(c)

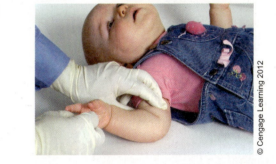

Figure 5-6 (a) Checking a carotid pulse on an adult. (b) Checking a carotid pulse on a child. (c) Checking a brachial pulse on an infant.

(the thyroid cartilage and largest cartilage of the larynx) on the side closest to you. Then slide the fingers down into the groove of the neck. Leave your other hand on the patient's forehead to keep the head back. You may have to vary the depth and location slightly during the pulse check, which should not be more than ten seconds. For an infant younger than one year old, use two fingers to check the **brachial pulse** (located in the inner aspect of the arm between the elbow and shoulder). Figure 5-6 illustrates checking a pulse on an adult, child, and infant.

If no pulse is found on an unresponsive patient who is not breathing or not breathing normally such as gasping, begin chest compressions, and continue following the AHA guidelines for **Cardiopulmonary resuscitation (CPR)**. (See Appendix for 2010 guidelines) CPR is an emergency procedure consisting of external cardiac compressions and pulmonary resuscitation (ventilations). The purpose of CPR is to circulate oxygenated blood to sustain life.

Another component in assessing circulation, is to check for bleeding. If additional personnel are available direct them to assess and manage major bleeding (see Chapter 8).

To perform chest compressions, make sure the patient is lying on a hard surface and then expose the patient's chest by removing the patient's clothing from the chest area. If there are bystanders available, have them encircle the victim facing outward to protect the patient's privacy. According to AHA guidelines, "push hard and push fast" is recommended for chest compressions. Compress the chest 2 inches for an adult, 2 inches for a child, and 1 ½ inches for an infant. Make sure there is recoil after each compression. Recoil is the rebounding of the chest back to baseline and allows blood to refill the heart chambers. Perform 30 compressions at a rate of 100 compressions per minute. Figure 5-7 demonstrates compressions on an adult.

Chest compressions of appropriate depth, rate, and quality are of the utmost importance. Fatigue of the responder is a factor in poor quality compressions. To maintain adequate compressions, it is beneficial to have more than one rescuer perform CPR and switch positions from compressions to ventilations at approximately two-minute intervals or sooner if fatigued.

A—Airway

After performing chest compressions, open the airway. To open the airway, use the **head-tilt, chin-lift method** (see Chapter 7). This method of tilting the head back and lifting the jaw up, is demonstrated in **Skill 5-1** at the end of the chapter. If the MOI indicates a possible spinal injury, perform a jaw thrust maneuver. This maneuver, which minimizes head movement and helps maintain stabilization of the cervical spine, is demonstrated in **Skill 5-2**. If a chest rise cannot be seen with ventilations and the jaw thrust maneuver, you may slightly extend the neck according to AHA guidelines.

B—Breathing

After compressions and opening the airway, two ventilations are given at one second per breath. **Rescue breathing**, or ventilating, is the act of assisting respirations for a person who is not breathing or not breathing normally.

Ventilations may be accomplished by applying a barrier device over the mouth and nose or over a tracheostomy. Your agency will require a protective barrier to prevent potential exposure to pathogens. This topic is discussed further in Chapter 7.

Too much ventilation could force air into the stomach and cause vomiting. To reduce the risk of vomiting, ventilate the patient *only* until you see the chest rise (Figure 5-8). If the patient starts vomiting, particularly **projectile vomiting** (vomiting which is ejected with force), the vomit could obstruct the patient's airway, and you could be exposed to pathogens. If vomiting occurs, turn the patient to his side, and if needed, use a gloved hand to clear substances out of the mouth in order to obtain an open airway for adequate ventilations. Provide suction if needed (discussed in Chapter 7).

"Hands-only CPR" also called "compression-only CPR" are terms for performing chest compressions without providing ventilations. This technique is a choice of the rescuer if a protective barrier is not available for use. Some research indicates that the blood may maintain oxygenation for several minutes without providing ventilations. If additional rescuers are available, it may be beneficial while performing only chest compressions to have someone open the airway using a head-tilt, chin-lift, or jaw thrust maneuver in order to provide passive air movement.

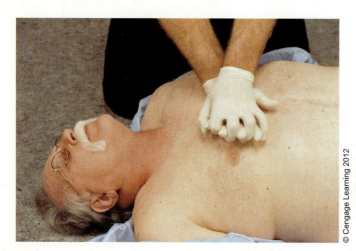

Figure 5-7 Chest compressions on an adult.

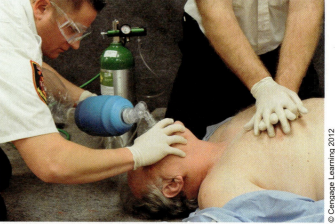

Figure 5-8 Ventilate the patient only until you see the chest rise.

Defibrillation

When the AED arrives, continue CPR while another rescuer places the pads on the adult, child, or infant's chest. If pediatric pads are needed but not available, adult pads can be used, but they should not touch each other (Figure 5-9). Alternate pad placement is addressed in the AHA guidelines. Next turn on the machine and follow the prompts of the AED. Before using the AED, make sure the patient's chest is dry and that the patient is not lying in water. Snow and ice do not impede use of the AED. Wearing gloves, look for and remove medication patches from the chest. If noticeable hair, shave the chest in the areas where the pads will be placed for adequate pad contact. Palpate the chest and observe for any implantable medical devices. Keep pads at least one inch away from internal or external medical devices. Be familiar with your agency's AED and make sure it is properly maintained (Figure 5-10).

Automated chest compression devices can also be used to help deliver chest compressions. These devices have been designed to provide consistent compressions that can be adjusted to each patient and reduce the fatigue caused by performing manual compressions. As demonstrated in Figure 5-11, this machine along with plunger type devices gives the EMR freedom to perform other functions at the same time.

Rapid Survey

If time allows and additional EMRs are available as CPR is in progress, a rapid survey can be done. A **rapid survey** also called a head-to-toe assessment is performed rapidly on an unstable or potentially unstable patient. This survey takes approximately one to two minutes. A rapid survey is discussed under the responsive patient later in this chapter.

Transport

An unresponsive patient requires a rapid transport. Patients with spinal injuries should be carefully stabilized if possible as the patient is transferred to a long backboard. Follow the local protocols set up by your medical director.

(a)

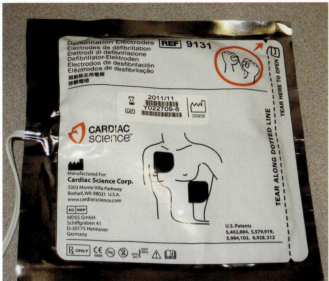

(b)

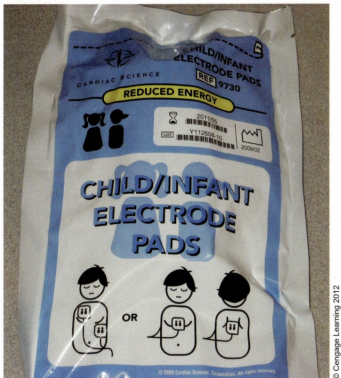

Figure 5-9 Adult (a) and pediatric (b) automated external defibrillator pads showing proper chest placement.

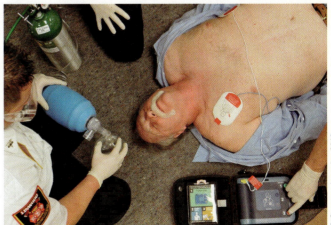

Figure 5-10 Automated external defibrillator.

(a)

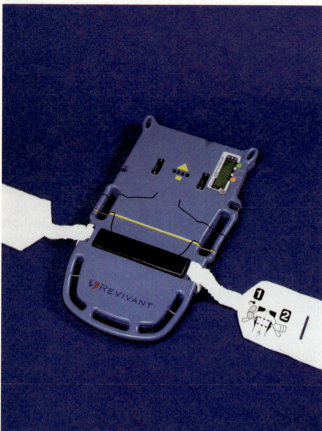

(b)

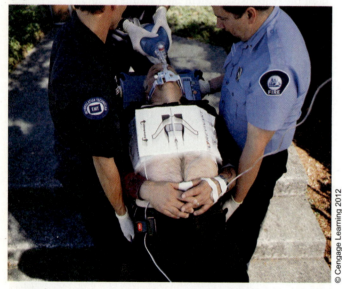

Figure 5-11 (a) The Autopulse device. (b) The Autopulse in position and performing compressions.

Responsive Medical or Trauma Patient

A responsive medical or trauma patient may have varying degrees of responsiveness. Breathing and pulse are evident, but in some cases, there may be inadequate perfusion,

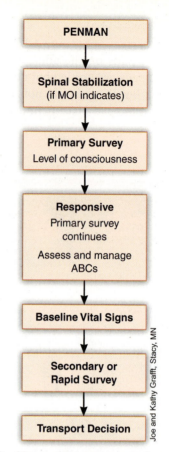

Figure 5-12 Managing a responsive patient.

which could lead to a life-threatening event. The EMR must continually monitor the patient's status. The last flow chart, illustrated in Figure 5-12, provides the steps that guide the EMR in responding to responsive medical or trauma patients.

Primary Survey

After completing PENMAN and spinal stabilization (if MOI indicates), the EMR starts the primary survey with a check for responsiveness using AVPU. In an alert patient who is not compromised with airway, breathing, or circulation (ABCs), the EMR can proceed with additional LOC assessments.

Orientation

To establish the patient's LOC in regard to orientation, ask her questions relating to person, place, and time.

- **Person:** Ask the patient to state her full name.
- **Place:** Ask the patient to state her current location.
- **Time:** Ask the patient to state the day, month, and year.

If the patient responds to all three correctly, she is said to be alert and oriented times three. This can be documented as A & O × 3. If she has only two correct responses, she is A & O × 2. If she states only her name correctly, she is A & O × 1. If the patient's orientation decreases at any point, she may have a life-threatening event and needs to be transported immediately. Try to confirm accuracy of answers with the family, friends, or bystanders. This confirmation is especially useful with a special-needs patient and in some older adults to determine a normal baseline orientation for that person.

The patient's **chief complaint**, the main reason for seeking medical services, can assist the EMR in determining LOC and be a vital piece of information in the assessment process. If the patient is alert and verbalizing appropriately, ask for the chief complaint.

ABCs for Responsive Patients

Orientation and chief complaint is assessed later on a responsive patient who is noticeably compromised with airway, breathing, or circulation, the ABCs. In this case, after assessing LOC using AVPU, you will immediately assess ABCs starting with the airway.

A—Airway

If the airway is open the patient can breathe, speak, or cough, and you will next assess for breathing. If the patient shows signs of an obstructed airway; is conscious but not able to breathe, speak, or cough; or becomes unconscious from an obstruction, follow the AHA guidelines for foreign body airway obstruction

B—Breathing

To evaluate the patient for breathing or respirations, assess the respirations for rate, rhythm, and quality.

Rate

To determine the number of respirations per minute, or **respiratory rate (RR)**, position yourself and the patient to check for a radial pulse as you count respirations, as shown in Figure 5-13. Lay the supine or sitting patient's hand over his chest and, while looking at your watch, count each time his chest rises. This method makes the EMR appear to be taking a pulse, so the patient is less likely to unintentionally change his breathing pattern. Count the number of respirations in 30 seconds and multiply by two to obtain a one-minute rate. If you see or hear ten respirations in 30 seconds, the total number of breaths per minute is 20. Document it as "RR 20." Table 5-1 shows normal RRs by age. A faster than normal RR is called **tachypnea**, and a slower than normal RR is termed **bradypnea**.

Rhythm

When counting respirations, note if the rhythm is regular or irregular. If the timing of the respirations is varied, consider them as being irregular.

Quality

To determine breathing quality, assess whether the patient is having labored breathing or is using accessory muscles during respirations. **Accessory muscles** are the muscles that are not normally involved in breathing. When a patient is in respiratory distress and accessory muscles are used,

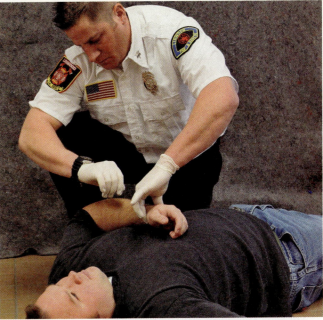

Figure 5-13 The EMR should position himself and the patient while checking respirations and pulse rate.

Table 5-1 Normal Respiratory Rates by Age

Age	Normal Respiratory Rate (breaths/min)
Adult	12–20
Adolescent (11–14 yr)	12–20
School-aged child (6–12 yr)	15–30
Preschool-aged child (1–5 yr)	20–30
Infant (1 mo–1 yr)	20–40
Newborn (0–1 mo)	30–50

© Cengage Learning 2012

you will observe the chest sinking in, clavicle retractions, nasal flaring, breathing through pursed lips (Figure 5-14), or use of neck muscles (strap muscles) during breathing (Figure 5-15). Children with respiratory distress will use their intercostal muscles to assist in breathing. The EMR can actually see the skin being retracted between the ribs and sometimes above and below the sternum with each breath (Figure 5-16).

Respirations should also be assessed for sounds such as high pitched wheezing, harsh, snoring, whistling, gurgling, or grunting. The EMR should look at the chest to see if the rise and fall is shallow (hardly visible) or deep. Check for symmetry of the chest rise. See if it rises equally on both sides or if it rises differently on one side, which is called **paradoxical respiration**. Observe the sitting position the patient takes. A patient in significant respiratory distress may sit in a **tripod position,** as shown in Figure 5-17, leaning forward propping his hands on his knees or a table or,

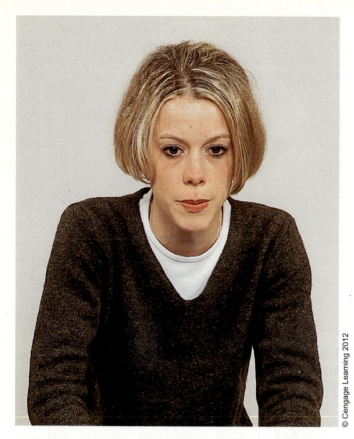

Figure 5-14 Breathing through pursed lips is a sign of respiratory distress.

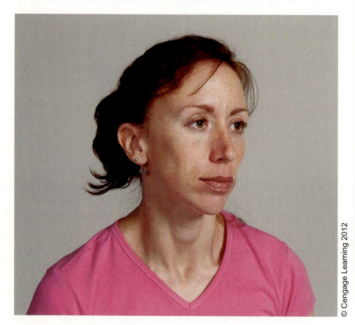

Figure 5-15 The strap muscles of the neck assist in respirations in times of distress.

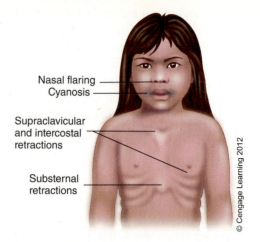

Nasal flaring
Cyanosis
Supraclavicular and intercostal retractions
Substernal retractions

Figure 5-16 Child with respiratory distress using accessory muscles.

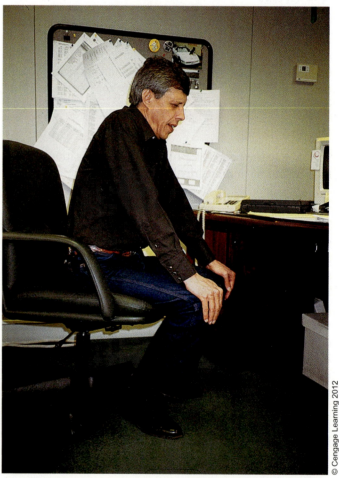

Figure 5-17 Patients with significant respiratory distress may be found in the tripod position.

if standing, he will prop himself up with his hands. Do not make the patient lie down but assist him to a **position of comfort** if he can tolerate the change in position. A position of comfort is a position that the patient independently assumes to assist him in breathing.

If you observe a fast RR, shortness of breath, irregular breathing patterns, labored breathing, or unusual sounds or if the patient is exhibiting anxiety or stating she cannot get enough air, you will need to provide supplemental oxygen before further assessment. (This is covered more thoroughly in Chapter 7.)

A complete description of breathing can be as documented as simply as "RR 16" if the rhythm and quality are not compromised. If any abnormalities of breathing are noted, documentation can look like this: RR 28/irreg/deep.

C—Circulation

It is vital to observe for major bleeding and control it (discussed in Chapter 8). If there are no signs of a major bleed or if you have controlled the bleed, assess the peripheral pulse by rate, rhythm, and quality.

Rate

The **peripheral pulses** are pulses farther away from the core of the body, such as the radial or brachial pulses. On adults and children, the **radial pulse** is usually used to assess the heart rate. The brachial pulse is used on infants younger than one year of age. The radial pulse is located on either arm in the inner aspect of the wrist on the thumb side (Figure 5-18). Check the pulse immediately after checking respirations, maintaining the same position as described for checking respirations. Use two to three fingers to locate and count the radial pulse for 30 seconds and multiply by 2 to obtain a one-minute rate. If you feel 35 beats in 30 seconds, the total number of beats per minute is 70. Document it as "P 70." A faster than normal heart rate is called **tachycardia,** and a slower than normal heart rate is called **bradycardia**. Table 5-2 lists the normal pulse rate ranges for different age groups.

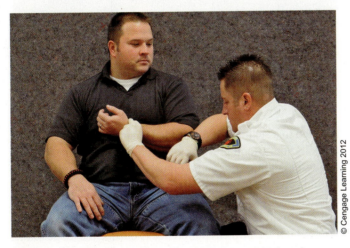

© Cengage Learning 2012

Figure 5-18 The EMR checking a radial pulse, located in the inner aspect of the wrist, thumb side.

Table 5-2 Normal Pulse Rates by Age

Age	Pulse Rate (beats/min)
Adult	60–100
Adolescent (11–14 yr)	60–105
School-aged child (6–12 yr)	70–110
Preschool-aged child (1–5 yr)	80–120
Infant (1 mo–1 yr)	90–140
Newborn (0–1 mo)	120–160

© Cengage Learning 2012

Rhythm

If the pulse is irregular, weak, or extremely slow check the rate for a full minute (this number is not multiplied) and document this number along with a notation that the pulse is irregular.

Quality

When taking the pulse, assess whether it is difficult to feel or if it is weak, **thready** (weak and rapid), or **bounding** (strong and forceful).

A complete description of the pulse can be documented as "P 70" if the rhythm and quality are not compromised or as detailed as "P 70/irreg/weak."

Capillary refill time (CRT) is another indication of adequate circulation unless factors exist such as cold exposure, age, and medical conditions. CRT has been found to be more reliable in infants and children. To check for capillary refill, note the color of the nailbed (Figure 5-19A) and then quickly squeeze and release pressure on the thumbnail. As shown in Figure 5-19B, the nailbed should go blanch (pale) and then return to pink within two seconds of release (Figure 5-19C). If it takes longer than two seconds for the nailbed to return to pink, the patient may be hypoperfused.

Skin Assessment

Skin is a good indicator of perfusion (circulation and oxygenation). Briefly expose appropriate skin areas of the patient to assess the skin for color, temperature, and moisture.

- *Color*: Check for color, noting both external skin areas and internal areas such as mucous membranes of the lower eyelids and inside the lips. Check whether the skin is pink, red, pale, grey (ashen), cyanotic, purplish red, or mottled in any area. To check skin color on a dark-skinned patient, mucous membranes may be more reliable.
- *Temperature*: Check the temperature of the skin by placing the back of your hand on the patient's forehead or abdomen to see if it is hot, warm, cool, or cold to touch.
- *Moisture*: Check the moisture of the skin. Assess if the skin is "wet" appearing or wet to touch (clammy). Notice if the patient is sweating profusely (diaphoretic) or if the skin is very dry.

Documentation of skin assessment might include "Skin: pale, cool, and clammy." Skin assessment along with vital sign readings provide important information that may indicate hypoperfusion or shock.

Baseline Vital Signs

At this point, you have already assessed the pulse and respirations while performing the primary survey. Unless the patient needs reassessment or interventions because of a change in status, the blood pressure is the next step for a responsive patient.

(a)

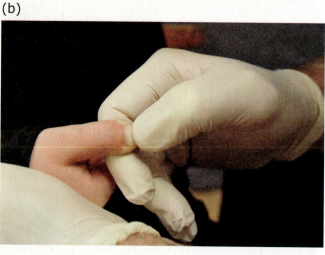

(b)

(c)

Figure 5-19 (a) First note the color of the nailbed. (b) Then squeeze the nailbed to obtain blanching. (c) Note the seconds when initial color returns to the nail bed.

Blood Pressure by Auscultation

Two numbers or readings are obtained when taking a blood pressure by **auscultation** (listening with a stethoscope), the systolic reading and the diastolic reading. A blood pressure cuff, in

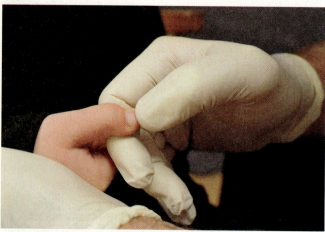

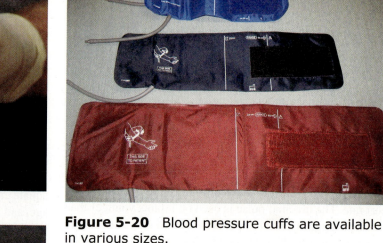

Figure 5-20 Blood pressure cuffs are available in various sizes.

© Cengage Learning 2012

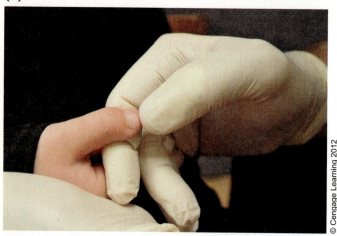

© Cengage Learning 2012

Figure 5-21 Blood pressure cuff range markings for arm circumference.

SELECT SMALLER CUFF   MIN   RANGE   MAX   SELECT LARGER CUFF
ADULT SIZE
25.4 TO 40.6 CM CIRCUMFERENCE

addition to a stethoscope, is needed to take a blood pressure by auscultation. Blood pressure cuffs come in different sizes for adults, children, and infants (Figure 5-20). A proper-sized cuff should cover more than half or less than two-thirds of the upper arm, elbow to shoulder. Follow the range markings indicated inside the cuff for circumference measurement of the arm (Figure 5-21). If the arm circumference is outside the range (either too small or too large), you will need to change cuff sizes for an accurate reading. An automatic cuff can be placed on the forearm or calf of a large person. The blood pressure is to be taken with the patient's arm in a position level with the heart, if possible. The head of the stethoscope is placed on the brachial artery to listen to the blood pressure. **Skill 5-3** at the end of the chapter illustrates the procedure of taking a blood pressure by auscultation. A blood pressure reading by auscultation is reported and written as two numbers such as "BP 120/80" and indicate which arm was used. Table 5-3 shows normal blood pressure values for adults and children.

A blood pressure should not be taken in the arm with a dialysis access, which is not always evident because these accesses are placed under the skin in an upper or lower arm.

Table 5-3 Normal Blood Pressures

Age	Systolic (mm Hg)	Diastolic (mm Hg)
Adults	90–150	60–90
Children	Approximately 80 + [2 × Age (in years) for children older than 1 yr]	Approximately two-thirds systolic

© Cengage Learning 2012

Also avoid taking blood pressures in an arm of a cancer patient who has had lymph nodes surgically removed from that arm or where there is a noticeable intravenous line. Palpate the extremity and observe for devices before taking the blood pressure. For accuracy, wait one or two minutes between blood pressure readings when using the same extremity.

Blood Pressure by Palpation

If the scene is very noisy and it is difficult to get a blood pressure by auscultation, the EMR may need to do a palpation blood pressure. To do this, palpate the radial pulse. Place the cuff as usual and pump it up until the pulse is no longer felt; then pump approximately 20 mm Hg higher and slowly release the pressure. When the pulse is felt in the wrist again, look to see the gauge reading and write down that number. When using palpation to get a blood pressure, only the systolic pressure can be obtained. A palpation reading is reported and written with one number such as "BP 120/P" and indicate which arm was used. Skill 5-4, at the end of this chapter, illustrates how to obtain a blood pressure by palpation.

Secondary Survey or Rapid Survey

After vital signs are taken, conduct a secondary survey or rapid survey using palpation and visualization. This assessment can be used on both trauma victims and medical patients and provides valuable information. Pay close attention to the patient's verbal and nonverbal cues while performing the assessment. All secondary surveys begin at the adult or older child's head. Make sure neck and spinal stabilization are maintained if the MOI indicates. Fractures are to be maintained in the position found. Only move a fractured body part to further assess the patient if the fracture is manually stabilized proximal and distal to the injury on the posterior side as well as supporting the adjacent joints.

If a patient is unstable or if further complications are suspected, a rapid survey will need to be performed. A rapid survey is a secondary survey performed in the shortest time possible, approximately one or two minutes. Sometimes a rapid survey is performed only if additional rescuers are present. A more detailed secondary survey should be completed on the stable patient.

Starting the assessment at the feet of a responsive young child or infant gives the pediatric patient time to gain confidence in the EMR. Perform the survey slowly and allow the pediatric patient to touch the assessment equipment if possible. Do not palpate the injured part until you have completed the remainder of the survey. A pediatric patient will quickly lose confidence in an EMR who scares or hurts him.

Assessment Tools

Assessment tools using acronyms have been established to help the EMR do a systematic and thorough head-to-toe assessment of patients. The assessment tools and the applications of those tools for conducting a survey and rapid survey follow.

SAMPLE

The acronym **SAMPLE** is a guide for the EMR to gather basic information:

S—Signs and symptoms: A sign is something that can be objectively observed; a symptom is a sign of illness or injury reported by the patient or discovered on examination.

A—Allergies: Note allergies to medications, insects, foods, or products. Note any seasonal allergies reported by the patient or family such as dust, trees, or pollen.

M—Medications: Obtain a list of medications the patient is taking, including any prescription medicine, vitamins, herbs, or over-the-counter (OTC) medications. Ask if the patient has missed a dose. Any medications found on the scene should be taken to the hospital with the patient.

P—Past pertinent medical history: Ask whether the patient has previously had this medical condition and if so, what helped them the last time this event occurred. Ask about other medical diagnoses the patient might have. Check the patient for medical identification jewelry on the neck, wrist, or ankle (Figure 5-22).

L—Last oral intake: Ask the patient when she last ate or drank, what she ate, and the amount consumed.

E—Events: Inquire about events leading up to the patient's current illness or injury.

DOTS

DOTS is an assessment tool used by the EMR during a secondary survey for both the medical and trauma patient. Look for:

D—Deformities
O—Open wounds
T—Tenderness
S—Swelling

TIC

TIC is another acronym assessment tool mostly used with muscular or joint trauma:

T—Tenderness
I—Instability
C—Crepitus (grating sound of two bone ends rubbing together)

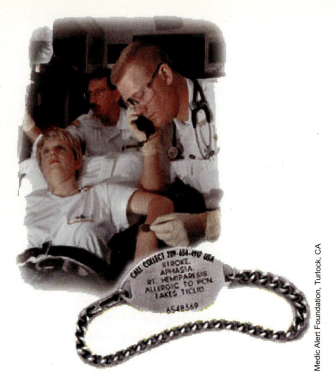

Figure 5-22 Always check for a medical identification bracelet or necklace on the patient.

Medic Alert Foundation, Turlock, CA

CMS

CMS is an assessment done on the extremities, usually the hands and feet. See Figures 5-23 and 5-24 for illustrations of CMS assessment. Both extremities should be assessed and compared:

C—Circulation: Assess the skin for color, temperature, and moisture. Check distal pulses in both wrists by checking the radial pulses and in feet by checking the posterior tibial pulse (tibial pulse) or dorsalis pedis pulse (pedal pulse).

M—Motor: Assess motion by asking the patient to wiggle her toes, squeeze your hand, or move her legs. Strength can be assessed, if no pain or deformity is present, by having resistance applied to the motions.

S—Sensory: While making sure the patient is not looking, check for sensation to touch by asking if she can tell where you are touching her. Ask if there is any numbness, tingling, burning, or pain.

PERRL

PERRL is an acronym used to assess the pupils of the eyes. A change in the pupils can indicate a brain injury or involvement:

P—Pupils, the dark part in the center of the eye
E—Equal—Observe if both pupils are equal in size
R—Round—Observe if both pupils are round
RL—Reactive to light—Observe reaction to light of both pupils (Discussed later in this chapter)

(a)

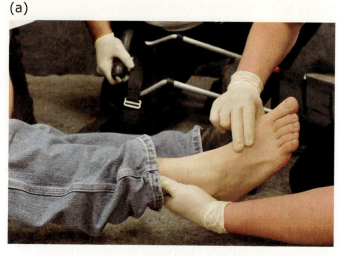

(b)

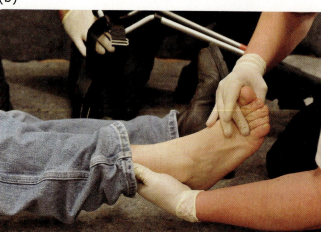

(c)

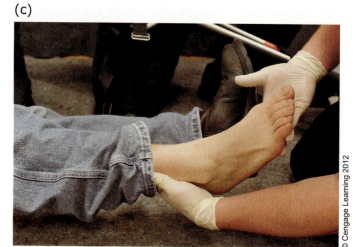

© Cengage Learning 2012

Figure 5-23 (a) Assess circulation of the lower extremities by checking the pedal pulses of the feet. (b) Ask the patient to wiggle his toes or move his legs to determine motor function. (c) Assess for sensation by asking the patient if he has any numbness, tingling, burning, or pain in his feet.

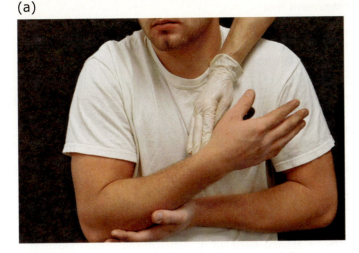

(a)

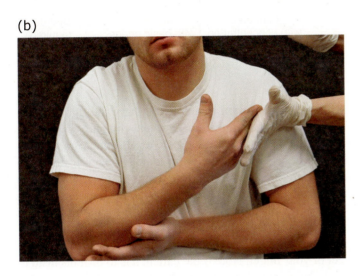

(b)

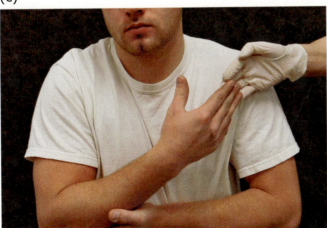

(c)

© Cengage Learning 2012

Figure 5-24 (a) Check circulation in the upper extremities by assessing skin for color and appearance. Check the radial pulse. (b) Have the patient apply resistance to your hand to assess for upper extremity motor strength. (c) Check for sensation by asking the patient if he can tell where you are touching him.

DRGERM

DRGERM is a guide for the EMR to perform an assessment on all four quadrants of the abdomen:

D—Distension (swelling, enlargement) of the skin

R—Rigidity (hardness, stiffness) of the muscle

G—Guarding (noted when the patient refuses to have you touch a tender area by pushing your hand away or tightening up her abdominal muscles)

E—Evisceration (visibly protruding organs)

R—Rebound tenderness (pain noted after you press down on the patient's abdomen and release the pressure)

M—Pulsating masses in the abdomen

OPQRST

The acronym **OPQRST** is used by the EMR to perform a more complete pain assessment. If the patient verbalizes pain or discomfort, ask about the following:

O—Onset: Ask the patient what he was doing when the event occurred.

P—Provoking: Ask what makes the pain worse or what makes it better.

Q—Quality of the pain: Ask what their pain feels like and only if they need choices offer descriptions of sharp, dull, stabbing, aching, burning, or crushing.

R—Radiation: Ask if the pain radiates anywhere or if it is localized (staying in one place).

S—Severity: Ask the patient to rate his pain using a pain scale of zero to ten, with zero being no pain at all and ten being his worst pain ever (Figure 5-25). When reassessing, ask how the pain compares with the last time it was reported. If the patient cannot understand the numbers on the chart, a face scale can be used to obtain a rating. When either the number or face scale is not possible due to age or special needs, document behaviors such as: tensing muscles, drawing up legs, arching, or difficulty to console.

T—Time: Ask the patient when the pain started and if she has had this type pain before, when, and how long it lasted.

Applying Assessment Tools

Referring to the acronyms discussed, you can now use palpation and visualization to perform a secondary survey. Areas to be assessed include the head, eyes, face, ears and nose, mouth, neck, chest abdomen, pelvis, legs, arms, and back. While palpating alternate your gloved hands as you go down the sides of the body in order to determine which side is involved. If the patient verbalizes pain in any area, do a more detailed pain assessment using OPQRST. Use SAMPLE on responsive patients. Both objective data and subjective data are important to a complete assessment.

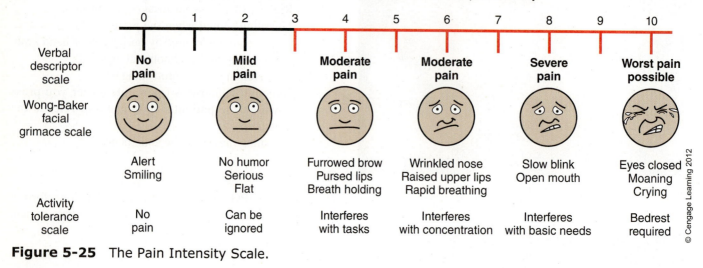

This pain assessment tool is intended to help patient care providers assess pain according to individual patient needs. Explain and use 0–10 Scale for patient self-assessment. Use the faces or behavioral observations to interpret expressed pain when patient cannot communicate his/her pain intensity.

	0	1	2	3	4	5	6	7	8	9	10
Verbal descriptor scale	**No pain**		**Mild pain**		**Moderate pain**		**Moderate pain**		**Severe pain**		**Worst pain possible**
Wong-Baker facial grimace scale	Alert Smiling		No humor Serious Flat		Furrowed brow Pursed lips Breath holding		Wrinkled nose Raised upper lips Rapid breathing		Slow blink Open mouth		Eyes closed Moaning Crying
Activity tolerance scale	No pain		Can be ignored		Interferes with tasks		Interferes with concentration		Interferes with basic needs		Bedrest required

© Cengage Learning 2012

Figure 5-25 The Pain Intensity Scale.

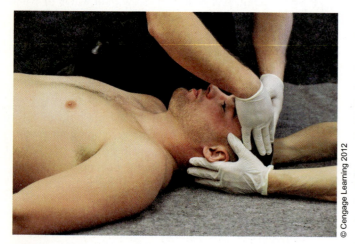

© Cengage Learning 2012

Figure 5-26 Check the head for bleeding, bruising, DOTS, and TIC.

Head

Check the skull for bleeding, bruising, DOTS, and TIC. Palpate all areas, including the back of the head, by checking your gloves for blood and feeling for uneven areas or depressions (Figure 5-26).

Eyes

Check the pupils for PERRL. The pupils should be equal, round, and reactive to light. The pupils may be constricted, dilated, or unequal if there is a head injury or specific medical condition, as shown in Figure 5-27. Reaction to light is assessed by covering and uncovering an eye or by shining a pen light or flashlight into one eye, as shown in Figure 5-28. Note if there is a change in the size of the pupil and the speed of the change. Reaction to the light will appear also in the other pupil that does not have the light source. Check for the reaction in each eye and compare. Determine if the reaction is brisk, sluggish, or absent. A normal response is brisk when the pupil changes back to baseline after approximately one second. If there are no abnormalities noted, document "PERRL." Check for tracking by having the patient look at your finger or a thin object as you move it in different planes. Assess whether the eyes follow smoothly in the various planes or jerk as they track an object or your finger. Note if the patient has to turn his head to track the object. Note any verbalizations of blurry or double vision. Table 5-4 lists some other terms that can be used to describe the pupils.

Face

Check the face for DOTS, TIC, drainage, bleeding, and symmetry. This is demonstrated in Figure 5-29.

Ears and Nose

Check the ear and nose for open wounds and for drainage such as fluid or blood. Use a flashlight or penlight if needed. Do not stop the flow of this fluid because it may be cerebrospinal fluid (CSF). Look behind the ear for bruising that might indicate a skull fracture. Check to see if the cartilage and bone are intact. Look in the nose for possible burns to the nasal hairs. Figure 5-30 demonstrates checking the ears and nose.

Mouth

Check the mouth for swelling, vomit, blood, foreign objects and broken or missing teeth. Check for open wounds on the tongue and inner cheeks. Check the breath for any unusual odors. Checking the mouth is shown in Figure 5-31.

(a)

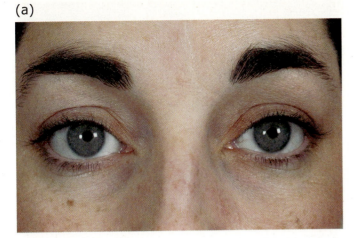

(b)

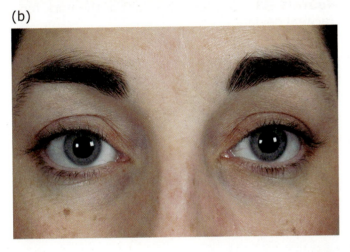

(c)

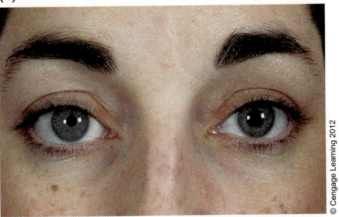

Figure 5-27 (a) Constricted pupils. (b) Dilated pupils. (c) Unequal pupils.

Table 5-4 Descriptive Terms for the Pupils

Pinpoint	Tiny pupils, usually smaller than 2 mm diameter
Constricted	Small, usually 2–3 mm
Midposition	Medium sized, usually 4–5 mm
Dilated	Large, usually 6–8 mm
Blown	Huge, usually greater than 8 mm

© Cengage Learning 2012

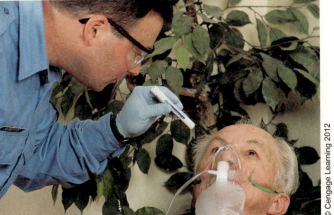

Figure 5-28 A pen light can be used to assess for pupil size and reaction to light.

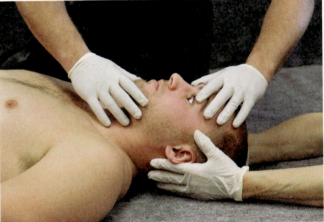

Figure 5-29 Checking the face for DOTS, TIC, drainage, bleeding, and symmetry.

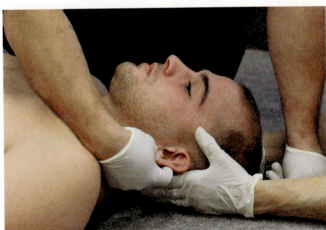

Figure 5-30 Checking the ears and nose.

Neck

Check the neck for TIC and DOTS. Check the back of the neck for pain, which could indicate a possible neck injury (Figure 5-32). Observe the anterior side for any **tracheal deviation** (movement of the trachea from the midline), indicating a severe lung problem. (Figure 5-33). Look for **jugular venous distension (JVD)** of the neck (extended jugular veins in the sides of the neck), which could indicate serious heart conditions. (Figure 5-34). Look for medical identification jewelry around the neck. See if there is a telephone number listed on the jewelry to call for information regarding the patient's medical history and contacts.

Chest

Check for symmetry of the chest as it rises and falls during respirations. Follow DOTS and TIC as you palpate the collar bone, sternum, and ribs. Check for penetrations or punctures (Figure 5-35).

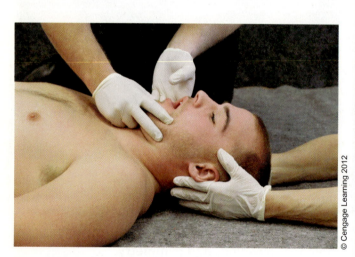

Figure 5-31 Checking the mouth.

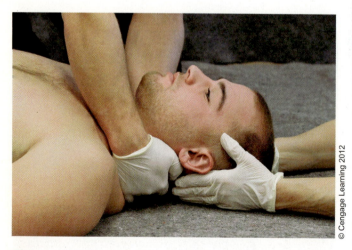

Figure 5-32 Palpation of the posterior neck for point tenderness.

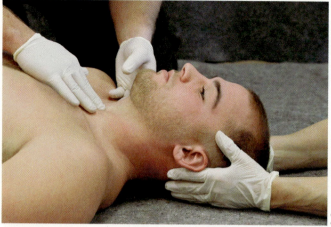

Figure 5-33 Checking the front of the neck for tracheal deviation.

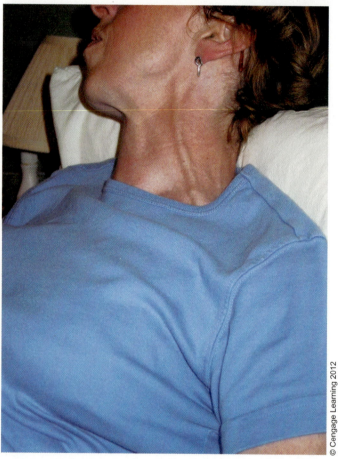

Figure 5-34 Jugular venous distension is a sign of excess fluid buildup, often seen in patients with chronic congestive heart failure.

Abdomen

Assess the abdomen using DOTS and DRGERM. Do not press too hard on the abdomen and do not attempt to reinsert eviscerated organs. Check all four quadrants of the abdomen (Figure 5-36). Look for possible pregnancy or ask the patient if she could be pregnant.

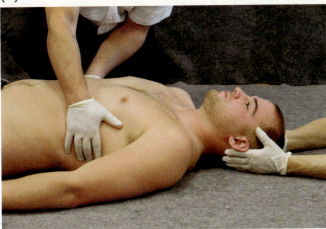

(a)

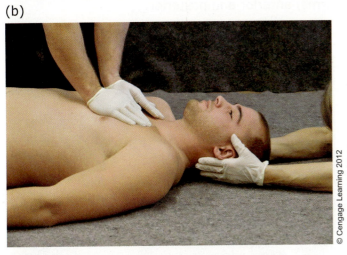

(b)

Figure 5-35 (a) Checking the chest for symmetry and rib injury. (b) The EMR must look at and feel the sternum for DOTS and TIC.

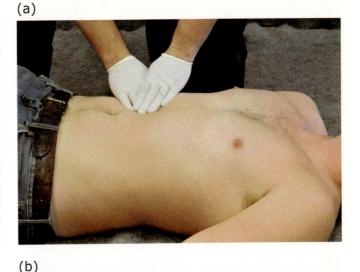

(a)

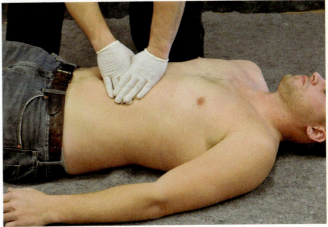

(b)

Figure 5-36 (a) An EMR can use DOTS and DRGERM to assess the patient's abdomen. (b) The EMR should check all four quadrants of the abdomen.

Pelvis

Assess for TIC and DOTS in the pelvic area. Use only gentle downward and inward pressure because of the potential hazard of worsening a pelvic fracture or severing the large vessels in the pelvic region and causing a major bleed (Figure 5-37).

Legs

Check the legs also called the lower extremities for TIC, DOTS, and CMS. Check the pedal or tibial pulses on both feet. You do not need to document a rate but note the quality of the pulses and note whether the pulse quality is equal in both feet. Palpate the back of the legs next. Assess the entire length of both legs, posterior and anterior (Figure 5-38). Look for medical identification jewelry on the ankle.

Arms

Check the arms also called the upper extremities for TIC, DOTS, and CMS (Figure 5-39). During the primary assessment, the rate, quality, and rhythm of a radial pulse rate was

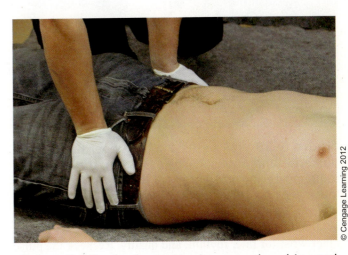

Figure 5-37 Apply gentle downward and inward pressure on the iliac wings when checking the pelvis.

(a)

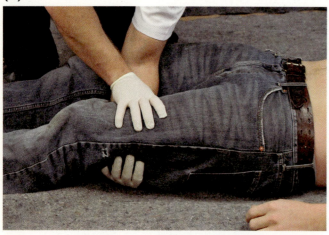

(b)

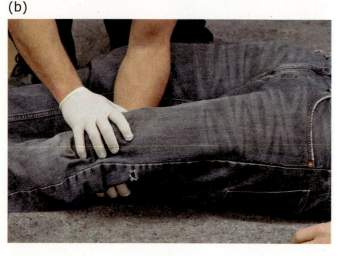

(c)

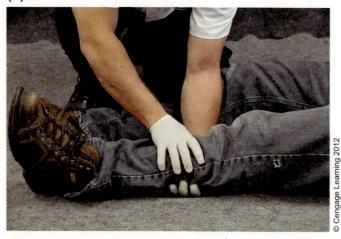

Figure 5-38 (a) Assessing the upper leg, posterior and anterior. (b) Assessing the knee and joint, posterior and anterior. (c) Assessing the lower leg, posterior and anterior.

obtained from one arm. Now check the radial pulse in the other wrist for rate, rhythm, and quality. Recheck the pulse in the initial arm if necessary and note if the pulse quality is equal for both arms. Look for a medical identification bracelet or watch on the wrists.

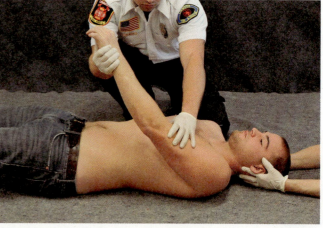

Figure 5-39 Assess the entire length of both arms, anterior and posterior.

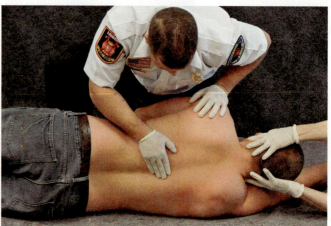

Figure 5-40 The back can be examined when the patient is logrolled onto his side.

Back

Carefully roll the patient onto his side and check the upper shoulder girdle, spine, ribs, and posterior pelvis and buttocks for TIC and DOTS (Figure 5-40). Using gloved hands, start at the upper back, and with gentle pressure, move down to the pelvic girdle and buttocks. If the patient cannot be turned onto his side because of a possible spinal injury, pain, or fracture, use palpation while they are lying supine. You will also use visualization by checking your gloves at intervals for blood.

Reassessment

The EMR has the responsibility to reassess patients periodically using primary survey, vital signs, and rapid or secondary survey to determine if his status is improving or declining. Unstable patients require reassessment every five minutes or less. A stable patient should be reassessed every 15 minutes unless the EMR notices a change in the patient's status. If there is any question as to whether a patient is stable or unstable error on the side of caution and reassess them every 5 minutes. An EMR reassesses a patient to identify changes in the patient's condition to evaluate if interventions are working and to determine if rapid transport is needed. Maintaining a dialogue with the patient is an essential part of the reassessment process. Remember, if more than one patient needs your assistance change your gloves in between patients.

Transportation Decisions

An EMR must make the decision to rapidly **package** (prepare for transport) or take time to further assess and stabilize a patient before transport. The method of packaging depends on the MOI, the patient's condition, resources available, and any environmental issues. Before transporting, request that the patient or family take the patient's prescriptions, OTC medications, herbal treatments, patient insurance card, and any pertinent legal documents to the hospital such as a health care directive.

Critical Thinking

Throughout patient assessment, an EMR will need to use critical thinking skills to assess, treat, communicate, and make transportation decisions. **Critical thinking** is the identification and evaluation of evidence to guide decision making. Critical thinking components are your knowledge base, experience, skills, and protocols.

The following is an example of how critical thinking works. When working with a patient who is unable to move an arm or leg on one side of her body, the EMR's *knowledge base* would help him recognize that this could be a symptom of a stroke. From *experience*, he has witnessed similar symptoms in a previous situation. His competency in EMR *skills* tells him to apply oxygen and place the patient in a semi-sitting position. He knows that time is of the essence and *protocols* indicate a need to transport this patient to the hospital as soon as possible. Because of critical thinking, he was able to increase the possibility of a favorable outcome for the patient.

Skill 5-1 Head-tilt, Chin-lift Method

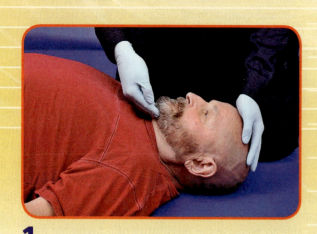

1 After donning the appropriate PPE, positions yourself at the side of the patient's head.

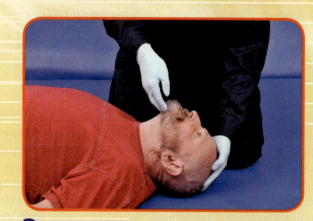

2 Place the palm of one hand on the patient's forehead and place the fingertips of the other hand on the patient's jaw.

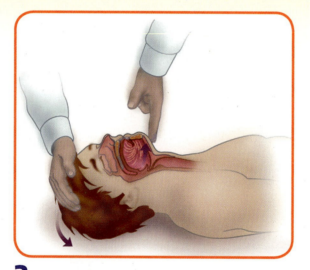

3 Tilt back the patient's head using a firm pressure on the forehead while gently lifting up the jaw to pull the tongue off the back of the throat. Care should be taken not to push backward on the jaw because doing so will only force the patient's mouth closed.

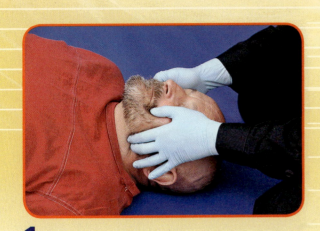

1 After donning appropriate PPE, position yourself above the patient's head.

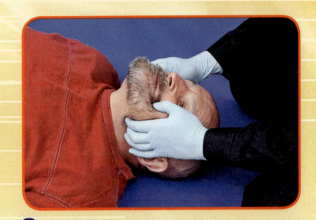

2 Place your middle and index fingers on the angles of the patient's jaw and your thumbs on the patient's cheekbones.

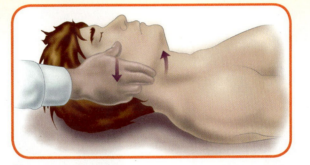

3 With the middle and index fingers, lift the jaw and the tongue up. Use your middle and index fingers to lift the jaw and the tongue up off the back of the throat while avoiding any movement of the neck.

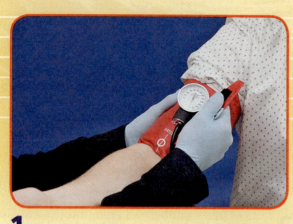

1 Place the blood pressure cuff around the patient's upper arm snugly. The cuff should cover more than half but less than two-thirds of the length of the upper arm.

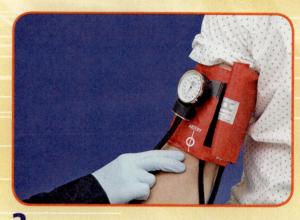

2 Find the brachial pulse (usually found on the medial side of the elbow).

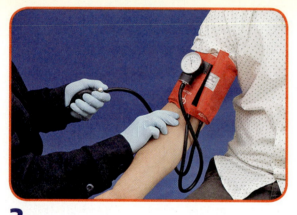

3 Close the valve on the cuff and inflate the cuff until the brachial pulse is no longer felt; then continue inflating for 20 mm Hg higher.

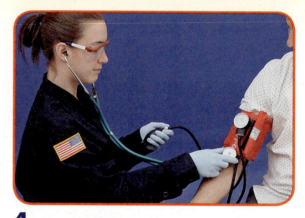

4 Place the head of the stethoscope on the brachial pulse and the ear tips in the ears.

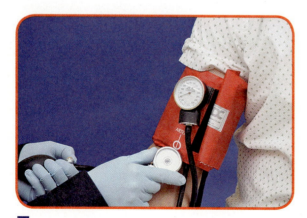

5 Deflate the blood pressure cuff slowly, at about 12 mm Hg per second, using the relief valve next to the bulb.

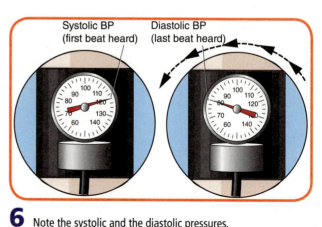

Systolic BP (first beat heard)   Diastolic BP (last beat heard)

6 Note the systolic and the diastolic pressures.

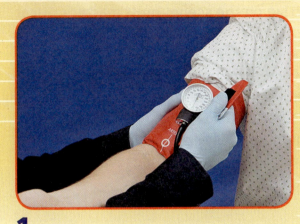

1 Snugly place the blood pressure cuff around the patient's upper arm. The cuff should cover more than half but less than two-thirds of the length of the upper arm.

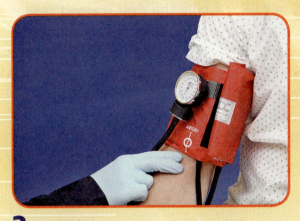

2 The EMR then finds the brachial pulse (usually found on the medial side of the elbow).

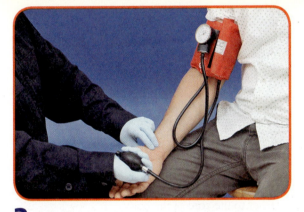

3 Close the valve on the cuff and inflate the cuff until the brachial pulse is no longer felt. Then continue inflating for 20 mm Hg higher.

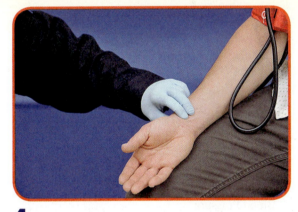

4 Place your fingertips over the radial pulse.

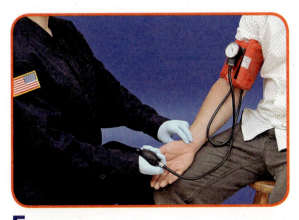

5 Slowly deflate the blood pressure cuff and note the pressure on the valve at the time you feel the return of the radial pulse.

© Cengage Learning 2012

SUMMARY

An EMR, usually the first trained responder to arrive on the scene, must master critical skills needed to successfully care for medical and trauma patients. That care is based on a complete and accurate assessment of the patient's condition. An EMR can use components of assessments such as PENMAN, spinal stabilization, patient assessment, proper interventions, reassessment, and transportation decisions to provide care. Following proven systematic assessment tools, such as DOTS, CMS, DRGERM, and OPQRST, and using critical thinking skills help the EMR obtain pertinent patient data that can be used to give appropriate, life-saving medical treatment decisions for the medical and trauma patient.

▶ REVIEW QUESTIONS

1. The P in PENMAN refers to
   a. Prevention
   b. Personal Safety
   c. Priority
   d. Provokes

2. The A in AVPU is?
   a. Airway
   b. Ambulance
   c. Advanced
   d. Alert

3. The primary survey begins after
   a. The secondary survey
   b. PENMAN
   c. Blood Pressure
   d. Skin Assessment

4. Auscultation blood pressure requires
   a. Listening with a stethoscope
   b. Feeling the pulse
   c. Listening to the apical pulse
   d. Feeling for air exchange

5. In the acronym TIC the T refers to
   a. Talk
   b. Tenderness
   c. Touch
   d. Traction

6. In the acronym PERRL the P refers to
   a. Pupils
   b. Provokes
   c. Protect
   d. Personal

7. The O in the acronym DOTS refers to
   a. Oxygen
   b. Obstruction
   c. Overdose
   d. Open injuries

8. Peripheral pulses are pulses
   a. Farther away from the core of the body
   b. Commonly called central pulses
   c. Closer to the core of the body
   d. Found in the abdominal cavity

9. Baseline vital signs refer to
   a. The first set of vital signs
   b. Trending of vital signs
   c. Checking vital signs every 5 minutes
   d. Checking vital signs every 15 minutes

10. A secondary survey is:
    a. Performed on an unstable patient
    b. Performed after PENMAN
    c. Performed on a stable patient
    d. Performed as soon as possible

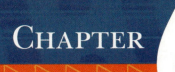

CHAPTER 6

DOCUMENTATION

LEARNING OBJECTIVES

By the end of this chapter, the reader should be able to:

- List and describe the components of the patient care report (PCR).
- Describe the difference between subjective and objective information on the PCR.
- Explain the acronyms SOAP and CHART.
- Define how the Health Insurance Portability and Accountability Act relates to Emergency Medical Responders.

INTRODUCTION

The field of Emergency Medical Services (EMS) is based on competent, compassionate care that must be carefully documented. Competency, professional compassion, and accurately documenting medical calls protect Emergency Medical Responders (EMRs). Good documentation begins with the EMR knowing the pertinent medical information that should be obtained from a patient and knowing the proper way to record and protect that information.

Patient Care Report

Documentation, commonly referred to as a **patient care report (PCR)**, is the legal record of the patient's condition and the care that was provided during the time spent with a patient. This report is important for continuity of care and treatment.

Legal Issues

If a lawsuit is brought against an EMR, the PCR for the incident in question should contain all of the necessary information to defend the EMR's actions. Therefore, complete, clear, and neat documentation is vitally important. If an EMR does not record care given to a patient, then for the purpose of the judicial system, the care was *not* given because it was not documented. Many agencies today have computer-generated PCR forms that assist EMRs in documenting services provided to a patient. Whether using a written form or a computerized form, EMRs must complete all components of the PCR because the patient data provide other health care providers a basis for continued care (Figure 6-1).

Components of the Patient Care Report

There are three components of the PCR: the call data, patient data, and the narrative. All components must be completed for every incident.

Call Data

The first component, the **call data**, contains information about the location of the call, call times, unit number, responding personnel, and date.

Patient Data

Patient data is the second component of the PCR. This component includes the following items:

- Name, sex, and date of birth
- Reason for the call; chief complaint
- Medical information, past and present
- Mechanism of injury (MOI), nature of illness (NOI), or both

- How the patient was found; help at the scene
- Primary survey
- Vital signs and trending
- Rapid or secondary survey
- Interventions
- Reassessment

An EMR may be delayed in obtaining some information from the patient because the first priority is performing primary and secondary surveys or providing immediate interventions. If an EMR cannot obtain all information necessary to complete the form, the EMR will need to write NA, meaning not available, in the space where missing information

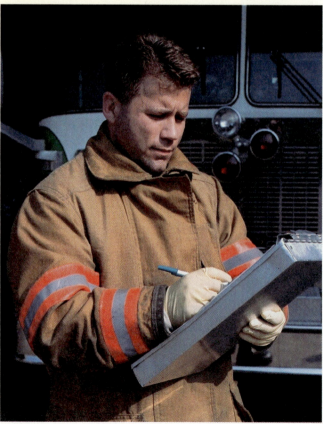

Figure 6-1 Documentation of patient data gives other health care providers a basis for continued care.

would have been recorded. Often law enforcement is on the scene and can assist in gathering information about the patient because they can search the patient for identification.

Trending Vital Signs

Trending is obtaining multiple sets of vital signs to determine if the patient is getting better, staying the same, or getting worse. Trending helps an EMR establish the urgency for transporting a critical patient. Trending is also essential to ensure that the care being given is working (Figure 6-2). If trending shows the care is not working, the EMR can make changes that give the patient a chance for a more favorable outcome.

Level of consciousness and vital signs must be taken every five minutes (at a minimum) for critical patients and at least every 15 minutes for stable patients. If a rapid transport is indicated, the EMR may have time for only an initial set of vital signs. Trending must be done with all patients, with the exception of rapid transport patients, to allow EMRs and other health care professionals to have more than a baseline set of vital signs for the patient's extended care.

Narrative Information

The narrative is the third component of the PCR. The narrative tells the story of everything that happened from the time the EMR arrived on the scene to the time that the patient is transported. The EMR must write clearly and concisely and avoid using slang rather than medical terms. The only abbreviations allowed are those used in medical terminology. Examples of some common approved medical terms include:

- NKA: no known allergies
- c/o: complained of

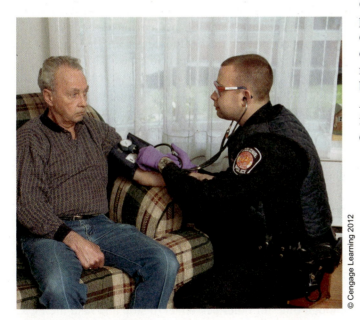

Figure 6-2 Obtain multiple sets of vital signs for trending to determine whether the patient is getting better, staying the same, or getting worse.

- Pt: patient
- Fx: fracture
- Dx: diagnosis
- R: right (R is usually encircled)
- L: left (L is usually encircled)
- lpm: liters per minute

Using slang or unrecognized abbreviations could cause confusion for other health care personnel during treatment or in a court of law where the EMR's competence could be questioned. The EMR should obtain a list of approved abbreviations and follow it. Always use military time when stating or documenting time, such as 1400 for 2 pm, 2000 for 8 pm, or 0000 for midnight. If a documentation error is made on the PCR, the EMR should draw a single line through the mistake, write in the correction, and then initial and date the correction as shown in Figure 6-3.

Objective Information

The narrative section of the PCR will contain information that can be observed and measured, called **objective information**. This is information that an EMR has personally seen upon physical examination and can testify in court that it is factual. An example of objective information would be "the patient has an open fracture to the anterior tibia of the right leg" or "the patient is vomiting." These data can be verified by everyone, including the patient.

Subjective Information

The narrative section of the PCR will contain information offered by the patient that is not objectively verifiable called **subjective information**. This information is based on the opinions or feelings of the patient, family, or bystanders. A patient provides subjective information when he complains of "back pain" or "nausea" or states, "I can't feel my feet" or "my chest feels as if it has a heavy weight on it." A family member provides subjective information when she says, "My brother is a diabetic" or "My husband has a heart condition." An EMR should never include her own opinions or feelings in the narrative, such as, "I believe this patient is lying and could have had a few six packs of beer before our arrival."

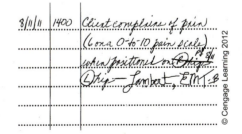

Figure 6-3 Cross out errors with a single line, write in the correction, and then initial and date the correction.

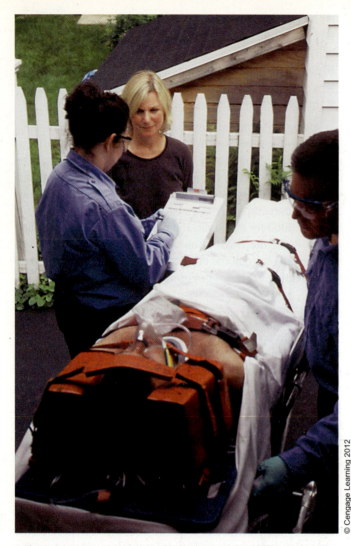

Figure 6-4 Subjective information provided by a family member can help the EMR assess and manage the patient.

This type of subjective information is guessing. However, subjective information provided by the patient, family members, or bystanders can be key to effectively assessing and managing a patient (Figure 6-4).

SOAP and CHART

Make sure the information obtained through SOAP or CHART is included in the PCR. It is not necessary, however, to repeat information fully recorded elsewhere. Use the narrative space in the PCR to give further details about the facts.

Acronyms developed to guide the EMR and other health care providers in obtaining useful information about the victim during an accident are particularly useful for recording information in the narrative section of the PCR. Two of these acronyms, **SOAP** and **CHART**, give the EMR a way to systematically approach the patient and carefully document changes to the patient's condition. See Figure 6-5 for a completed, written PCR.

SOAP:

- **S—Subjective information:** This is information the EMR obtains from the patient, a family member, or a bystander. This includes information obtained through a detailed pain assessment of OPQRST or finding out a chief complaint.
- **O—Objective information:** This is specific patient information obtained by the EMR and can include information obtained through DOTS and vital sign readings.
- **A—Assessment information:** The EMR forms an assessment from both subjective and objective information describing the patient's situation.
- **P—Patient care:** This is treatment or action that was taken based on the information at hand.

CHART:

- **C—Chief complaint:** The patient's main reason for calling emergency services.
- **H—History:** An account of the course of the illness or trauma.
- **A—Assessment:** A complete survey of the patient and vital signs.
- **R—Rx:** The treatment and interventions used.
- **T—Transport:** If the patient was transported, what agency was involved, and what time transportation took place.

Refusal of Treatment

Any competent adult may refuse medical assistance; however, the EMR should explain potential consequences of not receiving this assistance and advise the patient to call again if they change their mind. If the patient is unresponsive, is mentally challenged, has dementia, has a traumatic brain injury, or appears incompetent, the EMR assumes implied consent for treatment and must seek transport to a medical facility.

Most EMS systems have a separate patient refusal form for the patient to sign when treatment is refused (Figure 6-6). If the patient refuses to sign the refusal form, have another individual, preferably a family member or noninvolved party such as a law enforcement officer or firefighter, sign the refusal form as a witness indicating the patient refused care without threat or duress.

Transfer of Care

When transferring or "handing off" the care of a patient to EMS personnel with a higher level of training, it is important to communicate both verbally and by providing a copy of the PCR. In an emergency situation, there is often not enough time for other personnel to stop and read the PCR, so as packaging (preparing a patient for transport) is in process, the EMR will need to verbally communicate all pertinent information. A verbal report may consist of the SOAP or CHART format.

© Cengage Learning 2012

LINWOOD EMERGENCY MEDICAL SERVICES
FIRST RESPONDER REPORT

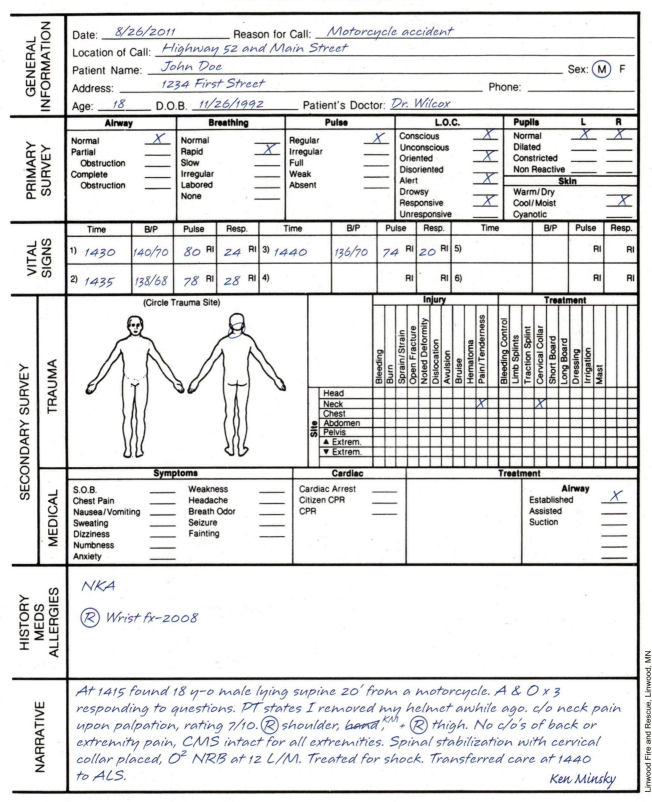

GENERAL INFORMATION

Date: _8/26/2011_   Reason for Call: _Motorcycle accident_

Location of Call: _Highway 52 and Main Street_

Patient Name: _John Doe_   Sex: (M) F

Address: _1234 First Street_   Phone: _____

Age: _18_   D.O.B. _11/26/1992_   Patient's Doctor: _Dr. Wilcox_

PRIMARY SURVEY

Airway		Breathing		Pulse		L.O.C.		Pupils	L	R
Normal	X	Normal		Regular	X	Conscious	X	Normal	X	X
Partial		Rapid	X	Irregular		Unconscious		Dilated		
Obstruction		Slow		Full		Oriented	X	Constricted		
Complete		Irregular		Weak		Disoriented		Non Reactive		
Obstruction		Labored		Absent		Alert	X	**Skin**		
		None				Drowsy		Warm/Dry		
						Responsive	X	Cool/Moist		X
						Unresponsive		Cyanotic		

VITAL SIGNS

	Time	B/P	Pulse	Resp.		Time	B/P	Pulse	Resp.		Time	B/P	Pulse	Resp.
1)	1430	140/70	80 RI	24 RI	3)	1440	136/70	74 RI	20 RI	5)			RI	RI
2)	1435	138/68	78 RI	28 RI	4)			RI	RI	6)			RI	RI

SECONDARY SURVEY

TRAUMA (Circle Trauma Site)

Site	Bleeding	Burn	Sprain/Strain	Open Fracture	Noted Deformity	Dislocation	Avulsion	Bruise	Hematoma	Pain/Tenderness	Bleeding Control	Limb Splints	Traction Splint	Cervical Collar	Short Board	Long Board	Dressing	Irrigation	Mast
Head																			
Neck										X				X					
Chest																			
Abdomen																			
Pelvis																			
▲ Extrem.																			
▼ Extrem.																			

MEDICAL

Symptoms		Cardiac		Treatment	
S.O.B.	___	Cardiac Arrest	___	**Airway**	
Chest Pain	___	Citizen CPR	___	Established	X
Nausea/Vomiting	___	CPR	___	Assisted	___
Sweating	___			Suction	___
Dizziness	___				___
Numbness	___				___
Anxiety	___				___

Symptoms (left list): Weakness, Headache, Breath Odor, Seizure, Fainting

HISTORY MEDS ALLERGIES

NKA

(R) Wrist fx—2008

NARRATIVE

At 1415 found 18 y-o male lying supine 20′ from a motorcycle. A & O x 3
responding to questions. PT states I removed my helmet awhile ago. c/o neck pain
upon palpation, rating 7/10. (R) shoulder, hand,ᴷᴹ + (R) thigh. No c/o's of back or
extremity pain, CMS intact for all extremities. Spinal stabilization with cervical
collar placed, O² NRB at 12 L/M. Treated for shock. Transferred care at 1440
to ALS.

Ken Minsky

Figure 6-5 An example of a completed, written patient care report.

COUNTY EMS
REFUSAL OF MEDICAL ASSISTANCE FORM

EMS Service: _____ Date: _____ Time: _____

Patient Name: _____ Age: _____ Phone # _____

Incident Location: _____ Incident # _____

Situation of EMS Call: _____ NON PATIENT: ☐
(see Non-Patient Encounter Form)

PATIENT ASSESSMENT:
Any current medical complaint: ☐ Yes ☐ No (If yes – describe:_____)
Suspected injury or illness based on patient history, physical examination or mechanism of injury: ☐ Yes ☐ No

Competency to Refuse Medical Assistance:

18 years of age or older: ☐ Yes ☐ No	Any evidence of:		
Patient Oriented to:	Suicidal? ☐ Yes	☐ No	
Person: ☐ Yes ☐ No	Head Injury? ☐ Yes	☐ No	
Place: ☐ Yes ☐ No	Intoxication? ☐ Yes	☐ No	
Time: ☐ Yes ☐ No	Any altered mental status? ☐ Yes	☐ No	
Event: ☐ Yes ☐ No	Mentally impaired in any way? ☐ Yes	☐ No	

Risks explained to patient: _____
Patient understands clinical situation and risks ☐ Yes ☐ No
Patient verbalizes understanding of risks: ☐ Yes ☐ No
Patient's plan to seek further medical evaluation:_____
Who will be with the patient after EMS departure?_____

BASE STATION CONTACT:
Physician: _____ BASE STATION: _____ TIME: _____
Base Physician spoke to patient: ☐ Yes ☐ No
Base Physician Orders: _____

PATIENT OUTCOME:
_____ Patient refuses transportation to a hospital against medical advice;

_____ Patient accepts transportation to hospital by EMS but refuses any or all treatment offered.

Treatment refused:_____

_____ Other: (Explain):_____

This form is being provided to me because I have refused assessment, treatment and/or transportation by EMS personnel for myself or on behalf of this patient. I understand that EMS personnel are not physicians and are not qualified or authorized to make a diagnosis and that their care is not a substitute for that of a physician. I recognize that there may be a serious injury or illness which could get worse without medical attention even though I (or the patient) may feel fine at the present time. I understand that I may change my mind and call 911 if treatment or assistance is needed later. I also understand that treatment is available at an emergency department 24 hours a day. I acknowledge that this advice has been explained to me by the EMS personnel and that I have read this form completely and understand its terms.

_____ _____ _____
Signature (patient or other)   Date   EMS Provider Signature

If other than patient, print name and relationship to patient

© Cengage Learning 2012

Figure 6-6 Many agencies use a separate patient care refusal form.

Patient Confidentiality

EMS professionals must remember that patient confidentiality and medical privacy is a legal requirement. The **Health Insurance Portability and Accountability Act (HIPAA)** encompasses many factors but specifically relates to the EMR regarding the protection of patient privacy, patient confidentiality, and security of health care information. EMRs must not divulge any patient information, verbal or written, to anyone other than health care providers directly involved in the continuation of a patient's care.

SUMMARY

Good initial documentation of patient care can lead to clues regarding the patient's condition through trending. Good documentation protects the EMR as well. The PCR is a legal document and may be used in a court of law. PCR information must be collected objectively, with subjective information from the patient, family, or bystanders noted as such. An EMR may use acronyms such as SOAP and CHART to provide a systematic approach for gathering and documenting patient medical information on the PCR and when transferring care. Remember that all verbal and written information collected is protected by law. EMRs are not allowed to give patient information to anyone except other health care providers.

REVIEW QUESTIONS

1. Name six elements of call data.
2. Describe why trending vital signs is useful in patient care.
3. Describe the difference between objective and subjective information.

4. State the components of SOAP and give examples of each.
5. What federal law regulates patient confidentiality?

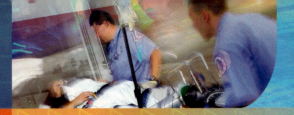

CHAPTER 7

AIRWAY AND OXYGEN MANAGEMENT

LEARNING OBJECTIVES

By the end of this chapter, the reader should be able to

- Explain how to determine if a patient's airway is open.
- Describe the use of suction devices for obstructed airways.
- Explain how to secure an airway with oropharyngeal airway and nasopharyngeal airway devices.
- Describe how to use a pocket mask or bag valve mask.
- List indications for supplemental oxygen.
- Explain differences between a nasal cannula and a non-rebreather mask for delivering oxygen.
- Explain pulse oximetry.
- Describe appropriate handling for oxygen tanks.

INTRODUCTION

The human body must have adequate oxygen to live. Lack of oxygenation eventually causes death. Under normal circumstances, the brain cells can survive approximately four to six minutes after the heart stops beating and then brain cells begin to die and irreversible brain damage or death occurs. However, in a cold environment, such as cold water, brain damage or brain death from lack of oxygen may be delayed beyond this typical timeline.

When confronted with a patient who has inadequate oxygen or no oxygenation, the Emergency Medical Responder (EMR) needs to work as quickly as possible to open an airway and administer oxygen to the patient. In an unresponsive patient with no breathing or no normal breathing such as gasping, follow the current American Heart Association (AHA) guidelines. This chapter focuses on techniques that an EMR can use to open and secure an airway, suction, ventilate, and deliver oxygen to a patient.

Airway

If a patient's airway is not open, oxygen cannot be delivered to the patient. An open airway is an adequate opening from the mouth and nose down the trachea to the lungs. After PENMAN and AVPU (see Chapter 5), the EMR should assess the ABC's starting with the airway in a responsive patient. If the airway is not open, as noted by the patient's not breathing, speaking, or coughing, the airway must be opened to prevent death or disability. Opening the airway may be as simple as performing a head-tilt, chin-lift maneuver or if a cervical spine injury is suspected, the jaw thrust maneuver (see Chapter 5).

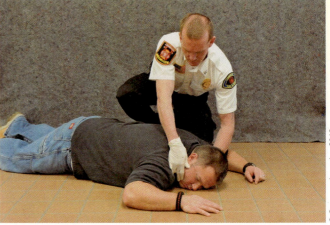

Figure 7-1 The patient in a prone position.

Positioning Considerations

If you find the victim in a car and if the mechanism of injury indicates, suspect a spinal injury. Opening the airway and ventilating the patient can be challenging. Seek entry to the vehicle, stabilize the victim's neck, and use the jaw thrust maneuver to open the airway. Many times this simple step will allow the patient to start breathing. If this maneuver fails, you must extricate (remove the patient) from the vehicle using spinal stabilization if possible.

If you find your patient in a trauma situation lying in a lateral recumbent or prone position and not breathing (Figure 7-1), try a jaw thrust maneuver while stabilizing the neck. If there is no breathing present, turn the victim as a unit if possible and proceed to open the airway. If the patient is still not breathing and ventilations have been attempted without chest rise, the airway may be obstructed.

Airway Obstructions

Determine if the patient's airway is **patent** (open) or obstructed. An airway can be obstructed by objects such as food, toys, dentures, or broken teeth. An airway can also be obstructed by secretions, such as blood, mucus, or emesis (vomit); by inflammation from a respiratory illness or allergic reaction; or by trauma to the face or neck. Additionally, spasms of the airway, such as asthma, can obstruct the airway. An airway can be totally obstructed or partially obstructed. In both cases, the patient will either be unresponsive or could become unresponsive.

When opening an obstructed airway caused by a foreign body (object or food), EMRs must follow current AHA guidelines for foreign body airway obstruction in a conscious or an unconscious person. Figure 7-2 illustrates two positions to relieve obstruction in a conscious patient.

Suctioning the Airway

If secretions are the cause of the obstruction, the EMR may need to suction the airway before ventilating. If secretions are in the airway, turn the victim's head to the side. Or if

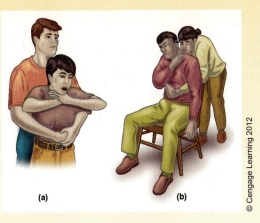

Figure 7-2 Abdominal thrusts performed on a conscious person while (a) standing and (b) seated.

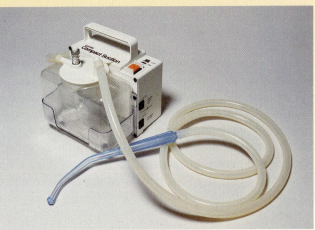

Figure 7-4 The mechanical suction machine has several disposable parts, including the suction catheter, the tubing, and the canister.

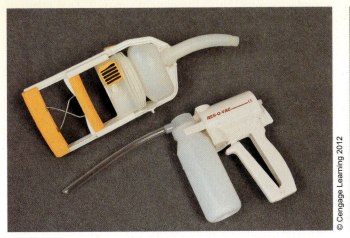

Figure 7-3 Manual suction devices.

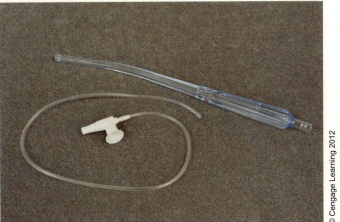

Figure 7-5 Rigid and flexible suction catheters.

there is a suspected spinal cord injury, turn the body as a unit. Use your gloved fingers to clean out the mouth. If this maneuver does not remove the secretions, suctioning will be necessary. By clearing secretions, you open the airway and prevent **aspiration,** which is the introduction of vomit, fluid, or other foreign material into the lungs. Aspirating secretions can further complicate good air exchange and possibly cause an infection such as pneumonia.

Manual and Mechanical Suctions

A **manual suction** is a suctioning unit that is inserted into the oral cavity and suctions secretions as the device is manually squeezed or pumped (Figure 7-3). This device is inserted only as far as it can be visualized in the mouth of the victim.

A **mechanical suction** unit is a suction device that is portable or mounted to the wall of an emergency response vehicle (Figure 7-4). Usually the battery-operated device stays plugged into a charger until time for use. It needs to be checked daily to make sure it is operating properly.

Mechanical Suctioning

A **suction catheter** is a long tube used to remove secretions from an airway. Suctioning a patient begins with selecting the proper size and type of suction catheter depending on the substance in the airway. There are two basic types of suction catheters, the rigid catheter such as the tonsil tip catheter or **Yankauer suction catheter** used to suction saliva, mucus, blood, or other secretions from the mouth, and the flexible longer catheter good for suctioning the nares (openings of the nose), or tracheostomy openings (Figure 7-5).

After the appropriate catheter is chosen, the catheter is attached to suction tubing on the suction machine and inserted into the mouth, nose, or trach. An EMR should then use suction *only* as the rigid or flexible catheter is being withdrawn and for a maximum of 15 seconds for an adult, 10 seconds for a child, and 5 seconds for an infant. When a patient is suctioned, oxygen is removed from the lungs. If possible, oxygen should be administered to the patient before and in between suction attempts. **Skill 7-1** at the end of this chapter illustrates suctioning the airway with a rigid catheter.

A patient may vomit if suctioning causes a gag reflex. If the patient vomits, the EMR should stop the suctioning, roll the patient to his side, and clear out the emesis. If there is a possibility of a spinal injury, roll the patient to his side while stabilizing the spine. If the suction catheter becomes clogged, place the catheter tip in water and turn on the suction to remove the debris. If the catheter still does not work, change catheters. Avoid going deeply for consecutive suctioning attempts and never force the suction catheter into the patient's mouth. When suctioning through a tracheostomy (Figure 7-6), the catheter needs to be sterile and requires specialized training. Follow your agencies protocols.

Recovery Position

The recovery position is used when a patient is again breathing without assistance. This position allows secretions to drain out of the victim's mouth and not into the back of the throat, causing another obstruction. In the recovery position, a patient is placed in a lateral recumbent position (Figure 7-7). Do not use the recovery position for patients with suspected spinal injuries.

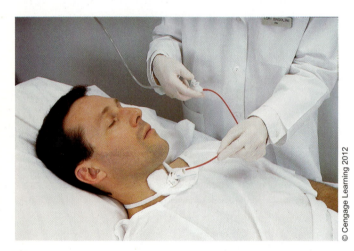

Figure 7-6 Tracheostomy tubes often become clogged with mucus and can be suctioned gently using a sterile flexible catheter.

Securing the Airway

Airway devices are used to maintain an open airway by keeping the tongue from obstructing the back of the mouth. However, even after insertion of an airway device, an EMR will need to use a head-tilt, chin-lift, or jaw thrust maneuver to help maintain the open airway. The two types of airway devices that an EMR may use are the oropharyngeal and the nasopharyngeal airway.

Oropharyngeal Airway

The rigid **oropharyngeal airway (oral airway or OPA)** is a medical device used to maintain a patent airway by preventing the tongue from partially or completely covering the epiglottis, which could prevent the patient from breathing. The OPA is placed in an unresponsive patient who does not have a gag reflex. The OPA comes in various sizes (Figure 7-8), and the proper airway size should be determined before placing an OPA in the patient's mouth. The length of the oral airway should match the distance from the angle of the jaw to the opening of the patient's mouth or front teeth or from the corner of the mouth to the earlobe. After selecting the correct size, open the patient's mouth and insert the airway with the tip of the OPA up. Follow the roof of the mouth until midway and then turn the airway 180 degrees. Never force an OPA into the oral cavity. If the patient vomits, suction the mouth. Do not reattempt to open the airway until the vomit is cleared. Most unconscious patients will need an airway placed, so it is important for the EMR to be proficient at properly inserting one. **Skill 7-2** at the end of this chapter illustrates how to insert the OPA.

Nasopharyngeal Airway

The **nasopharyngeal airway (NPA)** is a flexible tube designed to be inserted into the nasal passageway to secure an open airway. An NPA is used when an OPA cannot be used because the patient has damage to the mouth or has a gag reflex. Unresponsive patients with a gag reflex may include

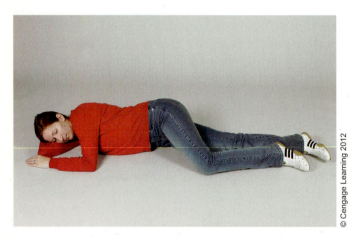

Figure 7-7 The recovery position allows natural drainage of airway secretions.

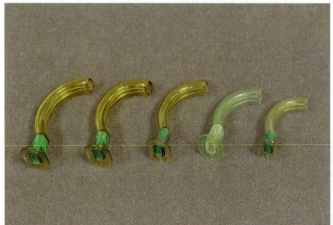

Figure 7-8 The correct oropharyngeal airway must be selected from the sizes available.

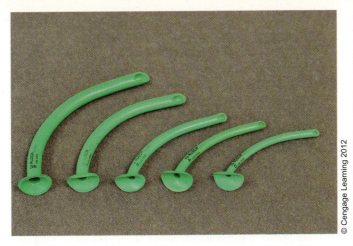

Figure 7-9 A nasopharyngeal airway, available in various sizes, must be properly fitted to the patient.

Table 7-1 Indications for Oxygen Administration

Respiratory distress or failure
Cardiopulmonary arrest
Chest pain
Stroke
Abdominal pain
Hypoperfusion (shock)
Altered mental status
Major trauma
Severe internal or external bleeding
Exposure to toxins (e.g., carbon dioxide, cyanide)
Near drowning or submersion
Suffocation or foreign body airway obstruction
Drug overdose

© Cengage Learning 2012

substance abusers, stroke victims, post seizure patients, and diabetics with hypoglycemia. The NPA is not indicated if the patient has a potential skull or facial fracture because of the risk for brain injury through the sinus cavities.

To find the correct NPA size (Figure 7-9), measure from the tip of the nose to the tip of the earlobe. Lubricate the airway with a water-soluble solution. Typically, the right nostril is larger, but either nostril can be used. Slide the airway gently into the patient's nostril with the beveled tip of the airway toward the septum of the patient's nose. Do not force the airway, which could damage vessels in the nose and cause bleeding. If resistance is met, the airway should be withdrawn and insertion attempted in the other nostril. An illustration of insertion of the NPA can be found in **Skill 7-3** at the end of this chapter.

Breathing

After the patient's airway is open, the EMR should assess the patient for air exchange to determine if the patient needs ventilation, adding oxygen if available, or if the patient needs supplemental oxygen.

Throughout the remainder of this text, the use of oxygen is discussed as it relates to specific medial and trauma conditions. Table 7-1 lists indications for oxygen administration.

Ventilating a Patient

A patient will need ventilation by a pocket mask or bag valve mask if the patient is:

- Unresponsive with apnea or periods of apnea
- Unresponsive with agonal breathing
- Bradypnea or tachypnea with signs of poor perfusion such as cyanotic, grey, or mottled skin

In most of the above situations the EMR will also be providing chest compressions along with two ventilations.

If there is a palpable pulse and the patient only needs ventilations, give one breath every 5–6 seconds for an adult and one breath every 3–5 seconds for a child or infant.

Pocket Mask

A **pocket mask** is a device used to deliver ventilations during a cardiac arrest, respiratory arrest, or with severe respiratory compromise. Typically, the air we breathe is made up of 21 percent oxygen. Human exhalation through a pocket mask delivers approximately 16 percent oxygen, which is adequate in most situations. Some pocket masks allow an oxygen source to be attached, therefore increasing the percentage of oxygen delivered. A pocket mask has a one way valve with a filter however it does not always protect the user from exposure to body substances, especially if the patient has projectile vomiting. If a pocket mask or other barrier device is not available, the EMR can choose to forgo performing ventilations. If ventilations are not given, and compressions are being performed, it may be beneficial for the EMR to keep the airway open with the head-tilt, chin-lift method for possible passive air movement. Figure 7-10 shows various types of pocket masks.

Pocket masks come in different sizes for adults, children, and infants. Choose the proper size mask so it covers the patient's mouth and nose while the head-tilt, chin lift method, or jaw thrust maneuver is used to open the airway. If located at the head of the patient, the EMR can use the C-E technique to obtain an adequate seal with the mask as shown in Figure 7-11. If located at the side of the patient, place your hand in a C position around the top of the mask and place the thumb of your opposite hand on the bottom of the mask. Then place your index finger under the chin, pressing the mask as you lift the chin and extend the neck (Figure 7-12). Breathe into the mask only until you see visible chest rise. As previously mentioned, over inflation of the lungs may cause vomiting.

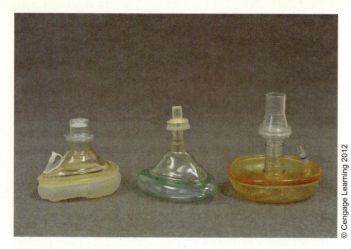

Figure 7-10 Various types of pocket masks.

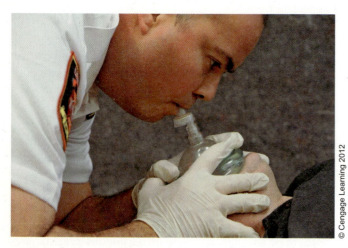

Figure 7-11 An Emergency Medical Responder using the C-E technique to obtain an adequate seal with a pocket mask.

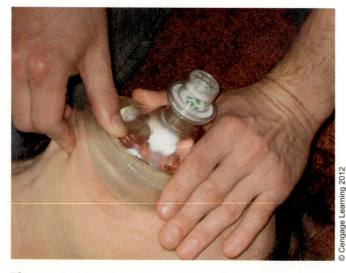

Figure 7-12 Pocket mask ventilation from the side of the patient using the C-E technique.

If the chest does not rise or air is escaping around the mask, the patient may have an obstruction, the mask may not have an adequate seal, or there may not be adequate head tilt. Reposition the head, increasing neck extension, and recheck the mask and hand position. If an adult mask is the only size mask available and an adequate seal cannot be made on an infant or child, turn the mask around with the nose portion on the infant's or child's chin. If a visible chest rise is still not present, consider suctioning or follow AHA guidelines for foreign body airway obstruction.

Bag Valve Mask

A **bag valve mask (BVM)** is a handheld device used to provide positive pressure ventilation to a patient who is not breathing or who is not breathing adequately (Figure 7-13). The BVM is used by squeezing a bag attached to a mask similar to a pocket mask. A BVM can be used with or without an oxygen source, but it is capable of providing up to 100 percent oxygenation when attached to a high-flow oxygen source. If using an oxygen source, provide at least 10 liters per minute (lpm) of oxygen flow. With a BVM, the EMR has little chance of being exposed to body substances when using proper PPE.

To use a BVM, place one hand on the mask to make a good seal over the patient's mouth and nose while tilting the head (if no spinal injury suspected). With your other hand, squeeze the self-inflating BVM only enough to see visible chest rise, as shown in Figure 7-14. If the patient has a suspected spinal injury and you do not see the chest rise, you may have to use slight neck extension until you see the chest rise.

If you do not see the chest rise, it may be because of an inadequate seal of the BVM over the mouth and nose. This can be remedied by increasing the head tilt, confirming mask and hand placement, or obtaining assistance from another individual to squeeze the bag or provide a C-E position on the mask (Figure 7-15). If a chest rise still is not visible after

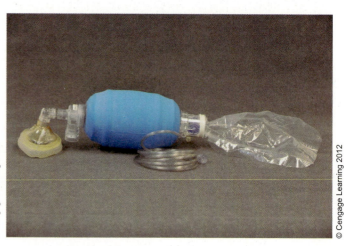

Figure 7-13 The bag valve mask device is used to ventilate the patient.

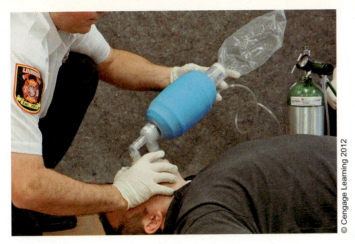

Figure 7-14 Bag valve mask with oxygen attached.

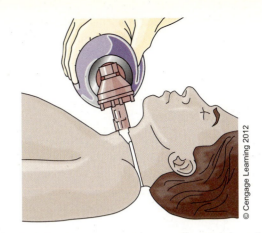

Figure 7-16 The bag valve mask attaches to all standard tracheostomy tubes. Caution should be taken because less volume is needed to ventilate the patient.

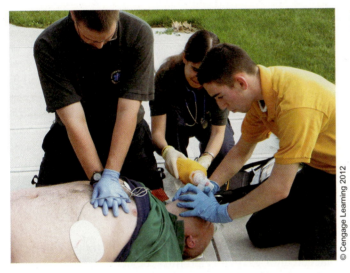

Figure 7-15 The Emergency Medical Responder obtaining assistance for the bag valve mask.

taking these steps, consider suctioning or performing the AHA foreign body airway obstruction technique.

A BVM can also be used on a patient with a tracheostomy. Disconnect the mask from the bag valve portion and attach it to the tracheostomy tube. Figure 7-16 shows how an EMR can ventilate a patient with a tracheostomy. If no BVM is available, a pocket mask can be used over the trach to provide ventilations.

Supplemental Oxygen Delivery

Supplemental oxygen is applied to patients with respiratory compromise. **Respiratory compromise** means that the patient is physically able to inhale and exhale air but is not receiving adequate oxygenation with her own effort. Supplemental oxygen is given via a nasal cannula or non-rebreather mask over the mouth, nose, or tracheostomy.

Indications of Respiratory Compromise

Indications of respiratory compromise in a responsive patient are:

- **Rate:** Tachypnea or bradypnea that does not provide adequate oxygenation.
- **Quality:** The patient requires effort to breathe or speak; maintains a tripod position or use of accessory muscles, including nasal flaring, pursed lips, abdominal breathing, head bobbing; or abnormally deep or shallow breaths.
- **Sounds:** Snoring; high-pitched grunting, barking, wheezing, or crowing breathing
- **Skin Color:** Pale, mild cyanosis, or duskiness
- **Verbalizations:** A patient may state, "I'm so short of breath" or "I can't catch my breath."
- **Altered mental status (AMS):** The patient shows signs of confusion or agitation.

Nasal Cannula

A **nasal cannula (NC)** is a soft, flexible tube with two nasal prongs that can be inserted into the patient's nostrils to deliver oxygen. Attach the cannula to an oxygen-tank regulator that is set between 1 and 6 lpm to provide approximately 25 to 45 percent oxygen concentration. Place the NC, prongs facing downward, into the patient's nostrils. With the slider loosened, loop the extra tubing behind the patient's ears and then cinch it loosely under the chin. Application of a NC is demonstrated at the end of this chapter in **Skill 7-4**.

Non-rebreather Mask

A **non-rebreather (NRB) mask** covers the nose and mouth of the patient and delivers oxygen at a rate of 10 to 15 lpm. At this rate, the patient receives 60 to 95 percent oxygen concentration. The mask has a one-way valve and a reservoir bag. The reservoir bag accumulates oxygen to obtain higher concentrations. The bag must be filled before the mask is placed on the patient. Place your finger over the valve in the mask and allow the reservoir bag to fill. Place the mask on the patient's face and then position and tighten the straps around the patient's head. Demonstration of the application of an NRB mask is found in **Skill 7-5**.

Blow-by Oxygenation

Some children and adults do not like the NRB mask and may feel as if they are suffocating with this mask on their face. When this situation arises, the EMR can use **blow-by oxygenation**, providing oxygen for a patient who cannot tolerate a mask by placing the mask or oxygen tubing near the patient's mouth and nose (Figure 7-17). For a young, agitated child, the mask can be disconnected from the tubing, and the end of the tubing can be placed in a toy, such as a stuffed animal, and placed close to the child's face.

Oxygen Delivery

Oxygen is used for a patient needing ventilation or experiencing respiratory compromise and needing supplemental oxygen. Oxygen given is measured by liters per minute, and the flow is adjusted by a knob on the regulator of the oxygen tank. The level of oxygen given to the patient is determined by the patient's signs and symptoms and, if available, a pulse oximeter.

Pulse Oximetry

A **pulse oximeter** is a device that measures the percentage of oxygen being carried by hemoglobin in the blood, as well as measure the heart rate (Figure 7-18). The oxygen-saturation percentage should be above 95 percent. A pulse oximeter is usually placed on a patient's finger, but a toe is acceptable. If a young child cannot tolerate the pulse oximeter on his finger, use a toe and place a large stocking over the plastic sensor to hold it in place.

When reading the pulse oximeter, check the appearance of the patient in conjunction with the saturation percentage and heart rate. A patient with a 96 percent saturation could also have tachycardia and be using accessory muscles to breathe. In this case, oxygen is needed even though the pulse oximeter reading indicates adequate oxygenation. The pulse oximeter may give an inaccurate saturation percentage if the person's fingers or toes are cold or in cases of carbon monoxide exposure. If the fingers or toes are cold, warm the site and try again later for a more accurate reading. If your general impression and the symptoms of the patient indicate the use of oxygen, do not wait or rely on the readings of the pulse oximeter.

The oxygen saturation reading along with your assessment may be helpful in determining what oxygen-delivering device should be used, as well as the oxygen flow rate. A properly assembled oxygen tank along with a pocket mask, BVM, NC, or NRB mask is needed to deliver oxygen. Always follow your medical director's protocols when using oxygen. Remember that oxygen is considered a medication.

Oxygen Tanks

An **oxygen tank** is a storage vessel for oxygen, which is either held under pressure in gas cylinders or as liquid oxygen in a cryogenic storage tank. Oxygen tanks are identified by their green color, the national color designated by the United States Department of Transportation. Many agencies carry either liquid oxygen or compressed gas oxygen in various tank sizes. The D-size cylinder is the most common size and when full has approximately 300 to 350 liters of oxygen with 2,000 pounds of pressure. The largest size of oxygen tank the EMR may use is the M-size, which has approximately 3,450 liters of oxygen and approximately 2,000 pounds of pressure.

Oxygen tanks have a pin configuration that allows for placement of **oxygen regulators**, devices placed on oxygen tanks to control the flow of oxygen to the tubing. The stems of the tanks have pin holes that accept only the pins of an

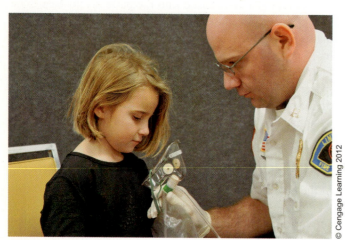

Figure 7-17 Blow-by oxygen provided to a young child.

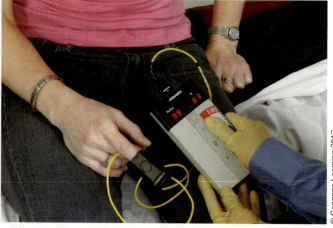

Figure 7-18 A pulse oximeter can be a valuable tool in assessing the patient but should never replace the Emergency Medical Responder's good judgment.

Table 7-2 Oxygen Tank Capacity

Use	Size	Capacity (L)	Factor	6 lpm	10 lpm	10 lpm
Portable	D	300–350	0.16	50 min	35 min	30 min
Portable	E	600	0.28	1.75 hr	1 hr 10 min	1 hr
Onboard	M	3.450	1.37	9.5 hr	7 hr	5.75 hr

lpm = liters per minute.
© Cengage Learning 2012

oxygen regulator. All regulators require a washer, or O-ring, to prevent oxygen leaks when the regulator and oxygen tank are joined together. New oxygen tanks come with a seal or O-ring attached.

To administer oxygen to a patient, the EMR must first assembly the oxygen regulator tank. The regulator is matched with the oxygen tank by comparison of their pins. Using a wrench, the EMR then quickly opens and closes the tank, often called "cracking the tank." After insertion of the plastic seal or O-ring to prevent leakage, the regulator and oxygen tank are put together and tightened. The tank can now be opened and the oxygen pressure within the tank noted. The EMR adjusts the liter flow by turning the knob in a counterclockwise motion until the correct liter flow appears. Complete oxygen tank assembly is illustrated in **Skill 7-6** at the end of the chapter.

Changing an Oxygen Tank

The EMR will need to monitor the amount of oxygen remaining in the oxygen tank and change the tank when the indicator needle on the gauge is in the shaded red area. Table 7-2 displays the liter volumes of each size of oxygen tank commonly used by EMRs. Each time you change an oxygen tank, you must also change the O-ring to ensure a good seal and prevent loss of oxygen. It is good practice to make sure there are additional O-rings and a wrench available. Table 7-2 displays the liter volumes of each size of oxygen tank commonly used by EMRs.

Oxygen Tank Safety

Oxygen tanks are pressurized and could become projectiles if improperly handled. Never carry an oxygen tank by the regulator or the stem. Never leave an oxygen tank standing upright while unsupervised. The tank should be placed on its side on the ground or floor in a position that protects the stem. Keep oil, grease, gas, adhesive tape, petroleum products, open flames, and cigarette smokers away from tanks. Giving oxygen to a patient creates a combustible atmosphere around the patient; thus, a spark or flame could easily cause fire.

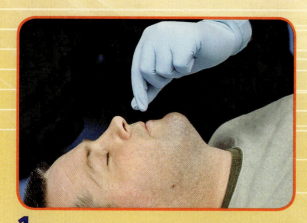

1 One EMR opens and assesses the airway using the technique appropriate to the patient's situation.

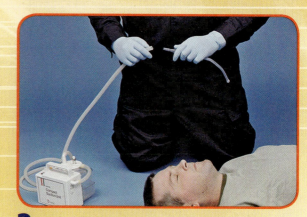

2 Another EMR removes the rigid suction tip from its protective covering, attaches the tip to the tubing, and then attaches the tubing to the intake of the suction machine. After the equipment is assembled, the EMR tests the machine's suction.

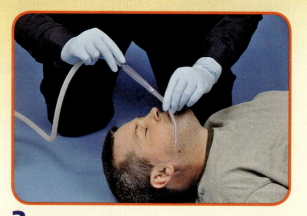

3 One EMR measures the length of the suction tip against the distance from the opening of the mouth to the angle of the jaw.

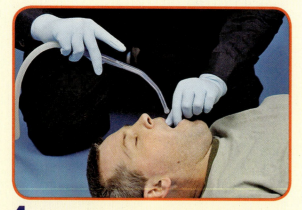

4 Open the patient's mouth with the nondominant hand. Placing the thumb on the lower teeth and the forefinger on the upper teeth or after tipping back the head, use your thumb on the mandible and open the mouth by pulling down the mandible.

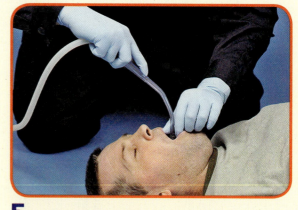

5 Insert the rigid suction tip to the depth of the measurement. Apply suction only as you withdraw the tip, usually by placing your thumb over a whistle port or releasing the kink of the suction tubing. Repeat suctioning as often as necessary but never for more than 15 seconds in an adult. It is important to oxygenate the patient between suction attempts.

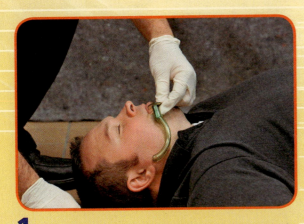

1 Choose an oral airway that fits the patient. The length of the airway should match the distance from the angle of the jaw to the opening of the mouth.

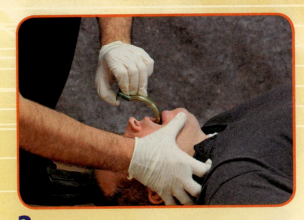

2 Open the patient's mouth and begin to insert the airway, curved portion downward, toward the jaw to about midway.

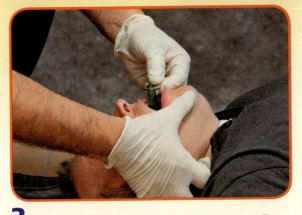

3 Rotate the airway 180 degrees so the airway naturally follows the curvature of the hard palate.

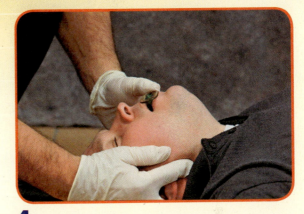

4 The airway is correctly placed when the flange of the airway rests on the patient's teeth.

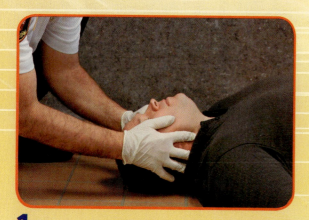

1 Examine the nostril opening to determine an approximate size of nasal airway that will be needed.

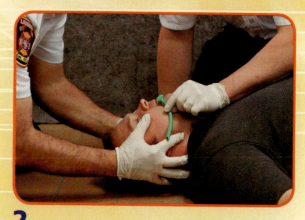

2 Compare the length of the nasal airway with the distance between the nostril and the tip of the earlobe.

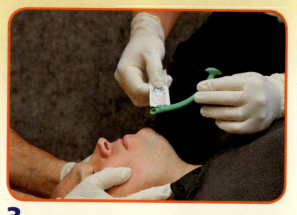

3 Apply a generous layer of water-soluble lubricant to the length of the nasal airway.

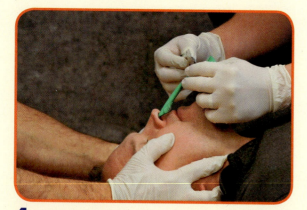

4 Gently introduce the nasal airway into the nostril using a gentle action, back and forth motion. The bevel of the airway should face inward toward the nasal septum.

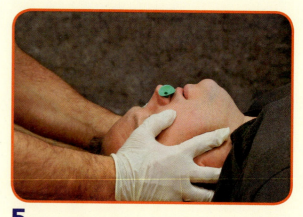

5 The airway is correctly placed when the flange of the NPA rests on the patient's nose.

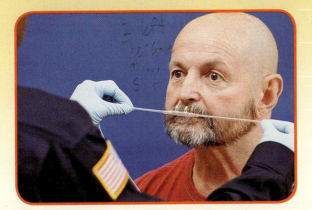

1 Choose the correct oxygen administration device. A nasal cannula is used when the patient cannot tolerate the NRB mask or when low concentrations of oxygen are required.

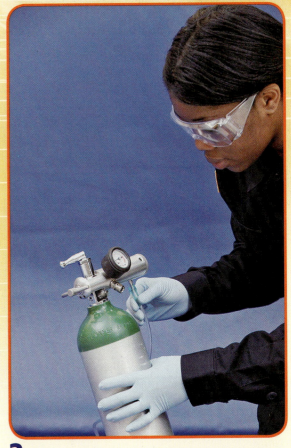

2 Ensure that the oxygen tank and regulator are correctly assembled. The oxygen tank should show sufficient pressure to provide continuous flow. Attach the oxygen tubing to the regulator and turn on the regulator. The regulator should be set from 1 to 6 lpm. A nasal cannula should never be used at a higher than 6 lpm flow rate.

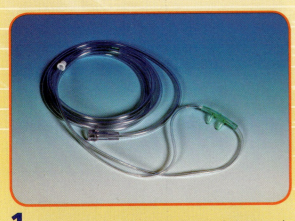

3 Gently introduce the nasal prongs into the nostrils so they appear to be lying on the floor of the nostrils and follow the natural curve of the nose. Some nasal cannulas have a molded tip that should point at the patient's lip.

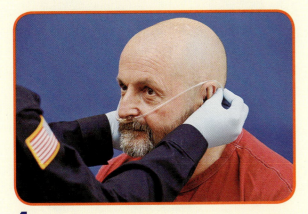

4 Drape the tubing over the ears with the tubing brought back to the front. The nasal cannula should not be draped over the head like a necklace because the danger of injury from strangulation is too great.

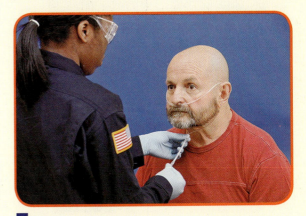

5 Cinch the tubing loosely under the chin with the ring or slider. Adjust the liter flow to ensure that the patient is receiving an adequate liter flow.

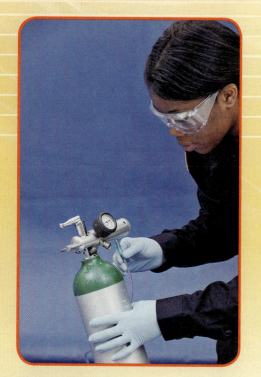

1 Ensure that the oxygen tank and regulator are correctly assembled. The oxygen tank should have sufficient pressure to provide continuous flow. To use the non-rebreather mask, attach the oxygen tubing to the regulator and turn on the regulator. As a rule, 10 to 15 lpm is sufficient. The regulator should never be turned below 6 lpm.

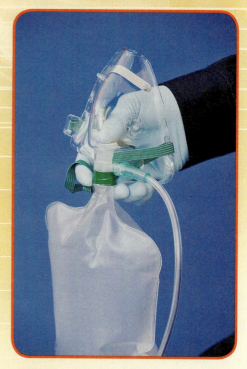

2 Place your thumb over the valve between the bag and the mask, permitting the bag to fill completely.

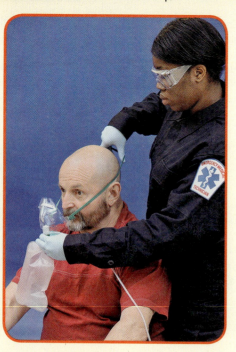

3 Grasping the mask in one hand and the elastic band in the other, seat the mask firmly on the bridge of the nose and drape the elastic band around the patient's head. Form the metal strip around the nose.

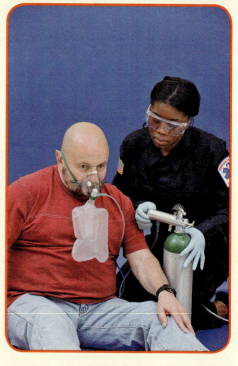

4 Adjust the liter flow to ensure that the oxygen bag is always filled to about one half.

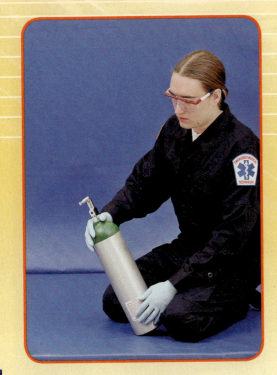

1 Confirm that the tank is an oxygen tank. By convention, all oxygen tanks are standardized with green paint.

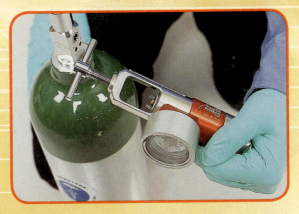

2 Compare the oxygen regulator's pins with the contacts on the oxygen bottle's stem. Again, by convention, oxygen regulators have a specific pin configuration that fits only oxygen bottles.

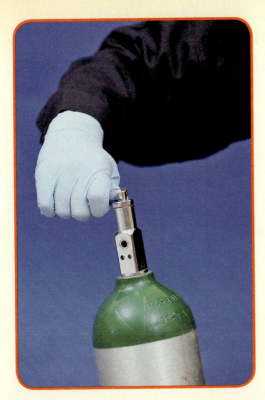

3 Using an oxygen wrench, mate the key to the latch and quickly open and close the oxygen tank. This procedure, called "cracking the tank," blows out any dirt and dust in the outlet.

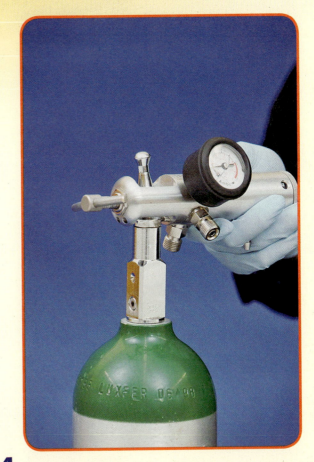

4 Mate the regulator to the oxygen tank, being sure to tightly seal the regulator. A plastic washer is always needed for an airtight seal.

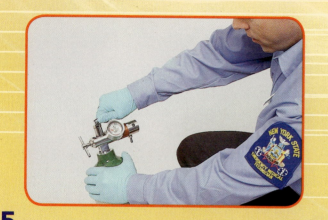

5 The oxygen tank may now be safely opened and the pressure within the tank noted.

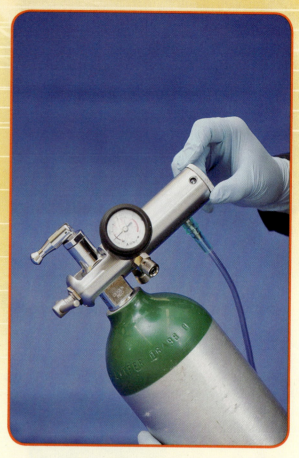

6 To adjust the liter flow rate, turn the knob in a counterclockwise motion until the correct liter flow appears.

SUMMARY

An EMR needs to effectively manage the patient's airway with positioning, suctioning, or airway devices. After the patient's airway is open, the EMR should focus on the patient's breathing. If the patient is not breathing or is getting inadequate oxygenation, the EMR needs to determine what oxygen delivery device to use, as well as the proper oxygen concentration. These basic and necessary skills must be mastered by the EMR to provide adequate oxygenation to the patient.

▶ REVIEW QUESTIONS

1. The air we breathe contains about _____ percent oxygen.

2. What percentage of oxygen is delivered with a pocket mask?

3. What size of oxygen cylinder is the most commonly size used by an EMR?

4. How many pounds of pressure per square inch does a full oxygen tank have?

5. When measuring the size of an oropharyngeal airway on a patient, the EMR measures from _____.

6. When attaching oxygen tubing to the BVM, the liter flow rate is at least _____.

7. When rescue breathing for an adult, the rate should be one breath every _____.

8. What airway would an EMR use when there is a gag reflex?

9. When a patient resumes adequate breathing on their own what position would you place them in if there is no spinal injury?

10. When would the EMR provide supplemental oxygen to a patient?

CHAPTER 8

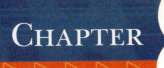

TRAUMA EMERGENCIES

LEARNING OBJECTIVES

By the end of this chapter, the reader should be able to

- Describe the principles of trauma assessment and management.
- Define shock and explain the assessment and management of a patient with shock.
- Define types of bleeding and explain methods for managing a patient with bleeding.
- Explain methods for treating a patient with burns.
- Describe methods for managing injuries to the skull, face, and neck.
- Describe different types of chest trauma.
- Explain assessment and management for different types of abdominal and pelvic cavity injuries.
- Explain assessment and management of patients with muscle injuries, joint injuries, and fractures.
- Define spinal cord injury and describe method for assessing a patient with a suspected spinal cord injury.

INTRODUCTION

Approximately 20 percent of Emergency Medical Responder (EMR) calls are for trauma. If a patient has experienced severe traumatic injury, an EMR must be able to quickly assess and care for the patient. The EMR in many cases will not be able to determine the severity of injury but will need to closely monitor for subtle changes in the patient's status. Trauma patients, particularly ones with more than one body system injured, must be treated aggressively and transported to a trauma center as soon as possible. This chapter will provide an overview of classifications, assessment tools, signs and symptoms, critical interventions, and management of various trauma emergencies.

Principles of Trauma Assessment and Management

An EMR should first perform all the components of an initial assessment, including PENMAN (see Chapter 5), spinal stabilization (if mechanism of injury [MOI] indicates), level of consciousness (LOC), and primary survey. Critical interventions are performed if indicated and include providing supplemental oxygen or ventilation, performing cardiopulmonary resuscitation (CPR), using an automated external defibrillator (AED), controlling major bleeding, and treating for shock. After performing critical interventions and the patient is stable the EMR will then obtain baseline vital signs and conduct a secondary survey or rapid survey, incorporating assessment tools when appropriate. Assessment tools assist in providing a more focused assessment. Using subjective information, objective information, and critical thinking skills, the EMR should then manage the patient and assist with preparing for transport if necessary.

Shock

Shock is a potentially life-threatening state in which the body experiences **hypoperfusion** (decreased blood flow through an organ), resulting in an insufficient supply of oxygen, glucose, and other nutrients to the body's cells, tissues, and organs. If left untreated, hypoperfusion may result in permanent damage to the cells and death. The body attempts to handle hypoperfusion by taking compensatory measures to prevent organ failure and death. This is done by sacrificing the perfusion of particular organs such as the skin to save others such as the vital organs (Figure 8-1). Blood flow to the brain is maintained at all costs because irreversible brain damage can result after four to six minutes of hypoperfusion to the brain cells.

Types of Shock

General classifications for causes of shock include inadequate blood or body fluids, an inability of the heart to pump adequately, and insufficient blood flow due to dilation of the blood vessels.

Hypovolemic Shock

Hypovolemic shock is a condition in which severe blood loss or a fluid deficit makes the heart unable to pump enough blood to the body. Fluid deficit can be the result of excessive vomiting, sweating, diarrhea, or inadequate intake of fluids. Hypoperfusion caused by a significant loss of blood is **hemorrhagic shock**, a specific type of hypovolemic shock.

Cardiogenic Shock

Another type of shock is **cardiogenic shock,** which results from inadequate cardiac pumping. The heart muscle fails to adequately perfuse the vital organs because of damage to the heart muscle. Cardiogenic shock is usually caused by heart damage from a severe heart attack.

Neurogenic Shock

Neurogenic shock is a hypoperfused state resulting from injury to the spinal cord. The injury results in the nerves' inability to constrict the blood vessels, and a generalized vasodilation (dilation of blood vessels) occurs. The vasodilation can cause a life threatening low blood pressure resulting in little or no oxygenated blood flow reaching vital organs.

Septic Shock

Septic shock is another hypoperfused state caused by a severe bacterial infection in the body. The toxins that the bacteria emit cause generalized dilation of the blood vessels.

Anaphylactic Shock

Anaphylactic shock (anaphylaxis) is an allergic reaction that causes a severe inflammatory response. This severe allergic reaction also results in blood vessel dilation.

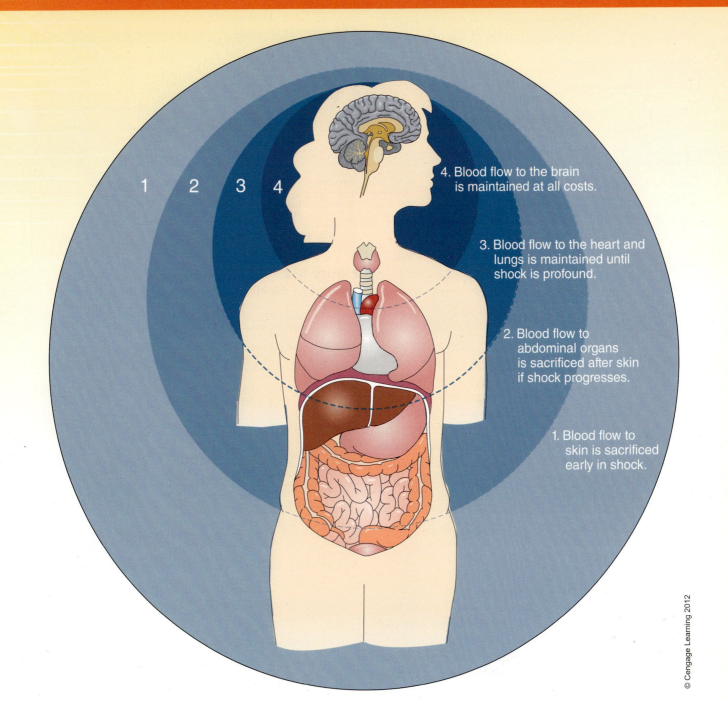

4. Blood flow to the brain is maintained at all costs.

3. Blood flow to the heart and lungs is maintained until shock is profound.

2. Blood flow to abdominal organs is sacrificed after skin if shock progresses.

1. Blood flow to skin is sacrificed early in shock.

© Cengage Learning 2012

Figure 8-1 When faced with hypoperfusion, the body sacrifices the perfusion of particular organs to maintain the blood supply to others.

Assessment Tools for Shock

After the initial assessment, providing critical interventions, and obtaining baseline vital signs use the assessment tool of SAMPLE to obtain subjective data from the patient, family, or friend. Ask the patient about

    S—Signs and Symptoms
    A—Allergies
    M—Current Medications
    P—Pertinent past medical history
    L—Last oral intake (food or fluids)
    E—Events leading up to the current situation

Signs and Symptoms of Shock

In the early stages of shock, the body tries to compensate for the loss of blood, insufficient blood flow, or deficit of body fluids. The EMR can look for the early warning signs of shock in the trauma victim such as confusion, agitation, anxiety, or restlessness. The vital signs can be used to ascertain whether the patient is having tachycardia or tachypnea. Other early signs of shock are cool, pale skin (except in spinal shock in which the skin will be warm and dry), nausea, thirst, or lightheadedness. Table 8-1 lists the signs and symptoms of compensated shock with the reasons for their presence.

Table 8-1 Signs and Symptoms of Compensated Shock

Sign or Symptom	Reason
Tachycardia	To maintain cardiac output
Tachypnea	To increase oxygenation
Cool, pale skin	Caused by shunting of blood to core of body away from the skin*
Nausea	Caused by shunting of blood to the core of the body away from the stomach and other abdominal organs
Thirst	Caused by the body's recognition of need for more fluid
Confusion, agitation	Caused by poor perfusion of the brain

*Patients with spinal shock will have warm and dry skin, an important distinction.

© Cengage Learning 2012

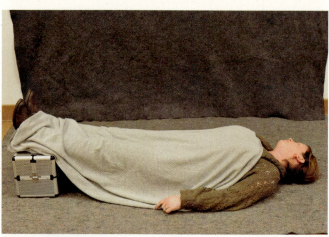

© Cengage Learning 2012

Figure 8-2 Treat for shock with the patient's legs elevated and blankets above and below the patient.

If the cause of shock in the victim is not treated or if the body is unable to continue compensating, the hypoperfusion will progress, and the shock will progress to a more critical state. The signs of shock at this stage will include dilated pupils, a drop in blood pressure, a thready or absent pulse, clammy skin, and skin color changes to a cyanotic or ashen appearance. Respirations will be shallow, rapid, labored, or absent. Deterioration of the patient's mental status will be obvious as the patient will exhibit signs of altered mental status (AMS). AMS is any significant change in the patient's awareness, behavior, emotions, cognition, or LOC.

Management of Shock

- Critical interventions: provide supplemental oxygen or ventilation, perform CPR and use an AED if indicated, control bleeding, treat for shock (see below), and seek rapid transport.
- Positioning is critical. Place the patient in the supine position to assist blood flow to the vital organs and brain. Raise the legs approximately 12 inches as long as there is no pain, evidence of fractures, head injury, or respiratory distress (Figure 8-2).
- If there is respiratory distress, elevate the upper body in a Fowler's position (Figure 8-3).
- Keep the patient from losing body heat by placing two blankets beneath the person and one on top.
- Reassess every five minutes.
- Look for medical identification jewelry regarding allergies or a heart condition.

Bleeding

The average adult has five to six liters of blood volume. If a major artery is severed, a person can bleed to death within minutes. Bleeding can be external or internal. External bleeding can be observed from body cavities or from breaks in the skin.

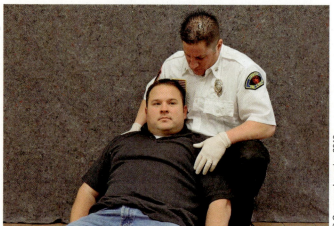

© Cengage Learning 2012

Figure 8-3 Fowler's position can be used to treat for shock with respiratory difficulty

Internal bleeding is not visible unless it is close to the surface in the form of a bruise. An EMR should look for symptoms of lightheadedness; AMS; skin pallor; pain upon palpitation; and changes in vital signs, including tachycardia, tachypnea, and hypotension. Loss of a significant amount of blood will result in further symptoms of uncompensated shock.

Three Types of Bleeds

The amount of blood loss depends on how much skin is damaged and how much force is behind the bleeding. There are three types of vessels that may be involved in bleeding. They are arteries, veins, and capillaries. Figure 8-4 demonstrates the different forms of bleeding.

In an arterial bleed, the arteries spurt a large amount of blood because they are under the greatest amount of pressure from the heart. Spurting correlates with each heart beat. Bleeding from an artery is the most serious form of bleeding.

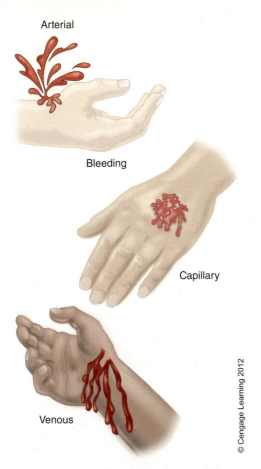

Figure 8-4 Arterial bleeding spurts, capillary bleeding oozes, and venous bleeding flows.

Veins return blood from the heart and have less pressure. Bleeding from a vein is usually steady and flows out of the wound. Unless the bleeding is coming from a deep vein, it is usually easier to control bleeding from a vein than bleeding from an artery.

Capillaries are small in diameter and have little pressure, so the blood flow from capillary bleeding appears to be slow and oozing. Capillary bleeding is usually not serious.

Assessment Tools for Bleeding

After performing the initial assessment, providing critical interventions, and obtaining baseline vital signs, the EMR should use the assessment tools of SAMPLE and a detailed pain assessment using OPQRST (see Chapter 5) to obtain subjective information from the patient. Have the patient rate their pain using faces or numbers of 1 to 10 with 1 being the least pain and 10 being the most severe pain. If unable to rate their pain take note of pain behaviors.

External Bleeding

A superficial open wound called an **abrasion** occurs when the uppermost layer of skin is scraped away and minor capillary bleeding occurs (Figure 8-5). This scraping away of the upper layer of tissue is the result of the skin on the body being rubbed on a rough, solid surface, such as in sliding

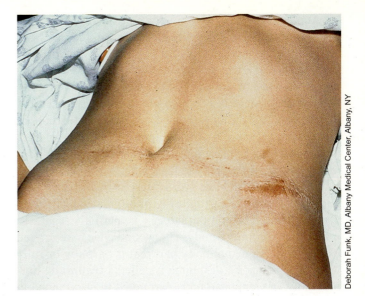

Figure 8-5 An abrasion usually oozes capillary blood.

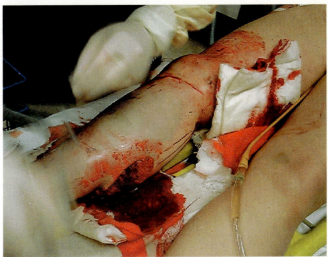

Figure 8-6 A laceration is a rip or tear in the skin.

across the asphalt during a motorcycle crash. Any time the body is in motion and rubs across a hard surface, an abrasion will likely occur.

An open wound described as a **laceration** occurs when a large amount of force is applied to the skin surface. The force can cause a full-thickness tear in the skin involving all the skin layers and veins and arteries (Figure 8-6). Typically, the edge of the laceration will be jagged or even stellate (star-like) (Figure 8-7), but if the victim was struck by a straight object, the wound edge may be straight.

An **incision** is another full-thickness open wound to the skin that can also involve veins and arteries. An incision is different from a laceration in that it has only straight edges usually made by a sharp object such as a knife or razor blade. Incisions can be life threatening because of the potential bleeding from veins and arteries under the skin (Figure 8-8).

Another type of open wound is a penetrating or **puncture wound**, a hole in the body caused by an object, such as a nail, bullet, or snake fangs. Some puncture wounds have exit wounds that are larger than the entrance wound. One example is a gunshot wound (GSW), as shown in Figure 8-9. An **impaled object** is a foreign object that has punctured the body and lodged in place and can be seen sticking out of the wound (Figure 8-10). An impaled object should not be removed from the face unless the object causes an airway obstruction and interferes with breathing.

An **avulsion** is a wound or flap of body tissue created by a forceful tearing away or separation of tissue from the body. The body tissue may be partially separated or fully torn from the body. The wound edges are ragged or shredded. An actual body part that is partially or fully pulled away because of trauma is called a **traumatic amputation**. An amputated body part needs to be wrapped in moist gauze, placed in a sealed plastic bag, and placed in a container with ice, as shown in Figure 8-11. Never place the part directly on ice.

Another type of avulsion occurs when the skin is forcefully separated or torn away from an extremity. This wound is called a **degloving avulsion** (Figure 8-12). A degloving avulsion can occur when a person gets trapped in a piece of machinery. Often the machinery will tear the skin off an arm or a leg.

Management of External Bleed

- Critical interventions: controlling major bleeding is paramount. If a major bleed is evident and there is more than one EMR available, one EMR should assess and intervene with the airway, breathing, and CPR using an AED if indicated while the other EMR controls the external bleeding. In addition to managing ABC's, the EMR will treat for shock, and seek rapid transport.
- Reassess every five minutes.

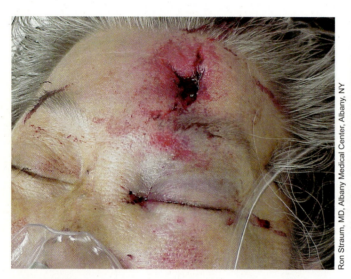

Figure 8-7 Blunt trauma can result in a stellate laceration.

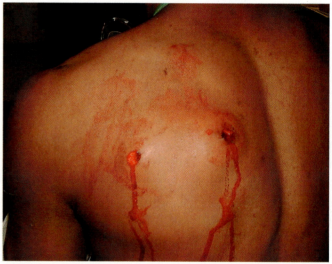

Figure 8-9 A gunshot wound is a puncture wound with an exit wound usually larger than the entrance wound.

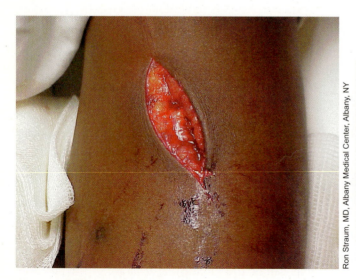

Figure 8-8 An incision made by a sharp object.

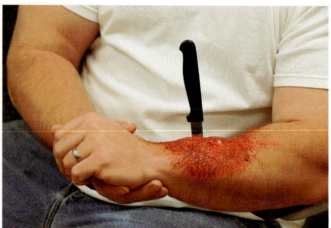

Figure 8-10 Impaled object in the arm.

Controlling an External Bleed

- Using a gauze or cloth, apply direct, firm, constant pressure to the site with gloved hands (Figure 8-13). Elevating the wound above the level of the victim's heart may help stop the bleeding.
- If bleeding continues through the gauze, apply an additional dressing directly on top of the first dressing and continue direct pressure. Do not take off the initial dressing because clotting could be disrupted. Apply a pressure bandage to secure the dressing and prevent further bleeding. (Figure 8-14).
- If the bleeding is life threatening and cannot be controlled by direct pressure, a tourniquet must be used. The EMR can use a commercial tourniquet as shown in Figure 8-15

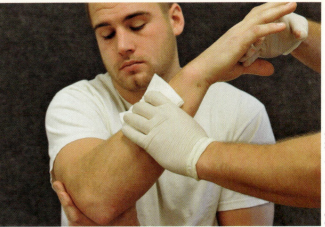

Figure 8-13 Apply direct, firm pressure to the site and elevate it to control bleeding.

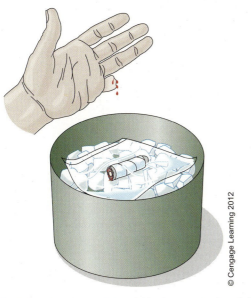

Figure 8-11 An amputated body part should be wrapped in moist gauze, placed in a plastic bag, and then placed on an ice pack.

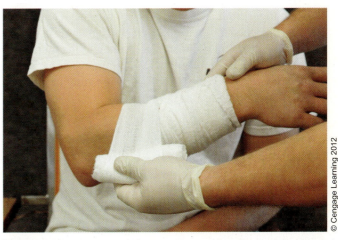

Figure 8-14 A pressure dressing can be applied after bleeding is controlled.

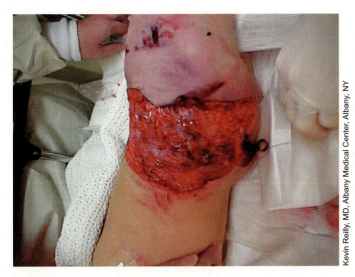

Figure 8-12 A degloving injury is seen most commonly around machinery.

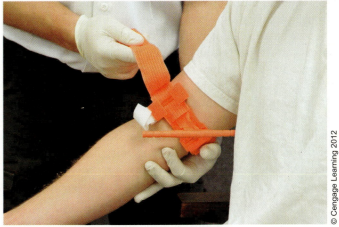

Figure 8-15 A tourniquet is used to stop life-threatening bleeding, such as that from an artery, when standard bleeding control methods are not effective.

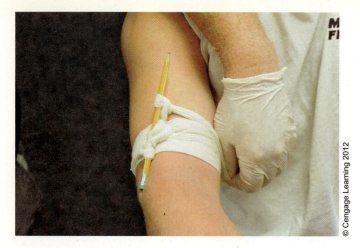

Figure 8-16 A tourniquet made from a cravat.

or one made from a cravat as shown in Figure 8-16. Applying a tourniquet stops the flow of circulation and oxygenation to the limb; however, studies show that a tourniquet can be applied for up to six hours without tissue or neurological damage. Document the location of the tourniquet and the time of application. Do not remove a tourniquet after it has been applied. Application of tourniquets will be discussed further in Chapter 9.

Internal Bleeding

A **contusion** or **ecchymosis** is a bruise that occurs when damage to tissue causes a slow bleed and blood pools under the skin (Figure 8-17). The bruise may not be visible for up to an hour after the point of impact. Bleeding from a blunt-force injury may produce a large, irregularly shaped area of blood under skin that is larger than the margin of the point of contact. Bruised areas, initially red, have a bluish tint after red blood cells break down. Sometimes a hematoma is formed when bleeding forms a pool of blood under the skin.

Internal bleeding can be deep, not visible and happen from an organ or cavity from vessels bleeding. Trauma causes include an impaled object, tear, rupture or a crushing injury. A crushing injury occurs when a body part is subjected to a great amount of force or pressure. Some or all of the following signs and symptoms of shock can be present upon assessment. The victim may have a weak, rapid pulse and a decreased blood pressure. The skin may be cool, moist, or pale. There may be swelling, tenderness, and pain at the site of the injury along with muscle rigidity. Lightheadedness and AMS may exist.

Management of Internal Bleeding

- Critical interventions: provide supplemental oxygen or ventilation, perform CPR and use an AED if indicated, treat for shock, and seek rapid transport
- Reassess the patient every five minutes.
- Assist with packaging for transport.

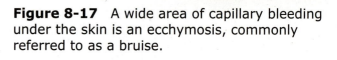

Figure 8-17 A wide area of capillary bleeding under the skin is an ecchymosis, commonly referred to as a bruise.

Burns

Burns harm the skin, destroy tissue under the skin, allow the entry of pathogens, cause loss of body fluids, and have an effect on body temperature. The severity depends on the depth, size, location, and source of the burn. An EMR can quickly estimate the body surface area that is burned in an adult by using the rule-of-nine formula. The adult body surface is divided into sections of 9 percent or multiples of 9 percent, with the genitals being assigned 1 percent. For example, if a patient is burned on his back and right anterior leg, the estimate percentage of body surface area burned that you would document would be 27 percent.

Children and infants have different body proportions, so the rule-of-nine formula is not used for them. See Figure 8-18 for a representation of the percentage of area burned for all ages.

Burn Classifications

There are three classifications of burns. A burn classification is determined by the depth of the burn to the skin tissue. A skin area that is burned may involve more than one classification of burn.

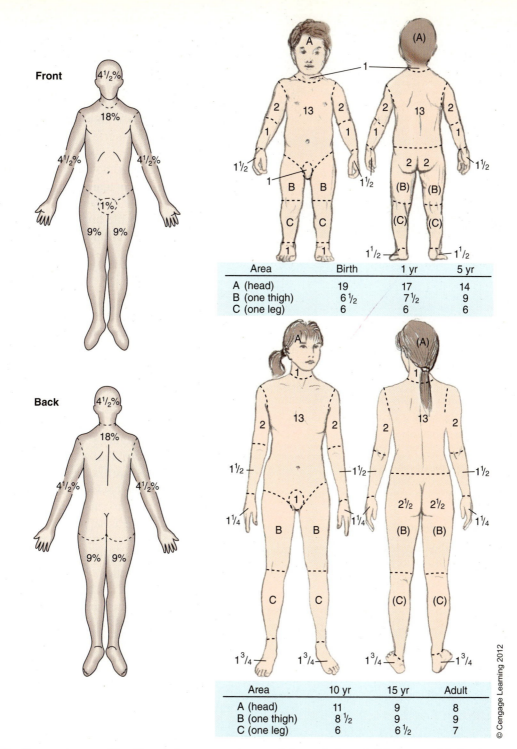

Area	Birth	1 yr	5 yr
A (head)	19	17	14
B (one thigh)	6 1/2	7 1/2	9
C (one leg)	6	6	6

Area	10 yr	15 yr	Adult
A (head)	11	9	8
B (one thigh)	8 1/2	9	9
C (one leg)	6	6 1/2	7

© Cengage Learning 2012

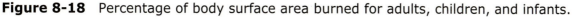

Figure 8-18 Percentage of body surface area burned for adults, children, and infants.

Superficial burns involve the topmost layer of skin or epidermis. The skin is reddened and painful. A mild sunburn is a common superficial burn.

Partial-thickness burns involve the epidermis and dermis layers of the skin. In addition to the skin appearing red, there will be blisters and swelling on the skin surface because of damage to vessels. A partial-thickness burn that covers 10 percent or more of the body is considered to be critical.

Full-thickness burns, the most serious burn, involves all of the layers of skin. Nerve endings, muscle, and fat can be involved and damaged so much that the skin surface becomes hard and inelastic and appears black. The patient will have little or no pain. See Figure 8-19 for a full-thickness burn.

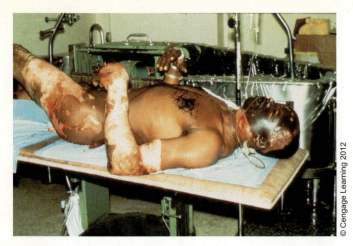
© Cengage Learning 2012

Figure 8-19 Full-thickness burns are frequently painless.

Assessment Tools for Burns

After performing the initial assessment, providing critical interventions, and obtaining baseline vital signs, the EMR should use the assessment tools of SAMPLE and OPQRST to obtain subjective information from the patient. Have the patient rate her pain using the pain scale of faces or numbers from 1 to 10 or noting pain behaviors.

General Burn Management

- Remove the victim from the burning source if the scene is safe.
- Critical interventions if indicated: provide supplemental oxygen or ventilation, perform CPR and use an AED, control major bleeding, treat for shock, and seek rapid transport.
- Loosely cover the burned area with a sterile (nonstick) dressing and secure with a bandage. For a large body area, cover with a sterile burn sheet or a clean bed sheet.
- Reassess the patient every five minutes.
- Assist with packaging.

Sources of Burns

Sources of burns are thermal, chemical, electrical, and radiation. The EMR needs to consider additional management with the different sources of burns.

Management of Thermal Burns

Thermal burns are caused by a heat source. The heat source can be fire, steam, hot objects, or hot water.

- If the victim is on fire, instruct the victim to stop, drop, and roll. If it can be done safely, wrap the patient in a blanket or an article of clothing to extinguish the fire.
- Cut away loose, burnt clothing. Do not pull clothing off the victim. If stuck to the skin, cut around it.

- Observe for inhalation burns by frequent reassessment of the airway.
- Most thermal burns can be treated by flushing the burned area with cold water. Flushing with cold water or placing cold packs (not ice) on the burn will relieve the swelling and pain. Do not, however, use this treatment method on an open wound or if more than 10 percent of body surface area is burned to prevent hypothermia.
- To prevent infection, do not break blisters caused by thermal burns. Do not apply ointments or lotions.
- Apply a dry, sterile dressing. If available, place non-stick dressings on the burn. Place dressing between each digit of involved fingers or toes. If possible, remove jewelry.

Management of Chemical Burns

Chemical burns are caused by acids, alkalis, and other wet or dry chemicals. Chemical burns can cause serious surface damage to skin. Identification of the chemical involved and chemical decontamination must be done before medical care is provided.

- Read the Material Safety Data Sheet (MSDS) for details on proper management of a specific chemical exposure. See the MSDS in Figure 8-20.
- The Department of Transportation free publication, *Emergency Response Guidebook (ERG)*, provides instructions regarding how to handle a chemical spill and provide appropriate first aid (Figure 8-21).
- If a victim's clothing is saturated with dry or wet chemicals, immediately remove the clothing while wearing proper personal protective equipment, including gloves, mask, and eye protection. Remember, dry chemicals can become airborne.
- Flush the contaminated area with clean or sterile water for 20 to 30 minutes.
- For dry chemicals, such as lime, brush off the powder first (Figure 8-22). Then flush the area with water for 20 to 30 minutes or as indicated by the MSDS sheet. Be aware that some dry chemicals should *not* be mixed with water and must be neutralized with some other agent.
- When flushing a chemical from an eye, remove contacts if possible, tilt the patient's head so the involved eye is lower than the other eye to avoid flushing the chemical into the unaffected eye (Figure 8-23).
- Apply a sterile dressing to areas burned by the chemical.

Management of Electrical Burns

Electrical burns are caused by an electrical current and usually have an entrance and exit point. An electrical current can severely injure or kill whether the source is a high-powered voltage or household electricity. As an electrical current

Material Safety Data Sheet

Version 1.7
Revision Date 05/16/2004

MSDS Number 300000000110
Print Date 07/28/2004

1. PRODUCT AND COMPANY IDENTIFICATION

Product name	:	Oxygen
Chemical formula	:	O2
Synonyms	:	Oxygen, Oxygen gas, Gaseous Oxygen, GOX
Product Use Description	:	General Industrial
Company	:	Air Products and Chemicals,Inc 7201 Hamilton Blvd. Allentown, PA 18195-1501
Telephone	:	800-345-3148
Emergency telephone number	:	800-523-9374 USA 01-610-481-7711 International

2. COMPOSITION/INFORMATION ON INGREDIENTS

Components	CAS Number	Concentration (Volume)
Oxygen	7782-44-7	100 %

Concentration is nominal. For the exact product composition, please refer to Air Products technical specifications.

3. HAZARDS IDENTIFICATION

Emergency Overview

High pressure, oxidizing gas.
Vigorously accelerates combustion.
Keep oil, grease, and combustibles away.
May react violently with combustible materials.

Potential Health Effects

Inhalation	:	Breathing 75% or more oxygen at atmospheric pressure for more than a few hours may cause nasal stuffiness, cough, sore throat, chest pain and breathing difficulty. Breathing pure oxygen under pressure may cause lung damage and also central nervous system effects.
Eye contact	:	No adverse effect.
Skin contact	:	No adverse effect.
Ingestion	:	Ingestion is not considered a potential route of exposure.

Exposure Guidelines

Air Products and Chemicals,Inc

Oxygen

Air Products and Chemicals, Inc.

Figure 8-20 The Material Safety Data Sheet contains a great deal of information important to Emergency Medical Responders.

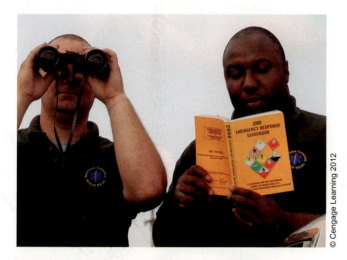

© Cengage Learning 2012

Figure 8-21 The *Emergency Response Guidebook* provides Emergency Medical Responders with initial instructions at a hazardous materials incident.

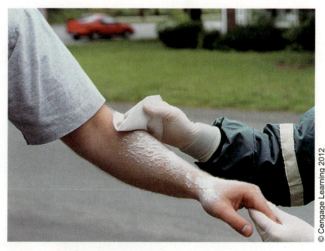

© Cengage Learning 2012

Figure 8-22 Dry chemicals should be brushed off first. Then large volumes of water should be used to rinse the residue off the patient.

passes through the body, it can burn and damage internal nerves, vessels, and tissues (Figure 8-24).

- Make certain the scene is safe.
- Make sure the power source is turned off. Do not touch the patient if they are in contact with the power source.
- If a downed line is involved, contact the local utility company to turn off the power. To avoid an injury, maintain a safe distance of at least eight feet from a downed power line.

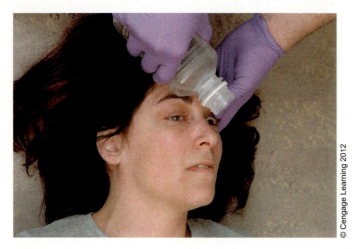

Figure 8-23 Flush the chemical from the eye with clean or sterile water.

- Have an AED ready for possible cardiac arrest.
- Assess for entrance and exit wounds on the victim.
- Apply a sterile dressing to wounds.

Management of Radiation Burns

Exposure to radioactive materials can result in radiation burns. Radioactive exposure can occur when a victim is involved in a vehicular crash in which one vehicle is carrying radioactive materials. Radioactive exposure can also occur during an accident at a nuclear power plant.

- Do not enter an area contaminated with radiation; wait for the specialized radiation team to secure the scene.
- Assess and manage the patient following the general burn management guidelines above after the patient has been decontaminated.

Rapid Transport for Burn Patients

Burns to the face and neck are considered life threatening because of their proximity to the airway and the potential for swelling and damage to the respiratory system. Observe for breathing difficultly, singed nasal hair, facial hair burns, and burns around the mouth. Rapid transport is advised for full-thickness burns. Rapid transport is also advised for partial-thickness burns if the involvement is more than 10 percent of the body surface area or if major joints, the hands, the feet, or the genitals are involved.

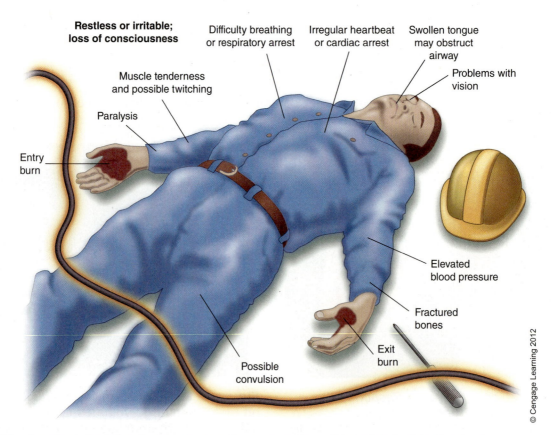

Figure 8-24 An electrical shock can cause a large number of injuries inside the body.

Injuries to the Skull, Face, and Neck

Injuries to the skull, face, and neck are common in crashes involving a motor vehicle, a bicycle, an all-terrain vehicle, a snowmobile, a motorcycle, or personal water craft. Injuries to the skull, face, or neck can lead to airway, breathing, and circulation issues for the patient. Additionally, if the MOI indicates, the cervical spine must be stabilized.

Skull Fracture

Blunt trauma can cause an open, or closed, fracture to the skull. In a **closed fracture,** the ends of the broken bone do not break the skin but depress the bones downward. A penetrating injury to the skull, such as a bullet or knife wound, can result in an **open fracture,** in which a bone end at any point has erupted the skin. Both types of fractures can cause brain injury. Radiography (X-ray) or computed tomography (CT scan) is the only way to determine the extent of a skull fracture injury.

Bruising or discoloration may indicate a skull fracture. Bruising behind the ears is called **Battle's sign,** and bruising around the eyes is called **raccoon eyes** (Figure 8-25). Both are indications of a skull injury.

Traumatic Brain Injury

A **traumatic brain injury (TBI)** is an injury to the brain from a direct cause (penetrating trauma), an indirect cause (blow to the skull, shaken baby syndrome), or a secondary cause (hypoxia). An indirect cause can be localized to the area hit or it can be a **contrecoup injury**. A coutrecoup injury occurs when the head is struck on one side and the brain strikes the opposite side of the skull. In this injury the CSF surrounding the brain is displaced so there is little or no cushioning for the brain when it hits the opposite side of the skull. The skull that encloses the brain is rigid and allows no room for excess fluid from bleeding or space for swelling. Therefore, bleeding and swelling in the brain cause increased **intracranial pressure (ICP)** on the brain that may cause brain damage. Increased ICP may cause the cerebrospinal fluid (CSF) to come out of an ear, the nose, or both to relieve pressure on the brain. CSF is usually clear fluid but may be tinged pink because of bleeding in the skull. An EMR can assume that change in LOC may indicate a brain injury and should look for physical findings that would suggest injury to the skull and brain (Figure 8-26).

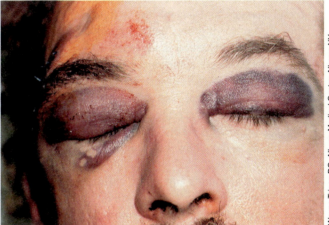

Figure 8-25 Raccoon eyes.

Wayne Triner, DO, Albany Medical Center, Albany, NY

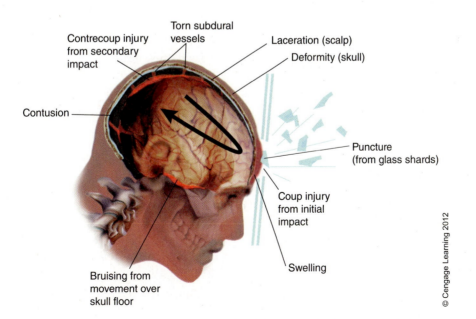

Figure 8-26 The Emergency Medical Responder should look for physical findings that indicate injury to the skull and brain.

© Cengage Learning 2012

Types and Symptoms of Traumatic Brain Injury

Concussions, contusions, and intracranial hematomas are three types of TBIs. The onset of symptoms can progress slowly or rapidly and the EMR will not know the full extent of the injury immediately. TBI symptoms can range from mild to severe depending on the location and extent of the bleeding. Categories of symptoms are described below:

- Mild brain injury symptoms include the following. Confusion or loss of consciousness for a few minutes or longer. The patient may exhibit irritability, restlessness, or combativeness and may resist medical treatment. A person with mild symptoms may not be able to recall the event or the time just before or after the event and may repeatedly ask what happened. Headache, nausea, and vomiting may follow. Subtle symptoms may continue hours later manifesting as fatigue, sleep disturbances, mood changes, and sensitivities to light and sound. Even though these symptoms usually resolve in 48 hours or less, medical evaluation is advised.
- Moderate to severe symptoms of a brain injury may include: Loss of consciousness, loss of memory, unequal pupils, visual changes, vomiting, changes in vital signs, profound personality changes, paralysis, incoordination, decreasing mental status, and visible CSF. Symptoms last hours to days however severe injuries can lead to disability or death.
- Symptoms of infants and young children unable to verbalize may include: irritability with difficulty to console, lack of interest in favorite toys or activities, change in sleep, change in nursing or eating habits, sad mood, and persistent crying.

Concussion

A **concussion** is a closed head injury caused by blunt force when the head hits an object or an object hits the head. The injury is not localized but disrupts the functioning of brain cell signals. Mild brain injury symptoms are present and are usually temporary. Symptoms depend on the location of disrupted signals.

Contusion

Blunt trauma can cause a **contusion** in the brain, causing the brain to bruise and swell. Symptoms of a contusion may be moderate to severe depending on the extent of injury and location of the involvement. A contusion can lead to disability or death depending on the amount of swelling.

Intracranial Hematoma

An intracranial hematoma occurs when a blood vessel ruptures and a collection of blood (hematoma) is trapped between the skull and brain. A **subdural hematoma** is a collection of blood within the subdural space of the skull that is caused by the tearing of small veins that run between the brain surface

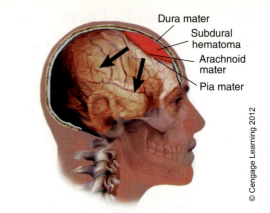

Figure 8-27 A subdural hematoma is usually the result of the tearing of small veins under the dura mater.

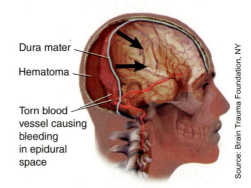

Figure 8-28 An epidural hematoma is often associated with a skull fracture and an arterial injury.

and the dura mater (Figure 8-27). An **epidural hematoma** is the collection of blood found outside of the dura mater just under the skull. The bleeding is usually caused by an injured artery, which results in bleeding and symptoms to progress more rapidly. The ICP from hematomas can damage brain cells and cause death or disability. Figure 8-28 illustrates this type of injury.

Assessment Tools for a Skull Fracture and Traumatic Brain Injury

After performing the initial assessment, providing critical interventions, and obtaining baseline vital signs use the assessment tools of DOTS, TIC, PERRL, (see Chapter 5), SAMPLE, and the Glasgow Coma Scale. If the patient is a child, use the Pediatric Glasgow Coma Scale. Obtain a detailed pain assessment using OPQRST if possible.

Glasgow Coma Scale and Pediatric Glasgow Coma Scale

The **Glasgow Coma Scale (GCS)** and **Pediatric Glasgow Coma Scale (PGCS)** are tools used to determine the extent of and urgency for transporting a patient with a TBI. The GCS is used to quantify a neurologically impaired adult patient's

Table 8-2 Glasgow Coma Scale Score

	Infants Younger Than Age 1 Year	Age 1 to 4 Years	Age 4 Years to Adult
EYES			
4	Open	Open	Open
3	To voice	To voice	To voice
2	To pain	To pain	To pain
1	No response	No response	No response
VERBAL			
5	Coos, babbles	Oriented, speaks, interacts, social	Oriented and alert
4	Irritable cry, consolable	Confused speech, disoriented, consolable	Disoriented
3	Cries persistently to pain	Inappropriate words, inconsolable	Nonsensical speech
2	Moans to pain	Incomprehensible, agitated	Moans, unintelligible
1	No response	No response	No response
MOTOR			
6	Normal spontaneous movement	Normal spontaneous movements	Follows commands
5	Withdraws to touch	Localizes pain	Localizes pain
4	Withdraws to pain	Withdraws to pain	Withdraws to pain
3	Decorticate flexion	Decorticate flexion	Decorticate flexion
2	Decerebrate extension	Decerebrate extension	Decerebrate extension
1	No response	No response	No response

Source: Brain Trauma Foundation, NY

level of responsiveness to stimuli. See Table 8-2 for the GCS and PGCS. The patient's reactions are recorded as numerical values in three categories: eye opening, verbal responsiveness, and motor responsiveness. The sum of the three scores is the total score. For an adult, a score of 13 to 15 indicates a mild TBI, 9 to 12 is a moderate TBI, and below 8 indicates a severe TBI. The total score on the PGCS ranges from lowest–3 (deep coma or death) to highest–15 (fully awake and aware).

The GCS and PGCS address abnormal positioning or posturing of the body, called decorticate or decerebrate posturing, that occurs with severe TBIs. In **decorticate posturing**, the patient's arms, elbows, wrists, and fingers are rigidly flexed over the chest on one or both sides of the body, and the legs are extended (Figure 8-29). Decorticate posturing may progress to decerebrate posturing if the TBI worsens. In **decerebrate posturing**, the head and neck are arched backward, and one or both arms or legs are rigid and extend and rotate internally (Figure 8-30).

Management of a Skull Fracture and Traumatic Brain Injury

- Spinal stabilization.
- Critical interventions: provide supplemental oxygen or ventilation, provide CPR using an AED if indicated, control major bleeding, and treat for shock.
- Reassess every five minutes. Include specific checks for swelling or bleeding inside the brain by checking for AMS, GCS, vital signs, behavior, seizure activity, movement, vision, eye tracking, and PERRL.
- If you notice CSF from the ears or nose, cover the area with a sterile dressing. Do not attempt to stop the flow of CSF.
- Do not remove an impaled object.
- If seizure activity occurs, protect the patient from harm.
- If perfusion is adequate, elevate the head and shoulders to no more than 30 degrees to decrease pressure in the

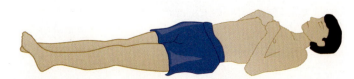

Figure 8-29 Decorticate or flexion posturing.
© Cengage Learning 2012

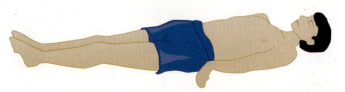

Figure 8-30 Decerebrate or extension posturing.
© Cengage Learning 2012

brain. If there is a potential spinal injury the backboard can be slightly inclined.

- Immediately seek transport to a trauma center for moderate to severe brain injury symptoms or if the adult patient has a systolic blood pressure reading below 90 mm Hg, a pulse oximeter reading below 90, and a GCS of 9 or lower.

Facial Injuries

The face is very vascular and bleeds profusely when injured. In most instances, the bleeding is not life threatening. Do not forget the big picture because facial bleeding can distract from other more critical issues.

Assessment Tools for Facial Injuries

After performing initial assessment, providing critical interventions, and obtaining baseline vital signs use the assessment tools of TIC, DOTS, SAMPLE, and OPQRST.

Management of Facial Fractures

Facial fractures can cause anatomical obstruction of the airway or swelling of the airway.

- Look in the mouth for broken teeth or dentures.
- Assess and manage airway and breathing. Facial fractures can cause anatomical obstruction or swelling of the airway.
- If you find an avulsed tooth, handle it by the crown, not the root. Keep the tooth moist in a gauze dressing (or in a cup of milk or clean water) and transport it with the patient.
- Do not insert a nasal airway into a patient with obvious facial injuries (Figure 8-31).

Management of a Nosebleed

A nosebleed or **epistaxis** can be controlled by the patient. Most nose bleeds should stop within minutes (Figure 8-32). If bleeding cannot be controlled, seek rapid transport.

- The patient should sit, leaning forward (assuming the MOI does not indicate a spinal injury). If supine roll the patient on their side using spinal stabilization to make sure bleeding does not cause aspiration into the lungs.
- Instruct the patient to pinch the soft part of the nostrils, keeping pressure applied for approximately 5 to 10 minutes.
- Apply a cold pack to the bridge of the nose to slow down the bleed.

Management of an Ear Injury

Ear injuries may consist of an avulsion, laceration, or an object in the ear.

- Keep avulsed parts moist and wrapped.
- If an object is in the ear, do not remove the object.
- Control bleeding. Dress and bandage any wounds, stabilize an impaled object.

Management of an Eye Injury

Eye injuries may be caused by a wound to the eye or a foreign object in the eye.

- Apply a light dressing or patch to both eyes, avoiding any pressure to the eyeball, to prevent further injury. Covering both eyes prevents excessive movement of the injured eye.
- If there is an impaled object in the eye, carefully stabilize the object (see Chapter 9), cover both eyes, and place the patient in the supine position with the upper body slightly elevated.
- A chemical in the eye should be flushed out with an appropriate solution indicated by MSDS for a minimum of 20 minutes. Remove contact lenses from the patient's eyes and position the patient with the head turned to the side so the involved eye is lower. This allows the irrigation fluid to run from the inside corner of the involved eye to the outside corner without touching the other eye.

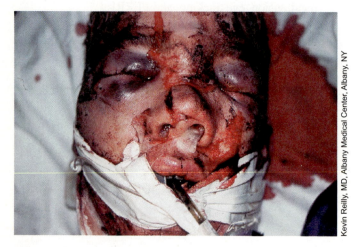

Figure 8-31 The presence of significant facial injuries is a contraindication to using a nasopharyngeal airway.

Kevin Reilly, MD, Albany Medical Center, Albany, NY

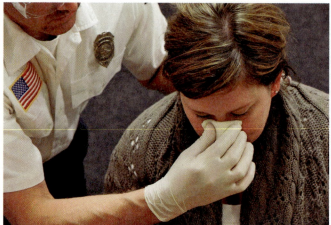

Figure 8-32 Controlling a nose bleed.

© Cengage Learning 2012

Neck Injuries

- Stabilize the spine for a potential neck injury.
- Be alert for and manage airway and breathing problems.
- If the large vessels of the neck, the jugular veins or carotid arteries, are severed, severe bleeding will result. Use direct pressure and when bleeding is controlled use a dressing and bandage without encircling the neck. Stabilize any impaled objects.

Chest Trauma

The chest or thoracic cavity contains several vital organs that affect breathing, oxygenation, and circulation. Some injuries to this area can be life threatening.

Assessment Tools for Chest Trauma

After performing an initial assessment, providing critical interventions and baseline vital signs, obtain information using the assessment tools of DOTS, TIC, SAMPLE, and OPQRST.

Rib Fractures

Rib fractures can be very painful but are not usually life threatening, unless the bone punctures an organ. A flail segment involves two or more adjacent ribs that are broken in two or more places. This produces a free-floating chest wall segment called a **flail chest** that may cause paradoxical movement, independent motion of the left and right sides of the chest (Figure 8-33). Pain resulting from the paradoxical motion causes the injured person to increase the respiratory rate but take more shallow respirations, thus decreasing air volume in the lungs. A rib fracture can also impale the underlying organs such as the lungs.

Signs and Symptoms of Rib Fractures

- Localized pain and tenderness near the fracture site
- Shallow breathing
- Pain increases when patient coughs, moves, laughs, or breathes deeply (Figure 8-34)
- Pain on palpation
- Guarding of the area
- Asymmetrical chest expansion
- Crepitus (the sound of bone ends grinding against one another)
- Deformity or discoloration at the injury site

Management of Rib Fractures

- Critical interventions: provide supplemental oxygen or ventilation, provide CPR and use an AED if indicated, control bleeding, treat for shock, and seek rapid transport.

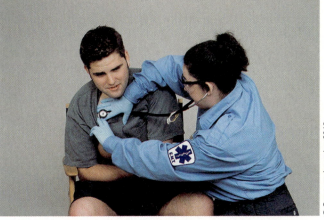

Figure 8-34 Breathing can be very painful with a fractured rib.

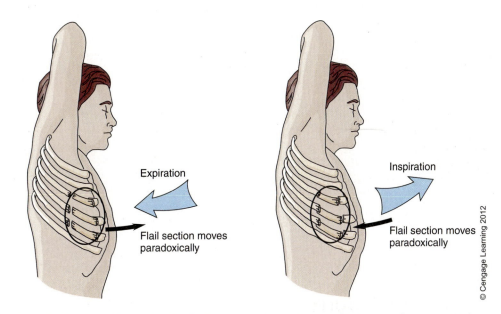

Figure 8-33 Paradoxical motion of a flail chest can impair ventilation and respiration.

- Teach the patient to "splint" the affected area for comfort by applying gentle pressure with a pillow, blanket, or article of clothing rolled up and placed on the center of the chest when deep breathing or coughing.
- Allow a position of comfort. This is a position in which the patient chooses to place himself for ease of breathing.

Pneumothorax

A **pneumothorax**, or collapsed lung, occurs when air enters the **pleural space**, the potential space between the lung and the chest wall (Figure 8-35). The buildup of this air creates pressure on the uninvolved lung and does not allow for the expansion needed for inspiration. A pneumothorax can be caused by a medical condition or a blunt or penetrating injury. A pneumothorax can be classified as a spontaneous, tension, or open pneumothorax.

Spontaneous Pneumothorax

A spontaneous pneumothorax occurs suddenly when an already weakened area of the lung breaks open. A partial or complete collapse of the lung may result. Nontraumatic events that can cause pneumothorax include physical exertion, coughing, flying at high altitudes, or scuba diving. This injury often occurs in young tall, thin males.

Signs and Symptoms of a Spontaneous Pneumothorax

- Sudden onset of chest pain
- Dyspnea (shortness of breath)

- Tachypnea
- Signs of shock

The severity of the symptoms depends on the size of the pneumothorax and the patient's health. The patient should be monitored for a possible tension pneumothorax.

Tension Pneumothorax

A **tension pneumothorax** is an increasing collection of gas in the pleural space, resulting in collapse of the lung on the affected side. It creates significant pressure inside the pleural cavity and is life threatening. The increased pressure causes the heart and vessels to be pushed away from the injured side (Figure 8-36). The vena cava can become blocked and cause decreased blood return to the heart. This will cause jugular vein distension (JVD), bulging veins in the side of the neck. A tension pneumothorax is usually caused by penetrating and blunt trauma.

Signs and Symptoms of a Tension Pneumothorax

- Extreme dyspnea and tachypnea
- Increasing resistance with bag valve mask ventilations
- Restless, anxious, and agitated
- Cyanosis
- Rapid and weak pulse (late stage)
- Hypotension
- Tracheal deviation
- JVD
- Hypoxia and shock

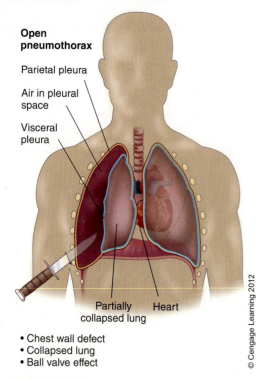

Open pneumothorax

Parietal pleura

Air in pleural space

Visceral pleura

Partially collapsed lung   Heart

- Chest wall defect
- Collapsed lung
- Ball valve effect

© Cengage Learning 2012

Figure 8-35 When air enters between the lung and the chest wall, pneumothorax is created.

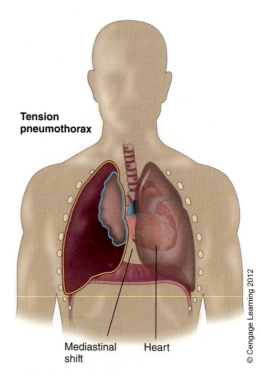

Tension pneumothorax

Mediastinal shift   Heart

© Cengage Learning 2012

Figure 8-36 Increasing pressure in the lung pushes the heart and great vessels to the opposite side of the chest.

Open Pneumothorax (Sucking Chest Wound)

A **sucking chest wound** is an open wound that allows air to pass in and out of the chest with each breath the victim takes. Bubbling or sucking sounds are created when outside air is sucked in through the wound opening. If air is not allowed out of the chest cavity, it can create a tension pneumothorax. GSWs, knife wounds, and other types of punctures can cause sucking chest wounds. A pneumothorax or sucking chest wound is shown in Figure 8-37.

Signs and Symptoms of an Open Pneumothorax

- Wound creates a sucking sound
- Symptoms of a tension pneumothorax
- Bubbling of blood around the wound

Hemothorax

The chest cavity contains major vessels such as the aorta and vena cava. If these vessels are lacerated by a penetrating object or ruptured by blunt trauma, bleeding occurs between the lung and chest wall. This accumulation of blood is called a **hemothorax**. It can be a simple bleed from a rib fracture, or a major vessel bleed resulting in hemorrhagic shock and death.

Signs and Symptoms of a Hemothorax

- Rapid or weak pulse
- Cool and clammy skin
- Restlessness and anxiety
- Hypotension
- Dyspnea, tachypnea
- Chest pain
- Coughing up frothy bright red blood

Management of Chest Trauma

- Critical interventions: provide supplemental oxygen or ventilation, provide CPR and use a AED if indicated, control major bleeding, treat for shock, and seek rapid transport.
- Spontaneous pneumothorax: monitor the patient for a possible tension pneumothorax.

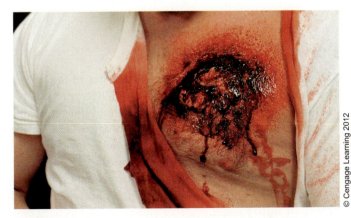

Figure 8-37 A patient with a pneumothorax, also called a sucking chest wound.

- Sucking chest wound: cover the opening with an occlusive dressing. Tape the perimeter of only three sides, leaving one side open.
- Leave an impaled object in place and secure it in the position found.
- Reassess every five minutes.
- Position the patient onto the injured side so the good lung is up to allow for greatest expansion of the uninjured lung. Place long backboard slightly on its side if a suspected spinal injury.

Abdominal Trauma

The abdominal cavity is divided into four quadrants and consists of the spleen, liver, gallbladder, stomach, pancreas, small intestine, large intestine, appendix, ovaries, uterus, and fallopian tubes. Injury to the abdomen can be caused by penetrating or blunt trauma including a deceleration injury. A **deceleration injury** occurs after impact when the forward movement of the body causes the organs to continue moving, causing tearing or rupturing. Blunt trauma also causes injury by the compression of organs against the spinal column. Although seatbelts in vehicles prevent a lot of serious injuries such as head and chest injuries, they can cause injuries to the abdominal organs. The EMR should look for bruising in the abdominal area called the "seatbelt sign."

General symptoms of abdominal injury include fever, pain, tenderness, distention, guarding, nausea, and vomiting. Rebound tenderness is caused from blood irritating the peritoneum, the lining of the abdominal cavity.

The EMR's role is not to diagnose which abdominal organ is involved but identify the location of the symptoms, potential for shock and urgency of transport. Assessment needs to be done every five minutes because life threatening symptoms may not be present initially.

Solid Organ Trauma

If solid organs are injured, they may bleed heavily and cause hemorrhagic shock. The solid organs of the abdominal cavity include the liver, spleen, and pancreas.

Liver Injury

The liver is the largest abdominal organ of the body and is located in the right upper quadrant of the abdominal cavity. Causes of liver injuries usually are blunt trauma or from a penetration of an impaled object such as rib fractures. All blood in the body flows through the liver. If the liver is injured, hemorrhagic shock can result. The patient may experience right upper quadrant pain as well as referred pain to the right shoulder.

Spleen Injury

The spleen is an organ located in the upper left quadrant of the abdominal cavity and is frequently injured with trauma. The spleen bleeds easily when injured; however, a capsule

© Cengage Learning 2012

surrounding the spleen tends to slow the development of shock. Rapid-onset hemorrhagic shock will occur if the capsule ruptures. The patient might experience not only upper left abdominal quadrant pain but referred pain to the left shoulder.

Pancreas Injury

Another abdominal organ is the pancreas, which lies across the back of the abdomen behind the stomach. Injury can be caused by blunt trauma but also from penetrating trauma with an impaled object. Because the pancreas lies deep within the abdominal cavity accidents most commonly seen are from seatbelts and handlebars from bicycles or motorcycles. Suspect an injury to the pancreas with vague upper and mid abdominal pain that may radiate into the back. Hemorrhage is possible and may result in shock.

Kidney Injury

The kidneys are located in the retroperitoneal area which is behind the peritoneum in the abdominal cavity. The kidneys are not completely protected by the ribs and can bleed into the retroperitoneal cavity. They can be injured by blunt trauma or by an impaled object, which produces sharp pain in the flank, (mid to low back). The patient may have blood in the urine.

Hollow Organ Trauma

The hollow organs of the abdominal cavity include the stomach, gallbladder, large and small intestines, appendix, and ureters. When these hollow organs are ruptured, content spillage and inflammation of the peritoneum can occur. This is extremely serious, and the patient must be transported to a medical facility as soon as possible. Intestine or other organs protruding through the abdominal wall is called an **evisceration**, as shown in Figure 8-38. The small intestine is most frequently injured because of its size and location. Intestinal rupture and spillage cause a rapid onset of burning, epigastric pain, rigidity, and rebound tenderness.

Assessment Tools for Abdominal Trauma

After performing an initial assessment, providing critical interventions, and obtaining baseline vital signs the EMR should gather information from a focused assessment, including DRGERM, OPQRST, and SAMPLE. During assessment, gentle to moderate pressure should be used when palpating all four quadrants.

Management of Abdominal Trauma

- Critical interventions: provide supplemental oxygen or ventilation, provide CPR and use an AED if indicated, control bleeding, treat for shock, and seek rapid transport.

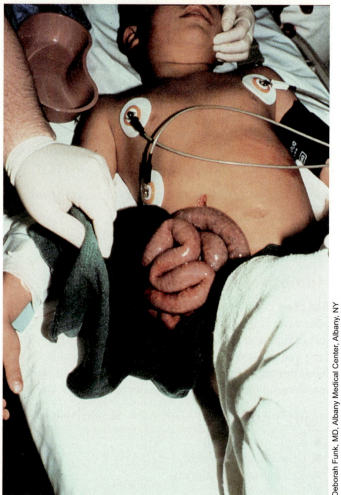

Deborah Funk, MD, Albany Medical Center, Albany, NY

Figure 8-38 Penetrating trauma to the abdomen can result in evisceration of intestines.

- Allow a position of comfort usually with the knees bent toward the chest.
- Do not put the eviscerated organs back into the cavity. Prevent further organ contamination by applying a sterile dressing.
- Reassess every five minutes.

Pelvic Cavity Trauma

The pelvic cavity is surrounded by the bones of the pelvis. The pelvic cavity contains the bladder, ureters, urethra, reproductive organs, and rectum. A fracture of the pelvis due to blunt trauma can be life threatening because some of the body's largest vessels exist there. If a vessel is severed, internal bleeding and hemorrhagic shock can result.

A soft tissue injury can occur to the genitals when they are impacted by a fixed object. This type of injury is called a **straddle injury** and may occur after a person has been on a bike or horseback riding. Bruising and swelling are evident, and wounds can bleed profusely.

Assessment Tools for Pelvic Cavity Trauma

After performing an initial assessment, critical interventions, and baseline vital signs, the EMR should obtain information using assessment tools of DOTS, TIC, OPQRST, and SAMPLE. Palpation needs to be gentle to prevent major bleeding caused by a possible severing of a blood vessel.

Signs and Symptoms of Pelvic Cavity Trauma

- Pain with palpation
- Tenderness or pain in lower abdomen, low back, or pubic area
- Pelvic bone crepitus
- Signs of hemorrhagic shock caused by internal or external bleeding

Management of Pelvic Cavity Trauma

- Critical interventions: provide supplemental oxygen or ventilation, provide CPR and use an AED if indicated, control external bleeding, treat for shock, and seek rapid transport.
- Avoid unnecessary movement.
- Reassess every five minutes assessing for signs of shock.
- Assist with packaging and placement on a long backboard.

Muscle and Joint Injuries

Muscles, tendons, and ligaments can be torn, bruised, cut, or crushed. Tendons attach muscles to bones, and ligaments are a fibrous tissue attaching bone to bone providing for joint stability. Muscle and joint injuries include sprains, strains, and dislocations. It is difficult during the EMR's assessment to discern one from another and there may be a combination of injuries including fractures.

- **Sprains** are injuries to ligaments that are caused by being stretched beyond normal capacity and possibly torn.
- **Strains** are injuries to muscles or tendons in which the muscle fibers tear as a result of overstretching, overuse, or a force
- **Dislocations** result when a bone or bones are displaced out of a joint (Figure 8-39). Vessels, nerves, tendons, and ligaments may also be involved in this injury.

Assessment Tools for Muscle and Joint Injuries

After performing an initial assessment, critical interventions, and baseline vital signs, the EMR should obtain information from a focused assessment using DOTS, TIC, OPQRST, and SAMPLE. It is vital to check and recheck the circulation, motor, and sensation (CMS) of the involved extremity and recheck it after an intervention or at intervals. Keep the area immobilized while assessing to prevent further injury.

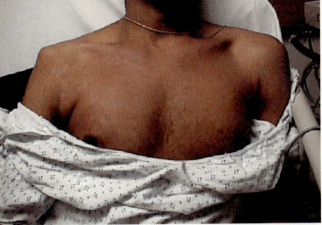

Figure 8-39 A dislocation is when a bone is forced out of a joint. Note the squared-off appearance of the dislocated shoulder.

Signs and Symptoms of Muscle and Joint Injuries

- Muscle spasms and pain
- Limited range of motion
- Decreased or absent CMS
- Guarding area injured
- Warmth, bruising, or redness in the injured area
- Joint deformity
- Swelling

Management of Muscle and Joint Injuries

- Critical interventions: control major bleed and seek transportation if indicated.
- Immobilize the affected area. Do not attempt to put a dislocated joint back in place (see Chapter 9).
- Apply a cold pack or crushed ice in an enclosed bag over the area for approximately 20 minutes to help reduce swelling and control pain. Avoid direct contact with the ice to the skin by placing a towel, cloth, or clothing article over the injured part and under the ice. Monitor the skin temperature.

Fractures

A fracture occurs when a bone is impacted by a force and breaks. Fractures can be divided into two categories, closed and open fractures. In either of these fractures bone ends can be displaced (ends not in alignment) or non displaced (ends in alignment). Fractures may cause damage to vessels, nerves, or soft tissue depending on the location and may result in mild to severe bleeding.

In a closed fracture, bone ends can be displaced or nondisplaced with the skin remaining intact (Figure 8-40). These fractures may be difficult to confirm because the area around the injury will be painful or swollen as with other injuries.

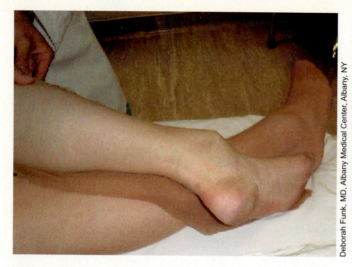

Figure 8-40 The area around a closed fracture may be painful, swollen, or deformed.

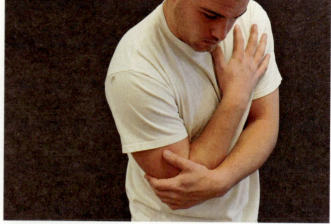

Figure 8-42 The patient may "self-splint" in an attempt to prevent further pain and injury.

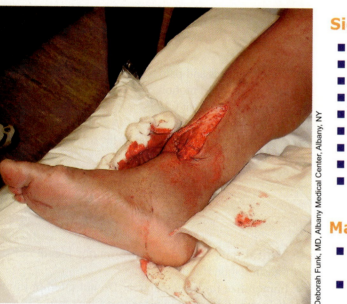

Figure 8-41 An open fracture occurs when the bone ends break through the skin.

In an open fracture, usually the ends of the broken bones have erupted through the skin; however, an outside force penetrating the skin and breaking the bone also causes an open fracture (Figure 8-41).

Assessment Tools for Fractures

After performing an initial assessment, critical interventions, and baseline vital signs the EMR should obtain information from the assessment tools of DOTS, TIC, OPQRST, SAMPLE, and CMS. It is vital to initially check CMS of an involved extremity and recheck it at intervals. Care must be taken not to move the fractured extremity while assessing unless proper stabilizing the extremity above and below the fracture and adjacent joints.

Signs and Symptoms of Fractures

- Swelling
- Deformity
- Pain
- Crepitus
- Contusion
- Decreased or absent CMS
- Guarding
- Self-splinting by the patient (Figure 8-42)
- Penetration of the skin by the bone or an object

Management of Fractures

- Critical interventions: control major bleeding, treat for shock, and seek transportation.
- Immobilize the limb with a rigid or flexible splint in the position found (see Chapter 9).
- Never try to move bone ends together.
- Manual traction may be necessary if there is loss of peripheral pulses. Manual traction consists of grasping the limb firmly and exerting a continuous gentle pull along the long axis of the bone. After manual traction is applied, you must use a traction splint (see Chapter 9). Do not continue manual traction if resistance is met or the bone is in alignment. Never apply manual traction for an open fracture.
- A closed fracture can become an open fracture and cause more damage to soft tissues, muscles, tendons, and ligaments if not handled properly.
- Cover open bone ends with a sterile dressing. Do not wrap a bandage tightly or directly over the exposed bone end.
- Apply cold packs or ice if available to a closed fracture.
- Reassess every five minutes.

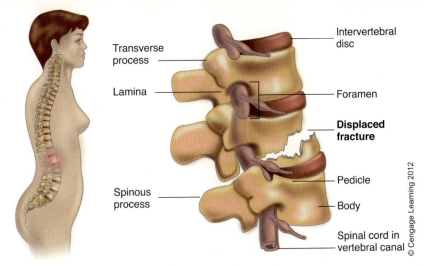

Transverse process

Lamina

Spinous process

Intervertebral disc

Foramen

Displaced fracture

Pedicle

Body

Spinal cord in vertebral canal

© Cengage Learning 2012

Figure 8-43 When supporting ligaments stretch or tear, the vertebrae may crack or be dislocated from their normal position and intrude into the narrow canal, causing significant injury to the spinal cord.

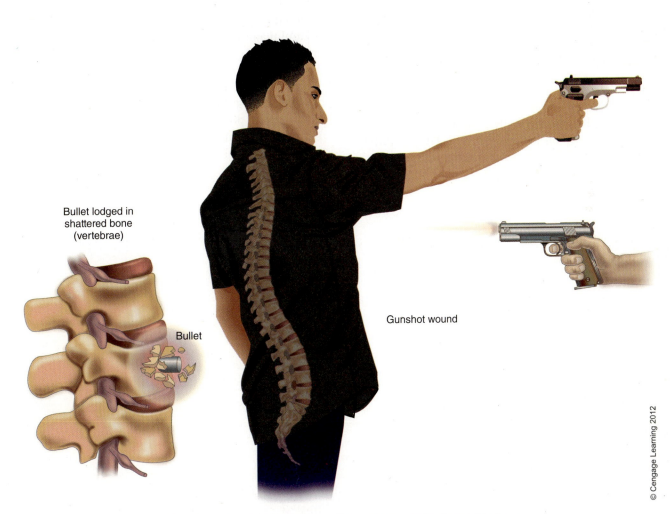

Bullet lodged in shattered bone (vertebrae)

Bullet

Gunshot wound

© Cengage Learning 2012

Figure 8-44 Penetrating injuries to the torso often cause spinal cord injury.

Spinal Cord Injury

A spinal cord injury (SCI) can result from swelling, bruising, or severing of the spinal cord from force to the vertebral column (Figure 8-43). SCI affects the body's ability to send and receive messages for movement and sensation. The vertebral column is divided into five sections of vertebrae. There are seven cervical, twelve thoracic, five lumbar, five sacral, and four vertebrae in the lower coccyx.

If the spinal cord is completely severed or damaged, the patient may become paralyzed and loose sensation below the level of fracture. **Quadriplegia** is paralysis of all four extremities, as well as affects other function below the fracture site, and can result from a cervical fracture or injury. **Paraplegia** is paralysis of the lower extremities, as well as affects other function below the fracture site, and results from a fracture or injury to the thoracic or lumbar spine.

A primary SCI results from impact, such as GSWs, knife wounds, or motor vehicle crashes. Primary SCIs caused by trauma may result in an immediate and often irreversible loss of motion, sensation, or both (Figure 8-44). A secondary SCI occurs when the spinal cord is not properly immobilized. There are six different movements of the vertebral column that cause damage to the spinal cord: flexion, extension, rotation, lateral bending, compression, and distraction (a hanging injury).

Assessment Tools for Spinal Cord Injury

After performing an initial assessment, critical interventions, and baseline vital signs, the EMR should obtain information from assessment tools including: DOTS, TIC, OPQRST, SAMPLE, and CMS. Use spinal stabilization while performing assessments.

Signs and Symptoms of Spinal Cord Injury

- Tingling or loss of sensation in the hands, fingers, feet, or toes
- Breathing difficulty
- Pain, tenderness, or pressure in the neck or in the back when palpating the spine
- Radicular pain (feels like electricity shooting through the body)
- Partial or complete loss of movement and sensation
- Signs of injury on the head or spine
- Patient found in the "hold-up position" (arms above the head)
- Priapism (sustained erection)
- Incontinence
- Muscle spasms
- Patient may tell you he heard a snap
- Neurogenic shock, bradycardia, or hypotension

Management of Spinal Cord Injury

- Provide spinal stabilization and place a cervical collar.
- Critical interventions: provide supplemental oxygen or ventilation, provide CPR and use an AED if indicated, control major bleeding, treat for shock, and seek rapid transport.
- Reassess every five minutes, including CMS.
- Assist with packaging by properly placing a patient who is lying on the ground on a long back board. If the patient is in a sitting position, place him on a short backboard before moving him to a long backboard (see Chapter 9).

SUMMARY

An EMR must be able to recognize different types of trauma in order to access and manage a patient in the best way possible. Making a proper assessment, knowing critical interventions, and general management for various trauma situations can help an EMR give appropriate care to patients until they can be transported to a facility for further treatment.

TRAUMA EMERGENCY SCENARIOS

The following trauma scenarios are designed to test the EMR student on the application of focused trauma assessment, critical thinking skills, and management. To enhance application, use simulation to practice these scenarios.

Scenario 1

At 2300, you arrive at the scene of a motor vehicle crash. A 22-year-old male victim is conscious and walking around. He says he is alone and that he lost control of his vehicle and hit a telephone pole. The patient has some facial bleeding and lacerations and abrasions on his forehead; however, he states he is "feeling fine." The windshield has "spider cracks" where the patient's head hit the windshield. The patient states he doesn't want to go to the hospital but will allow you to assess him. He is compliant with your instructions. Your initial assessment reveals the patient is A & O x 3.

At 2315, the patient tells you he is experiencing a throbbing headache rated at 8/10, neck pain, and nausea. He is now A & O x 1. ALS, Advanced Life Support, arrives at 2335.

Critical Thinking Exercise

1. List your initial actions at 2300.
2. What do you think may be happening to the patient?
3. How would you continue to manage this patient at 2315?
4. Write a patient care report (PCR) narrative for this patient using the principles of SOAP or CHART.

Scenario 2

Your agency receives a call concerning a 65-year-old woman who has fallen down the basement stairs. When you arrive at 1445, the patient's husband calmly points to the door leading to the basement and tells you she is down there. You find an elderly woman sitting against a wall with a large bump over her left eye. She is conscious and complains of pelvic and left lower leg pain. Your assessment reveals:

Initial Assessment	Reassessment at 1505
A & O x 3	Pulse: 110 beats/min
Respiratory rate: 18 breaths/min and labored	Respiratory rate: 20 breaths/min
Pulse: 96 and regular	BP: 120/70 mm Hg
BP: 150/90 mm Hg	She now complains of feeling cold

Temperature is warm and dry

Critical Thinking Exercise

1. List the findings of your primary assessment. What is her chief complaint?
2. What is significant about her chief complaint?
3. What will you do to manage this patient? Why?
4. Does this patient require rapid transport? Why?
5. Write a PCR narrative for this patient.

Scenario 3

Your agency receives a call at 1045 to respond to a construction site where a man has fallen. When you arrive on the scene, you find a 25-year-old man who fell approximately 15 feet to the ground. Several construction workers are attempting to assist the patient. He is found on his right side, and you are told by one worker that he pulled a rod out of the right side of the patient's chest. Upon examination of the wound, you see blood bubbling out of the opening. Your initial assessment reveals:

Respiratory rate: 24 breaths/min and labored	A & O x 2
Pulse: 120 beats/min	Difficulty breathing
Blood pressure: 160/80 mm Hg	Skin temperature: cool

Emergency Medical Services arrives, and you assist with packaging and transferring the patient to the rig at 1105.

Critical Thinking Exercise

1. What are your initial actions?
2. How would you mange this patient? List by priority.
3. What type of wound does the patient have? How would you bandage this wound?

4. Was it appropriate for the worker to pull out the impaled object? Why or why not?

5. Write a PCR narrative for this patient.

GLASGOW COMA SCORE EXERCISE

Score the following patients using the Glasgow Coma Score tool.

Patient #1

- The patient has his eyes open and looks at you.
- The patient speaks normally and answers your questions appropriately.
- The patient is able to follow commands such as: "Show me two fingers."

Score _____

Patient #2

- The patient's eyes are closed even when you apply a painful stimulus.
- The patient makes no sound even when you apply a painful stimulus.
- The patient does not follow commands and does not move even when a painful stimulus is applied.

Score _____

Patient #3

- The patient's eyes are closed even when you call loudly, but he opens his eyes when you apply a painful stimulus.
- The patient says, "Don't!" or "Stop!" when you apply a painful stimulus but does not speak in whole sentences and does not answer questions.
- The patient does not follow commands, but when you apply a painful stimulus, the patient pushes your hand away.

Score _____

REVIEW QUESTIONS

1. Define shock.
2. Name the three types of vessels that cause bleeding.
3. Name the three classifications of burns.
4. Define a concussion.
5. What condition is a collection of gas in the pleural space that causes the lung on the affected side to collapse?
6. When injured, what solid organ located in the upper left quadrant of the abdominal cavity exhibits referred pain to the left shoulder?
7. What type of fracture does not break the skin?
8. What is a secondary spinal cord injury?
9. Explain the difference between a sprain and a strain?
10. Describe steps to control severe bleeding.

REFERENCES

1. Adapted from Davis RJ, et al: Head and spinal cord injury. In Rogers MC (ed): *Textbook of Pediatric Intensive Care*. Baltimore, Williams and Wilkins, 1987; James H, Anas N, Perkin RM: *Brain Insults in Infants and Children*. New York: Grune and Stratton, 1985; and Morray JP, et al: Coma scale for use in brain-injured children. *Crit Care Med* 12:1018, 1984.

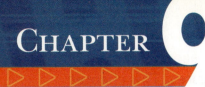

CHAPTER 9

DRESSINGS, BANDAGING, AND IMMOBILIZATION TECHNIQUES

LEARNING OBJECTIVES

By the end of this chapter, the reader should be able to

- Identify different types of dressings.
- Identify bandage types and methods for using bandages.
- Describe various types of splinting devices and the basics for using splinting devices.
- List the steps in properly splinting extremities.
- Describe methods for immobilizing patients.

INTRODUCTION

The EMR must be familiar with different types of dressings, bandages, and immobilization techniques to properly care for patients with wounds and fractures. This chapter discusses types of dressings, application of dressings, bandaging materials, and immobilization devices used by Emergency Medical Responders (EMRs).

Dressings

Dressings are sterile, absorbent materials placed directly over a wound to control bleeding and protect the open wound from further injury and contamination. Different types and sizes of dressings and bandages are displayed in Figure 9-1. Most dressings come in sterile packaging and ideally should be kept sterile. Keeping the dressings sterile may be difficult in certain environmental conditions. To keep the dressings as clean as possible, an EMR should wear proper personal protective equipment (PPE) when handling dressings. When applying a dressing to an open wound, use gloves to pick up the dressing at the corner and place it on the wound.

Gauze Dressings

Gauze dressings are the most common dressings that come in various sizes and thicknesses of sterile cotton weave material. These dressings are meant to be applied directly over a wound, and if they remain sterile, they prevent contamination and infection of the wound.

Trauma Dressings

Trauma dressings are large cotton dressings that usually consist of two layers of gauze with an absorbent cotton core. These dressings are large enough to cover major wounds and are used to control profuse bleeding.

Universal Dressings

Universal dressings are 9- by 36-inch or larger gauze dressings with several layers of absorbent cotton. This dressing is used along with direct pressure to control major bleeding and when large areas of the body need to be covered.

Occlusive Dressings

Occlusive dressings do not allow air or moisture into the wound. They often have a petroleum gel or thin plastic film that creates a barrier to the air. These dressings help block air from being drawn, causing an embolism, in open neck wounds where a jugular vein has been severed. They are also applied to an open pneumothorax to prevent air from entering the pleural space and enlarging the pneumothorax.

Non-adherent Dressings

Non-adherent dressings have a special coating that does not allow the dressing to stick to a wound. Non-adherent dressings are useful on burns and frost bite injuries. They can be placed between the fingers and toes of patients with burns or frostbite to keep the digits from sticking together.

Hemostatic Dressings

Hemostatic dressings contain powders or other substances that promote the clotting of the blood when applied directly on an open wound (Figure 9-2). These dressings should be used only for heavy bleeding that cannot be controlled by

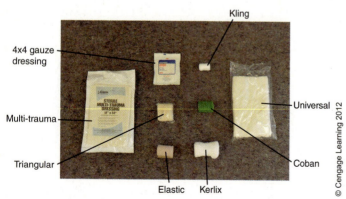

Figure 9-1 Various dressings and bandages.

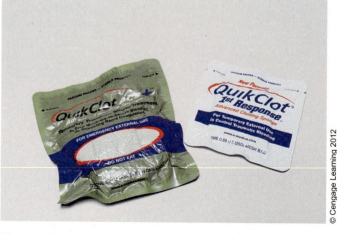

Figure 9-2 Hemostatic agents can be used along with direct pressure for severe hemorrhage to rapidly clot the blood.

direct pressure and traditional bleeding control measures. Follow your agency's protocols when using hemostatic dressings.

Improvisational Dressings

Improvisational dressings can be used if a packaged commercial dressing is not available. Use the cleanest item available such as a handkerchief or piece of clothing. Plastic wrap or foil can be used to create a nonsterile occlusive dressing.

Bandages

Bandages, generally made of strips of cloth, are used to hold dressings securely in place, provide pressure to control bleeding, and protect the wound from further injury. Bandages do not have to be sterile.

Roller Bandages

Roller bandages are made from cotton cloth rolled into cylinders for better control during application. Usually made of cotton gauze, they are designed to wrap several times around a dressing to hold it in place and provide pressure to the wound. Roller bandages come in various sizes from two to six inches wide and several feet in length.

Elastic Bandages

Elastic bandages secure dressing in place and can be self-adhering, secured with tape, or have Velcro or metal fasteners. When using an elastic bandage to secure a dressing, never stretch the bandage to its full length. Stretching out the bandage completely can impede blood flow and cause swelling. Stretch the elastic bandage only halfway when using it to secure a dressing.

Military Compresses

Military compresses contain a cotton dressing and bandage in one package. This compress dressing has attached "tails" to secure the dressing to the wound (Figure 9-3), allowing the EMR to apply the dressing and wrap the bandage around the wound at the same time.

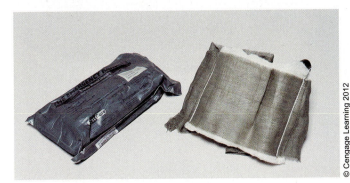

Figure 9-3 A military compress has a dressing integrated into the bandage, making it convenient to use in an emergency.

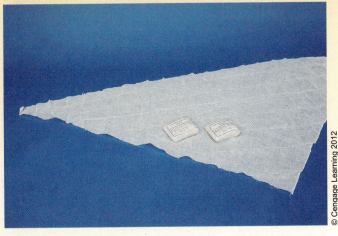

Figure 9-4 A triangular bandage has multiple uses.

Triangular Bandages

Triangular bandages are triangular pieces of muslin or cotton cloth used to hold dressings on the head or other large areas of the body in place. A triangular bandage folded to approximately a two-inch width is called a **cravat** and can be used to make a sling to secure an arm (Figure 9-4). Cravats can be used in many other circumstances, such as holding splints on extremities for fracture immobilization or making a tourniquet if necessary.

Tourniquets

Tourniquets are used when direct pressure, elevation of an extremity, or pressure bandages fail to stop bleeding. Tourniquets have been shown to be very effective in stopping heavy, uncontrolled bleeding and may be left in place for up to six hours with effective results. An inflated blood pressure cuff can be used as a tourniquet. A commercial tourniquet or a cravat can be used. After the tourniquet is applied, do not release it and prepare the patient for immediate transport to the hospital. The EMR must note the time the tourniquet was applied preferably on a visible area such as the forehead of the patient. Applications of a commercial tourniquet and cravat tourniquet are demonstrated in **Skill 9-1** at the end of the chapter.

Improvisation Bandage

An improvisation bandage can be made by cutting a T-shirt from the bottom up in one long spiral. These bandages do not need to be sterile because they do not go directly on a wound, but they should be as clean as possible because they will hold a dressing in place.

Methods of Bandaging

Wounds can occur anywhere on the body. Wounds must be dressed and bandaged according to the location of the wound. Accordingly, an EMR must be familiar with various methods of bandaging techniques. With most bandages you will need to initially anchor the bandage, use twists at intervals, and secure the ends of the bandage. These techniques are explained below:

- Anchor the bandage by using recurrent turns to hold the bandage in place or by angling the initial turn then folding it over and using a recurrent turn.
- Using twists at intervals will keep the bandage more secure and prevent sliding of the bandage. Twists on top of the wound will provide mild pressure to possibly prevent further bleeding from an open wound.
- After the area is covered, secure the end of the bandage by taping, tucking in the end, cutting the length in half and tying, or by tying off excess bandage material.

A demonstration of these techniques are shown in **Skill 9-2** at the end of the chapter.

Recurrent Bandage

A **recurrent bandage** is used to hold a dressing in place over a large area, such as the head, as shown in Figure 9-5. A roller or elastic bandage can be used as a recurrent bandage.

Anchor the bandage and place each wrap directly over the previous wrap use twists if determined, and secure the end.

Spiral Bandage

A **spiral bandage** is a roller or elastic bandage that can cover an entire extremity. It is started by anchoring the bandage with a wrap around the narrowest part of the limb. Each wrap should cover the previous one by one-half to ensure complete coverage of the dressing. Anchor the bandage initially with a recurrent turn. See Figure 9-6 for a demonstration of spiral bandaging of a leg.

Figure-of-Eight Bandage

A **figure-of-eight bandage** is an elastic or roller bandage that turns across itself like a figure of eight and is used for holding dressings on wounds of a joint and the palm of the hand or to secure an impaled object in place. Figures 9-7 through 9-9 demonstrate how a figure-of-eight bandage technique can be used on a variety of wounds.

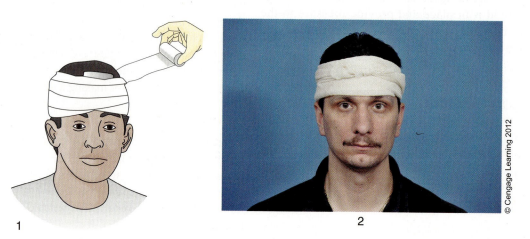

1   2

© Cengage Learning 2012

Figure 9-5 A recurrent bandage of the head can hold a dressing in place.

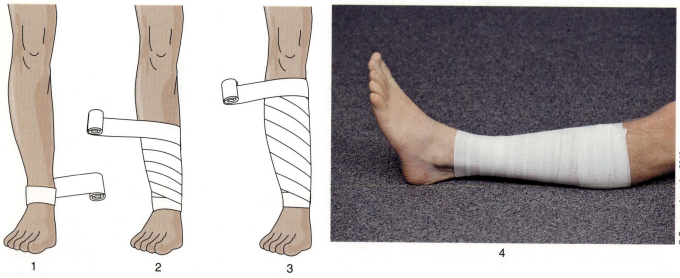

1   2   3   4

© Cengage Learning 2012

Figure 9-6 A spiral bandage is wrapped around the extremity in a spiral fashion.

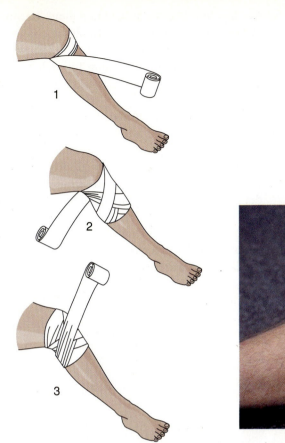

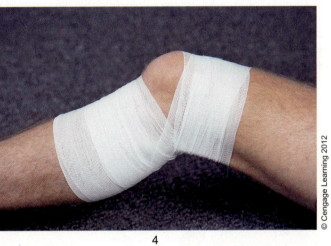

Figure 9-7   A figure-of-eight bandage of the knee.

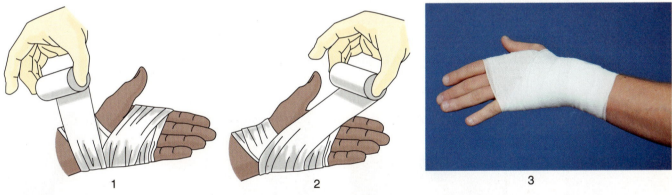

Figure 9-8   A figure-of-eight bandage on a dorsal hand wound.

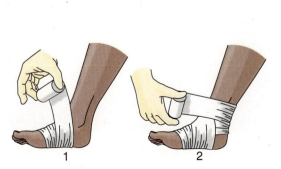

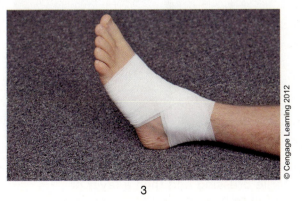

Figure 9-9   A figure-of-eight bandage of the foot.

Additional Bandaging Applications

The type and location of a wound often dictate that some bandages are more appropriate than others. Special conditions must be taken into consideration for dressing and bandaging neck wounds, eviscerations, straddle injuries, impaled objects, avulsions, amputations, eye and head wounds, and shoulder and hip injuries.

- *Neck wounds:* A neck wound can result in a deep cut or laceration. A dressing to a neck wound is held in place with a roller bandage or an occlusive dressing if the jugular vein or artery is severed. Be careful about securing any bandage around the neck because breathing could be affected (Figure 9-10).
- *Eviscerations:* The EMR should not attempt to place a protruding or eviscerated organ back into the abdomen

but should cover the area with a moist sterile dressing and then cover it with a layer of plastic or aluminum foil and secure it with a loose bandage, as shown in Figure 9-11. The plastic or aluminum foil helps to retain the patient's body heat. Never push *any* organ back into the body.

- *Straddle injuries:* A soft tissue injury to the perineal area or genitals can bleed profusely. Secure a trauma or universal dressing in place with cravats to stop the bleeding and stabilize the area (Figure 9-12). These injuries occur from bicycles, motorcycles, all-terrain vehicles, or other devices the patient was riding and in which genitalia or perineum are injured.
- *Impaled objects:* To stabilize an impaled object, use a donut made out of a cravat, a disposable cup, or a roller bandage placed around the object and bandaged in place.

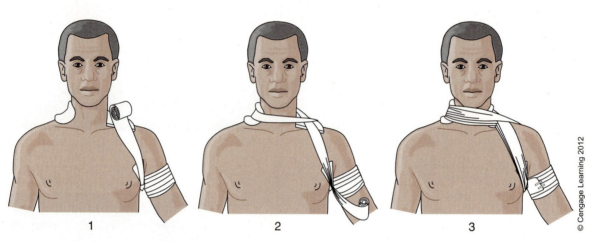

1   2   3

© Cengage Learning 2012

Figure 9-10   An occlusive dressing is held in place by a roller bandage.

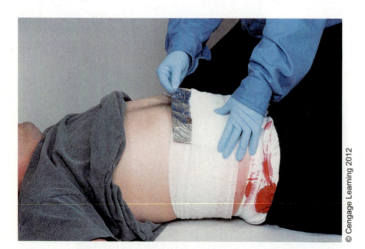

© Cengage Learning 2012

Figure 9-11   An evisceration should be covered with a sterile dressing and then a layer of aluminum foil to help retain the patient's body heat and protect the organs from injury.

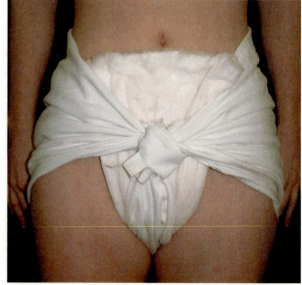

© Cengage Learning 2012

Figure 9-12   A diaper bandage made with triangular bandages is used to hold a trauma dressing for a straddle injury.

The only location where an impaled object can be removed is in the cheek of the patient if it interferes with breathing. See **Skill 9-3** for a demonstration of stabilizing an impaled object.

■ *Avulsions or amputations:* An avulsion or amputated limb usually occurs when the patient is entrapped in a machine or vehicle or injured in a sport activity. Areas of the body that are commonly affected are the nose, ears, fingers, and extremities. Figure 9-13 demonstrates a trauma dressing being held in place on a stump by a triangular dressing.

■ *Eye injuries:* Eye injuries commonly involve dust, chemicals, foreign substances, and impaled objects. The EMR must understand the delicacies of the eye and stabilize the object and handle it with care. Stabilization of an object can be provided with a donut, roller bandage, or a disposable cup, as shown in Figure 9-14. Application of an eye bandage for eye injuries is demonstrated in **Skill 9-4**.

■ *Head injuries:* Head injures tend to bleed freely and must be controlled by dressings and bandages. Use of a cravat or roller bandage secures a dressing after bleeding is stopped. The steps for bandaging the head using a triangular bandage are shown in **Skill 9-5**.

■ *Shoulder and hip injuries:* Shoulder injuries are common from motorcycle and bicycle accidents and other sporting activities. Shoulder and hip injuries are difficult to bandage and can be a challenge to the EMR. Use a trauma or universal dressing to cover the large affected area and secure it with a triangular bandage and cravat. An application of a dressing and bandage to a shoulder injury is demonstrated in **Skill 9-6**.

Basics of Dressing and Bandaging

■ Always use PPE. Use gloves and, if needed, wear a gown, mask, or eye shield.
■ Keep dressings as sterile or clean as possible.
■ Control bleeding by using pressure over the dressing. If the first dressing becomes saturated with blood, do not remove that dressing. Instead, apply additional dressings over the saturated ones.
■ Cover the entire surface of a wound with a dressing and cover the area above and below the dressing with a bandage.
■ Anchor the initial turn of a roller or elastic bandage.
■ For additional security of the bandage, use twists.
■ Secure the end of the roller or elastic bandage.
■ Do not wrap a bandage too tightly. After bandaging, check the distal extremity for circulation, movement, and sensation (CMS). Loosen the bandage if CMS is compromised. Keep the patient's fingers and toes exposed to assess and reassess circulation.
■ If a tourniquet is applied, seek rapid transport. Note the time the tourniquet was applied.

Splinting

A splint immobilizes an area of the body to reduce damage, decrease pain, and prevent paralysis caused by fractures. Be certain to check CMS before and after splinting an extremity.

Classifications of Splinting Devices

Splinting devices are used to immobilize a fracture, strain, sprain, or dislocation. Splinting can be grouped into five general classifications: slings and swathes, flexible splints, rigid splints, pneumatic splints, and traction splints.

Slings and Swathes

Slings are triangular bandages used to support injured arms. **Swathes**, triangular bandages or cloths folded into a band, are used to secure a sling in place. Used together, a sling and swathe support an injured arm or shoulder while holding it in place. The injured arm is suspended in a triangular bandage or sling and is firmly anchored to the body by a cravat used as a swathe. The swathe secures the sling in place, allowing the body to provide external support and needed rigidity. The

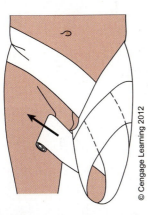

Figure 9-13 A trauma dressing is applied to a stump and then held in place by a triangular or roller bandage.

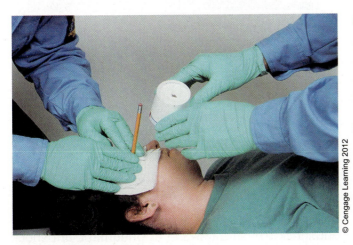

Figure 9-14 A cup helps stabilize an impaled object of the eye.

knots of the sling should not be placed on the side of the neck and need to be padded. Steps for performing a sling and swathe of the arm are demonstrated in Skill 9-7.

Flexible Splints

A **flexible splint** is made from a material that can be formed to fit any body angle and then made rigid. Various flexible splints are shown in Figure 9-15. These splints are particularly useful for joint injuries. A SAM and flexible ladder splint are examples of these types of splints (Figure 9-16).

Rigid Splints

Rigid splints are made of firm material, such as hard plastic, boards, or rigid cardboard that can be placed next to an injured limb to provide support. Rigid splints can be used on arm and leg fractures, and joint injuries. These splints must be padded, and CMS must always be checked before and after application of any splint. Skills 9-8 through 9-10 demonstrate application of a rigid splint on extremity fractures and a joint injury.

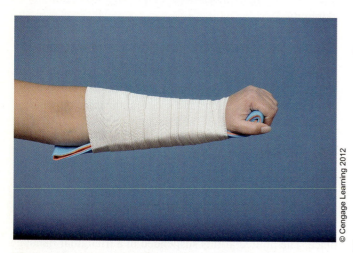

Figure 9-15 Various splints.

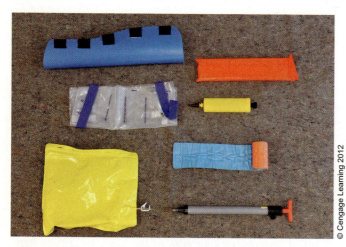

Figure 9-16 A flexible splint, similar to the SAM splint, is convenient for splinting a deformed extremity. Note the hand in the position of function.

Pneumatic Splints

A **pneumatic splint** immobilizes a fracture by inflating or deflating a device until the splint becomes rigid. A vacuum splint, shown in Figure 9-17, is a type of pneumatic splint. The military antishock trousers (MAST) or pneumatic antishock garment (PASG) is used to stabilize both femur and pelvic fractures. This garment can be applied to the patient's lower extremities by a trouser method or by a wrapper method, which is particularly useful when the legs have fractures or the pelvis is unstable, as shown in Figure 9-18.

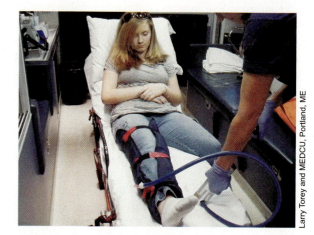

Figure 9-17 A vacuum splint is a type of pneumatic splint.

(a)

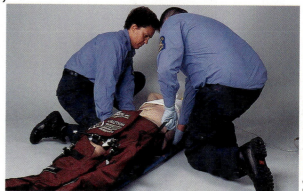

(b)

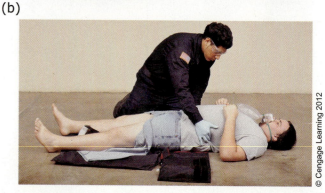

Figure 9-18 (a) The trouser method for military antishock trousers (MAST) or pneumatic antishock garment (PASG) application. (b) The wrapper method for MAST or PASG application.

Traction Splints

Traction splints stabilize closed femur fractures by providing a continuous pull along the axis of the bone. These splints decrease muscular spasm and pain, as well as preventing the bone ends from overriding. Remember that these traction devices cannot be used on an open femur fracture because bringing the bone ends back under the skin could cause further bleeding and contamination. Application of a traction splint to manage a closed femur fracture is demonstrated in **Skill 9-11**.

Improvised Splinting Techniques

There are times when the Emergency Medical Services response is delayed. If an EMR does not have equipment to stabilize a fracture, several improvisational techniques can be used to create a splint.

- Use a T-shirt to make a sling secure with safety pins while placing the hand in the position of function (Figure 9-19).
- Use a belt as an arm sling (Figure 9-20).
- Use magazines, a soft book, or newspapers as a splint (Figure 9-21). Follow splinting with sling and swathe.
- Place a blanket, sleeping bag, or ground mat between the legs with the legs bandaged together to stabilize a lower leg fracture (Figure 9-22). This is a splint for the lower extremities when no other rigid splinting materials are available.
- Use a pillow as a splint for an ankle injury (Figure 9-23). A pillow stabilizes and protects the ankle from further harm. Keep the knee stabilized also in case of potential knee fracture
- Use a bedroll or pillow for a dislocated shoulder (Figure 9-24). This is an effective immobilization for a dislocated shoulder.

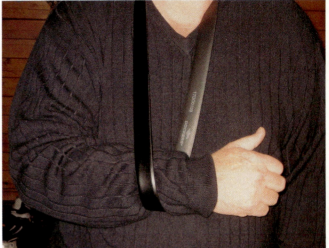

Joe Grafft, Stacy, MN

Figure 9-20 A belt can be used to make a sling for a shoulder injury. If used for the arm, splinting must be done first.

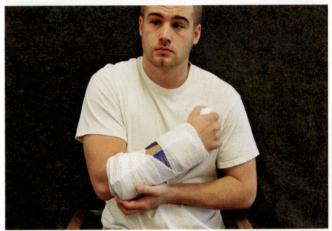

© Cengage Learning 2012

Figure 9-21 Use a magazine or soft cover book to stabilize a fracture of the arm. Check circulation, movement, and sensation before and after splinting. Follow with a sling and swathe.

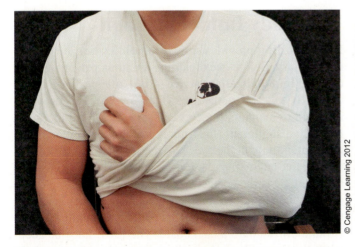

© Cengage Learning 2012

Figure 9-19 Use the patient's T shirt to stabilize a fracture of the forearm. Secure it with safety pins and place the hand in a position of function.

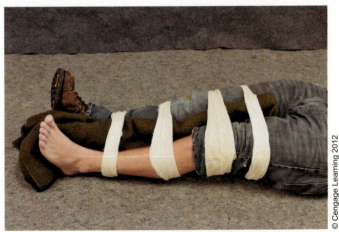

© Cengage Learning 2012

Figure 9-22 A blanket can be used between the patient's legs with the legs bandaged together to stabilize a fracture to the lower leg.

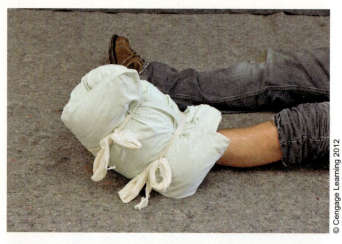

Figure 9-23 Using a pillow to splint an ankle fracture or sprain is an effective way to stabilize and protect the ankle from further harm.

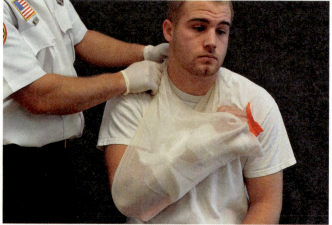

Figure 9-25 Elevate the extremity above the level of the heart after immobilizing a possible fracture.

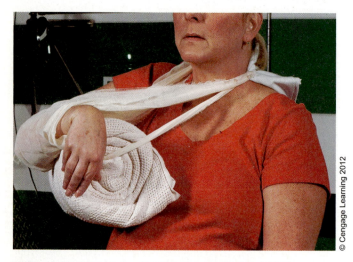

Figure 9-24 A bed roll, secured around the body by a cravat, maintains the arm in the position found. This is an effective immobilization for a dislocated shoulder.

Basics of Splinting

- Wear PPE.
- Expose the area by cutting away clothing without moving the extremity.
- Control bleeding at the fracture site.
- Manually stabilize a possible fracture above and below the fracture site and the adjacent joints before splinting. If possible, splint in the position found.
- Always assess for CMS distal to the fracture before and after splinting. Loosen the splint if the patient reports a change in sensation (numbness, tingling, or burning), increased pain, or increased swelling or if the fingers or toes become cold, pale, or blue. Also loosen ties on the splint when a decrease in pulse or movement occurs.

- If you do not feel pulses or signs of circulation in a long bone extremity, such as in a closed angulated fracture, gentle traction and slight rotation along the long axis of the bone may be necessary. If pulses have not returned, package the patient and seek transportation to the nearest medical facility.
- If possible, place the hand or foot of a fractured extremity in its natural position, the **position of function**. The foot should be bent at the ankle at a 90-degree angle, as in standing. The hand should be positioned with the wrist slightly extended and with a grip (for example, holding a roller-gauze).
- Never allow a patient to bear weight on an injured limb.
- After immobilizing, elevate a possible fracture above the level of the heart and apply cold packs (Figure 9-25).
- Pad gaps between the splint and limb as well as bony areas.
- Do not place cravats or other straps over a fracture site because this may cause further injury.

Full-Body Immobilization

Backboarding provides spinal immobilization for a traumatic injury. Before backboarding a trauma patient, apply a **cervical immobilization device (CID)**, often called a cervical collar, to stabilize the neck (Figure 9-26). This device is intended to maintain the cervical spine and head in a **neutral inline alignment** (the natural anatomical position of the head and neck with the eyes looking forward and the chin at a 90-degree angle from the long axis of the body). Make certain the CID is the correct size and placed according to the manufacturer specifications. Maintain manual neck stabilization at all times while the CID is applied and until the head is immobilized onto a backboard. The EMR must be adept when dealing with a potential cervical spine injury and applying the cervical collar. **Skill 9-12** demonstrates the placement of a cervical collar.

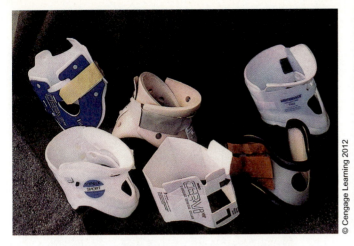

Figure 9-26 Several different sizes of cervical spine immobilization devices are available.

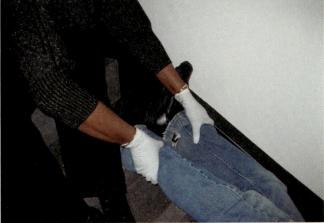

Figure 9-27 A patient who has fallen down the stairs must be held securely by the feet and legs while an assessment is done.

Short Backboard

Short backboards, or **short spinal immobilization devices (SSIDs)**, are used for immobilizing a patient with a possible cervical or other spinal injury who is found in a sitting position, such as in a motor vehicle. After the patient's neck is manually stabilized and a cervical collar is placed, the application of the SSID is used to temporarily stabilize the patient's spine during transfer to a long backboard. The SSID is always transferred to a long backboard for transport. See **Skill 9-13** for a demonstration of the application of a short spinal immobilization device.

Long Backboard

The long backboard is used when a patient requires a full-body spinal immobilization. The patient's nose, navel, and toes need to be in a straight line. With a cervical collar in place, one of the more difficult procedures an EMR can experience is immobilization of a potential spinal injury when the patient is found in the prone position. A demonstration of a full-body spinal immobilization is found in **Skill 9-14** at the end of the chapter.

Many times there are a limited number of EMRs responding to a patient with a possible spinal injury who is in a supine position. The method used most often in the field to move a supine patient to a long backboard is called the modified logroll. **Skill 9-15** demonstrates the modified method of performing a logroll on a supine patient.

If the patient has fallen down a flight of stairs or is found on a slope, the EMR will need to successfully move the patient to a long backboard without causing further injury. One EMR must grasp the feet of the patient to keep him from moving down the stairs or incline while another EMR stabilizes the head (Figure 9-27).

There are times when the EMR may be confronted by a patient who is in the standing position after an accident or vehicle crash and complaining of neck pain. The EMR will require a minimum of four people to transfer this patient from the standing position to the long backboard. First the EMR stabilizes the cervical spine of the patient. CMS is checked, and the cervical collar is placed on the patient. Other EMRs stabilize the backboard and secure the patient across the chest under the arms. The patient is then lowered to the floor and secured to the backboard. **Skill 9-16** illustrates the transfer of a patient from a standing position to the long backboard.

The seven-person lift is used when a patient has potential spinal injuries and is found supine. The lift requires seven EMRs and provides the best immobilization lift for the patient. Initially, the EMRs use spinal immobilization and placement of the cervical collar. Six EMRs position themselves over the patient, carefully placing their hands under the patient, while one EMR continues to hold the head for cervical stabilization. The patient should be lifted no more than three or four inches, just enough to slide a long backboard from the feet of the patient to the EMR at the head. When the long backboard is in place, the EMRs, on command, lower the patient and secure him to the long backboard. CMS is checked before and after the move. Figure 9-28 illustrates the placement of the EMRs and their hands during a seven-person lift.

Rapid Extrication

There are times when an EMR must make a decision to rapidly remove a patient from a vehicle. This will require manual stabilization of the spine of an unstable patient who may have a spinal injury as a result of motor vehicle crash. If time permits, move the SSID to the long backboard; if not, perform a rapid extrication as demonstrated in **Skill 9-17**, noting that CMS must be checked before and after extrication.

Pediatric Challenges

Because a child's head is larger in relation to the body than that of an adult, a child's neutral inline alignment may be compromised on a backboard, causing the neck to flex

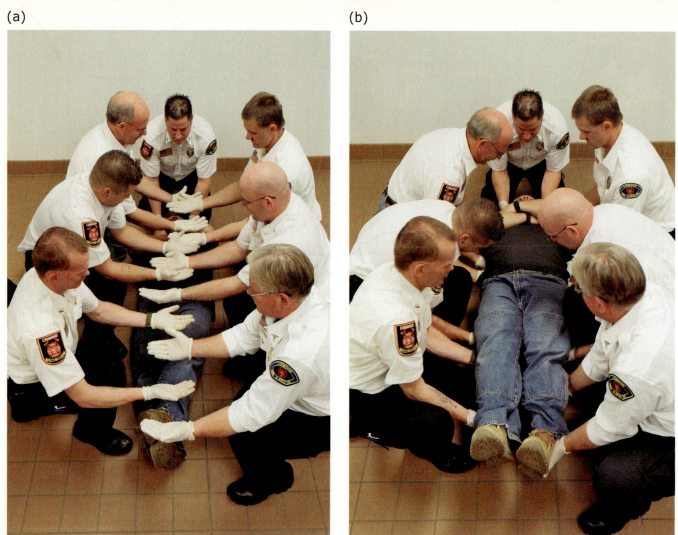

Figure 9-28 (a) Note the body and hand positioning of the men doing the lifting. (b) The Emergency Medical Responders carefully place their hands under the patient, lifting him no more than three or four inches off the floor, just enough to slide in a backboard.

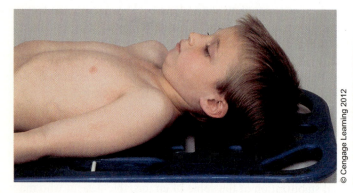

Figure 9-29 When lying flat, the child's head forces the neck into a flexed position.

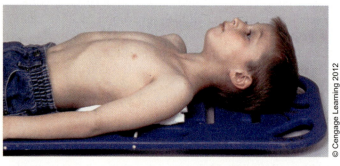

Figure 9-30 Padding behind the child's body from the shoulders to the heels puts the neck in a neutral position when the child is placed on a backboard.

significantly toward the chest. This flexed position is illustrated in Figure 9-29. To maintain a 90-degree angle of the jaw to the long axis of the body, you will need to use a pediatric backboard, which accommodates for the child's larger occiput (back of the head), or place padding beneath the child's shoulders to compensate (Figure 9-30).

Helmet Challenges

If a patient wearing a helmet is involved in a traumatic incident with a possible spinal injury, you must use special safety precautions before deciding whether to remove the helmet. If the patient's airway and breathing can be accessed and managed, you may choose to leave the helmet on the patient. If you leave on the helmet, the patient should be secured to the long backboard by placing extra padding under the shoulders similar to the method used with a pediatric patient.

If the patient's airway and breathing cannot be managed or if the patient has signs of apnea, obstructed airway, inadequate respirations, or vomiting or needs cardiopulmonary resuscitation, the helmet must be carefully removed. Helmets come in various types and styles. See **Skill 9-18** for the procedure of removing a motorcycle-type helmet with a full face shield from a patient with a possible spinal injury.

Application of a Commercial Tourniquet

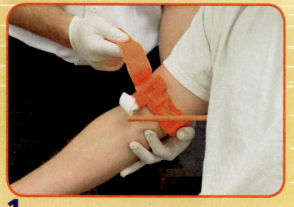

1 Place the commercial tourniquet just above the injury.

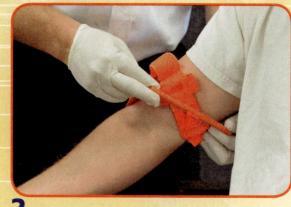

2 Tighten the windlass until bleeding stops.

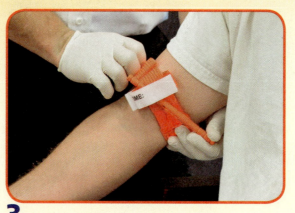

3 Secure the windlass. Note the time of placement.

Application of a Cravat as a Tourniquet

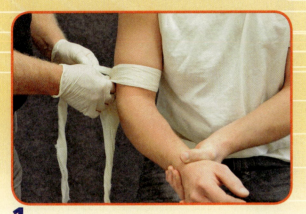

1 Make certain the cravat is at least two inches wide and placed above the injury.

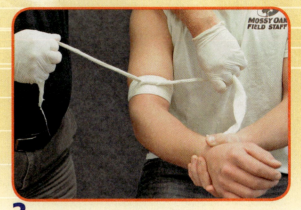

2 Make one wrap around the extremity; tie a knot tightly in the center of the cravat.

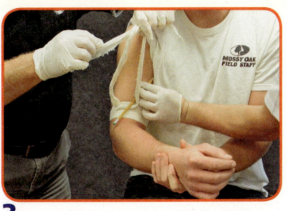

3 Place a windless on the center of the knot and tighten it to the cravat.

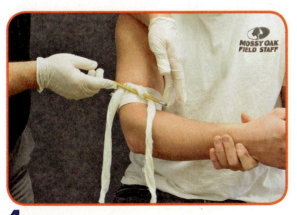

4 Tighten the windlass until bleeding stops.

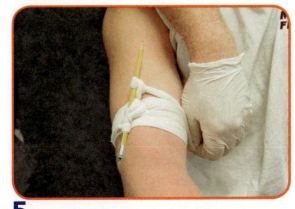

5 Secure the windlass. Note the time of placement.

© Cengage Learning 2012

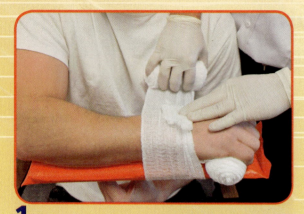

1 Anchor the bandage by angling the end of the first wrap using one recurrent turn.

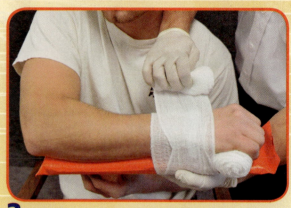

2 Fold the angled tab down and continue with a recurrent turn.

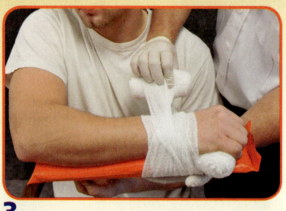

3 Use twists at intervals to secure the bandage and prevent further bleeding.

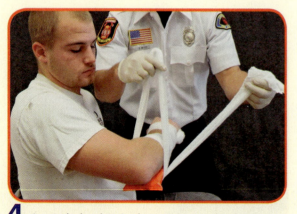

4 Secure the bandage in place using excess bandage material.

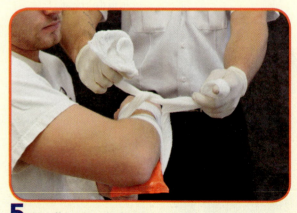

5 Tie off using excess bandage material.

Stabilizing an Impaled Object with a Roller Bandage

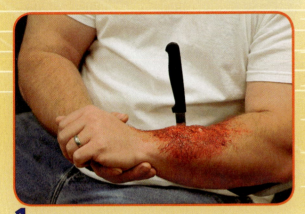

1 The patient is placed in a position of comfort.

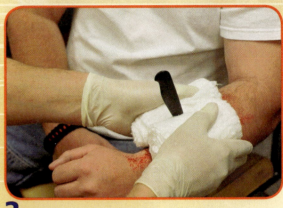

2 Place a roll of gauze on both sides of the object for support and stabilization.

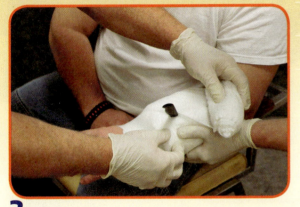

3 Wrap the gauze with recurrent turns and then use a figure-of-eight turn.

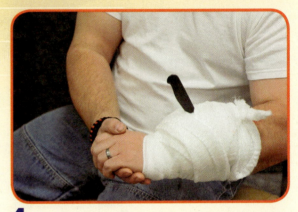

4 Continue wrapping around the object with figure-of-eight turns, ending with recurrent turns. Then secure the ends.

Stabilizing an Impaled Object with a Donut Made from a Cravat

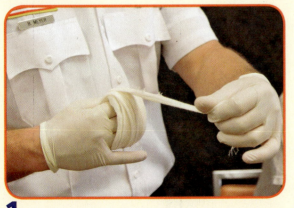

1 A cravat can be rolled around the fingers several times to form a donut-shaped bandage.

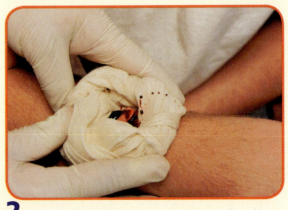

2 The donut can then be placed over the protruding object and secured to the body.

© Cengage Learning 2012

Skill 9-4 Application of an Eye Bandage

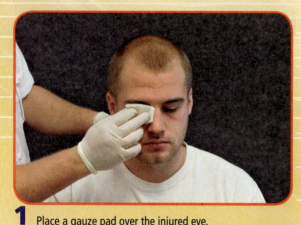

1 Place a gauze pad over the injured eye.

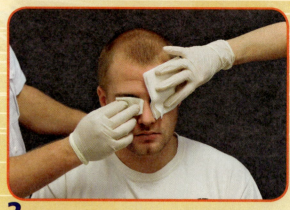

2 Place a second gauze pad over the uninjured eye to prevent movement.

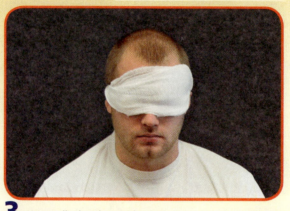

3 Use a roller bandage with recurrent turns to secure the dressings in place.

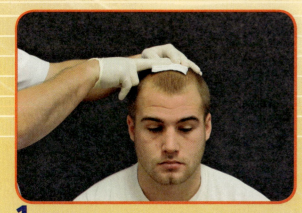

1 Place a gauze dressing over the head wound to control bleeding.

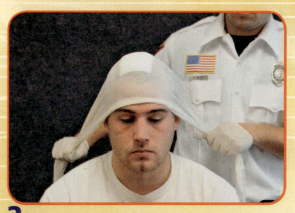

2 Place a triangular bandage on the head with the apex (pointed end) to the back of the head.

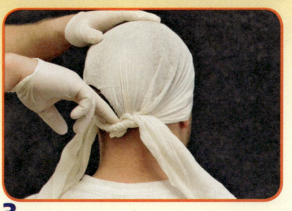

3 Tie the bandage low in the back of the head over the apex. Tighten and secure the bandage over the dressing by pulling on the apex.

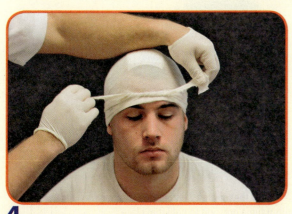

4 Bring the ends around to the front and tie in the middle of the forehead.

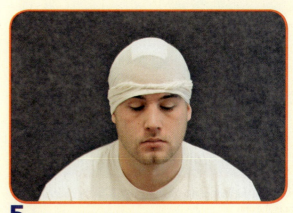

5 Secure the ends of the bandage.

© Cengage Learning 2012

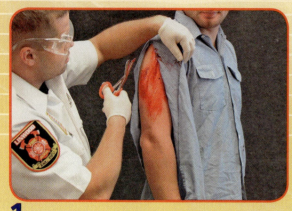

1 Cut the shirt, if necessary, to expose the wound to the shoulder.

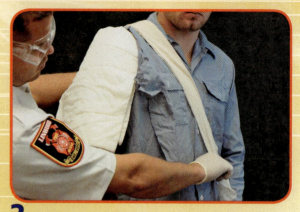

2 Place a multi-trauma dressing over the wound and a cravat over the shoulder.

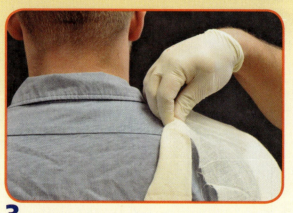

3 Place the apex of a triangular bandage at the top of the shoulder. Wrap it under the cravat three times to secure it.

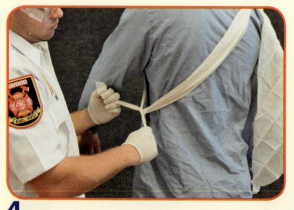

4 Bring the ends of the cravat to the side of the patient under the arm and tie the cravat.

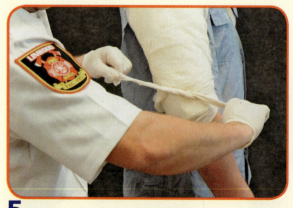

5 Wrap the tales of the triangular bandage around the multi-trauma dressing to hold it in place.

© Cengage Learning 2012

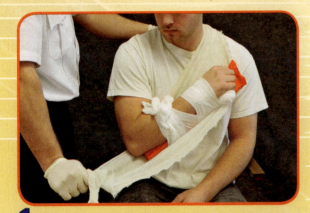

1 Place the triangular bandage, as shown, under the splint. Tie a knot in the apex to keep the elbow from slipping.

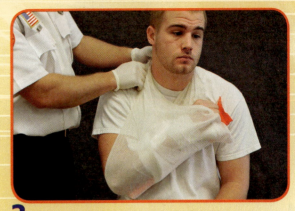

2 Cross the ends of the triangular bandage over the patient's shoulder and tie them. Be careful to pad the knot at the side of the neck.

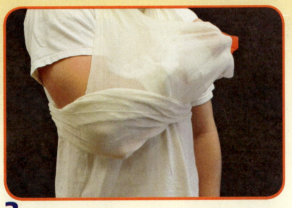

3 Secure the sling with a swathe that is wrapped around the body and tied on the patient's side. Part of the swathe can be pulled over the elbow to further immobilize the arm.

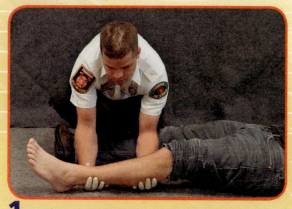

1 Check for CMS. Then with your hands under the patient's leg, support the patient's leg above and below the fracture site.

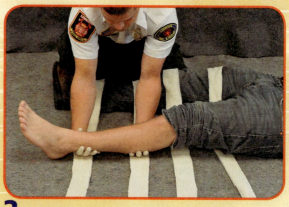

2 A second EMR can then place cravat bandages crosswise under the patient's leg.

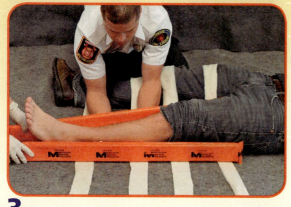

3 Place padded rigid splints on either side of the leg while it is still being supported.

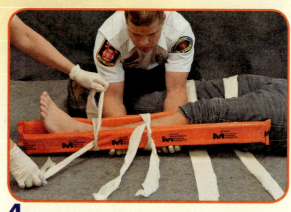

4 Tie the cravats above and below the fracture site. Tie any knots on the side of the splint, not over the fracture.

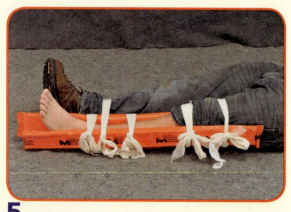

5 Tie the remaining cravats on the fractured leg. Secure the other leg to the rigid splint with a cravat.

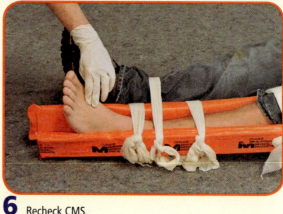

6 Recheck CMS.

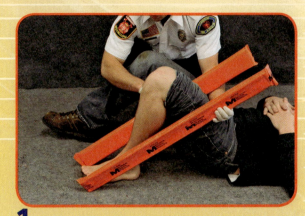

1 Check for CMS. Place a rigid splint on either side of the knee joint without straightening the leg.

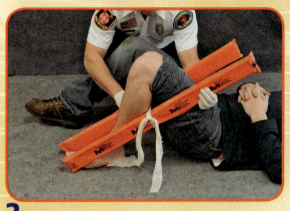

2 Place the center cravat underneath the knee and wrapped around the two splints. Tie together the splints at that point.

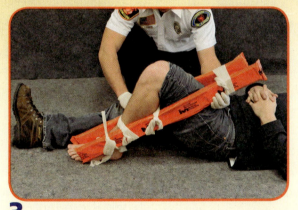

3 Using a cravat, tie the top of the rigid splints together and then the bottom of the splints together, as shown. When finished, tie the uninjured leg to the splint for immobilization. Recheck CMS.

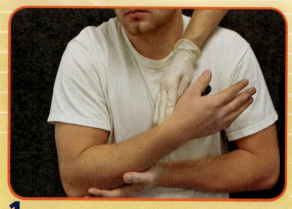

1 The patient is found self-splinting the forearm fracture. Check CMS.

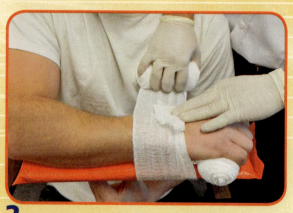

2 Place a rigid splint under the arm and anchors it with a roller bandage. Place the hand in the position of function.

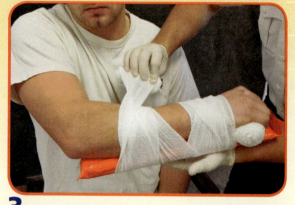

3 Secure the rigid splint with a reverse twist. Do not cover the fracture site.

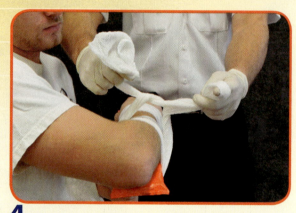

4 Prepare to tie off the roller bandage. After the rigid splint is secured to the arm, recheck CMS.

Skill 9-11 Immobilization of a Closed Femur Fracture with a Traction Splint

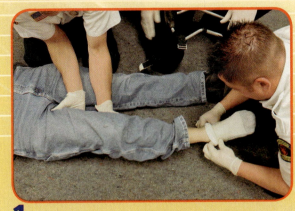

1 Manually stabilize the limb while another rescuer removes the sock; check CMS; and prepare to apply gentle traction.

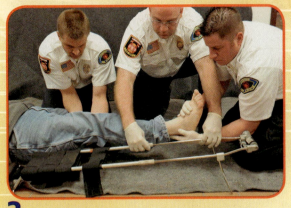

2 Prepare the traction device by measuring the splint against the uninjured leg first and then extending the splint about six inches longer than the uninjured leg.

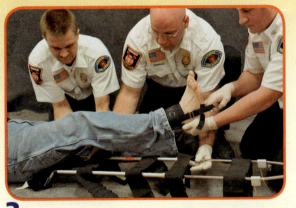

3 Apply the ankle hitch to the ankle and gently slide the traction splint under the leg.

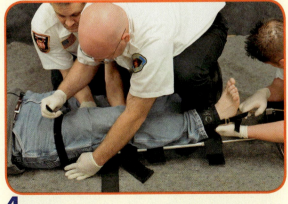

4 Secure the ischial strap across the thigh. Place the other straps so that one is above and one is below the fracture, one is at the knee, and the last is above the ankle. Do not secure these straps at this time.

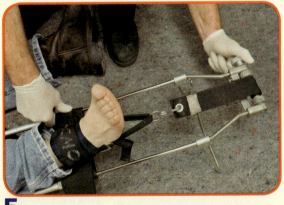

5 Attach the windlass to the ring on the ankle hitch and apply traction until the patient feels some relief, or if the patient is unconscious, until the calf muscle tightens. Secure the remaining straps in place and recheck CMS.

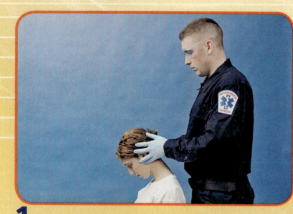

1 Move the patient's head into neutral alignment. If the patient complains of pain or you feels resistance, the patient's neck should be splinted in position found.

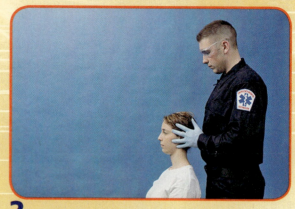

2 Maintain continuous manual stabilization of the patient's head throughout the rest of the procedure.

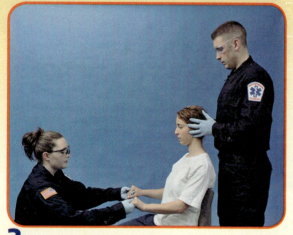

3 A second EMR checks for CMS.

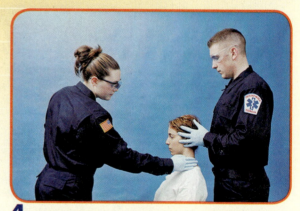

4 The second EMR then measures the patient's neck for a cervical collar, according to the manufacturer's recommendations.

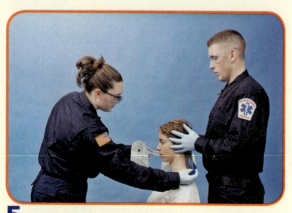

5 Slide the posterior portion of the collar into the void behind the patient's neck.

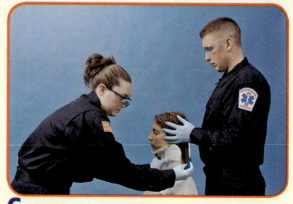

6 Cupping the chin piece in one hand, the second EMR slides the anterior portion of the collar up the chest until it captures the chin.

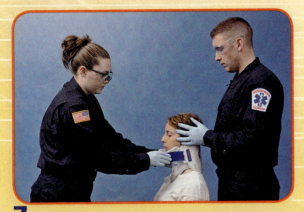

7 With the collar in place, fasten the Velcro securely in place.

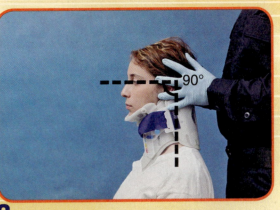

8 Checking for a proper collar fit, the second EMR mentally draws a line from the opening of the ear to the middle of the shoulder and from the opening of the ear to the eyes. The imagined angle should be 90 degrees.

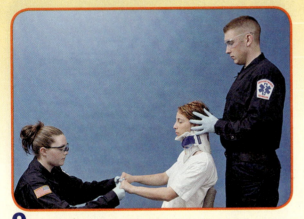

9 The second EMR rechecks CMS.

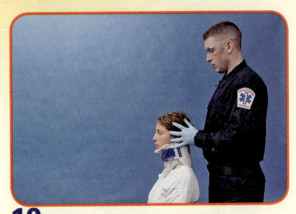

10 The EMR at the head must maintain continuous stabilization despite the presence of the cervical collar. The patient is now ready to be placed on a short spinal immobilization device.

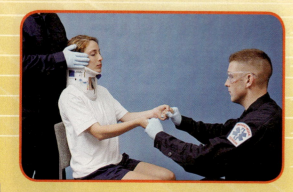

1 Manually stabilize the cervical spine. A second EMR applies the cervical collar. Check CMS.

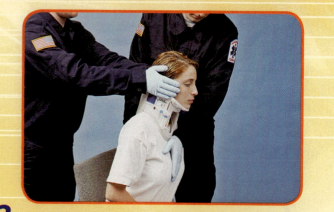

2 While one EMR maintains continuous manual stabilization, the other EMR places his arms along the anterior and posterior thorax. The patient may now be moved forward as a unit, keeping the spine in line.

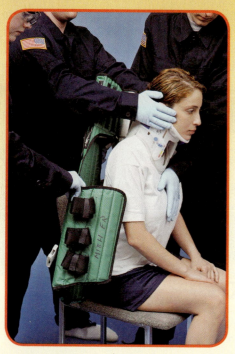

3 The SSID is then positioned carefully behind the patient, and the patient is moved back against the device.

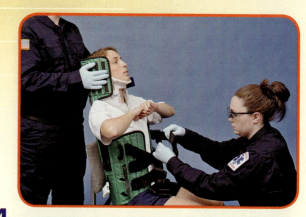

4 Secure the patient to the SSID with the middle strap first, abdominal strap second, and the top strap last, being careful not to tighten the top too much as it can impede breathing. Secure the leg straps if the SSID has them.

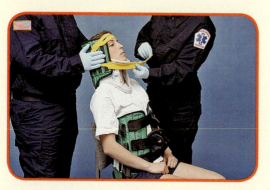

5 Pad the void behind the head, if needed, and then secure the patient's head to the SSID, fastening the top strap first and then the chin strap.

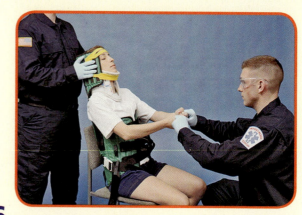

6 Reassess for CMS before transferring the patient to a long backboard.

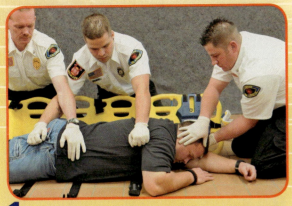

1 The EMR at the patient's head applies spinal stabilization as other EMRs position themselves to one side of the patient. The backboard is pushed up against the patient, and the straps are tucked under the patient. A check for CMS is done.

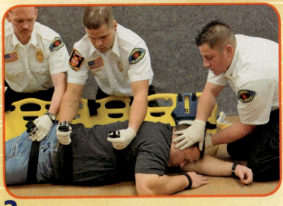

2 The EMRs tighten the straps to the patient while another EMR, at the end of the backboard, handles stabilization of the head.

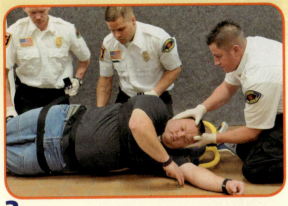

3 The EMR at the head gives the command to roll the patient from his stomach to his side against the backboard.

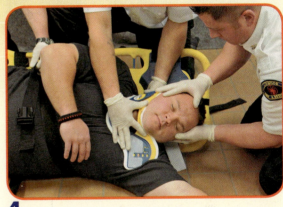

4 The cervical collar is placed on the patient.

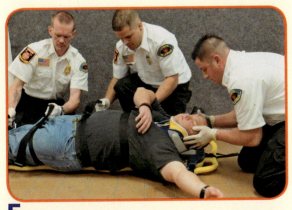

5 The EMR at the head gives the command to roll the patient as a unit onto the backboard into a supine position.

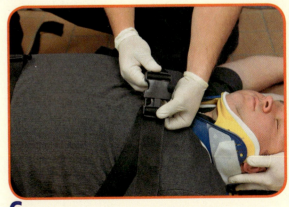

6 Straps are then readjusted and tightened, beginning at the chest, being careful not to tighten the chest strap too tightly as to impede breathing. Strapping is continued with the abdominal strap next followed by the upper legs and then the lower legs.

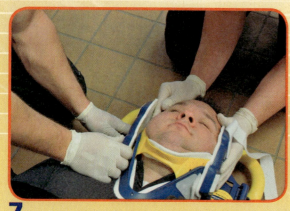

7 The EMR at the head places the head block in place.

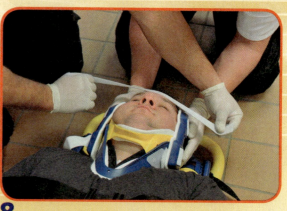

8 The head strap is placed on the patient.

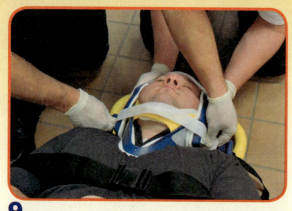

9 The EMR places the chin strap on the patient if protocol allows.

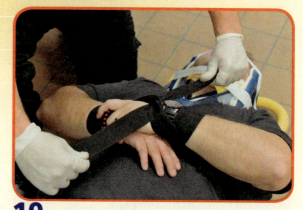

10 The EMR secures the patient's arms together and rechecks for CMS.

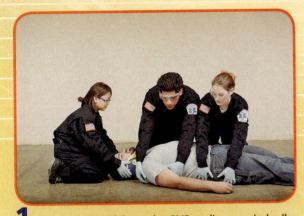

1 Check for CMS while another EMR applies a cervical collar. One EMR then holds manual stabilization of the neck while two more EMRs take positions at the patient's shoulder and pelvis, reaching across the patient and grasping the patient's shoulder and pelvis, respectively.

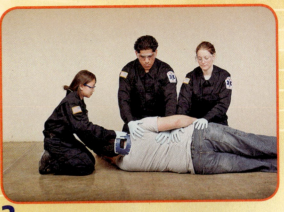

2 On command, the three EMRs roll the patient onto his side. The bottom arm should be extended away from the patient's side. Do not roll the patient on top of this arm.

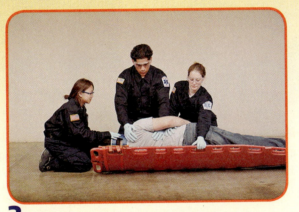

3 One EMR pulls the long backboard into place under the patient.

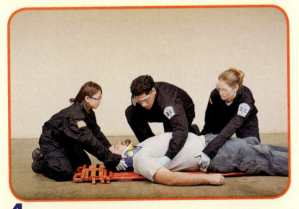

4 On command, the patient is rolled as a unit onto the backboard, and the patient is pulled up to the center of the board, using the long axis drag.

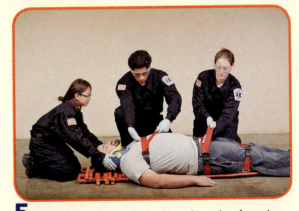

5 Secure the patient to the backboard in order of top, then middle, and then bottom straps. Place the head block and secures the patient's head to the block. Recheck for CMS.

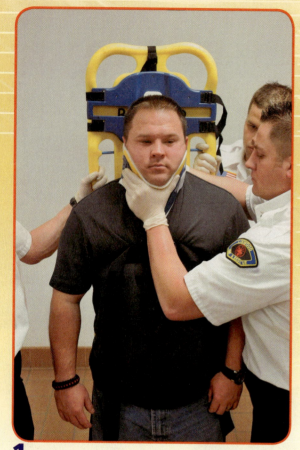

1 Stabilize the cervical spine of the standing patient; check for CMS and place the cervical collar.

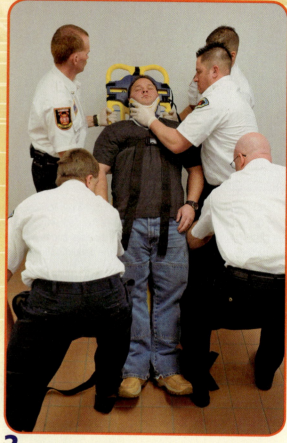

2 Secure the patient to the board while standing, at the chest area, then lowered to the floor on the backboard and completely secured before transfer.

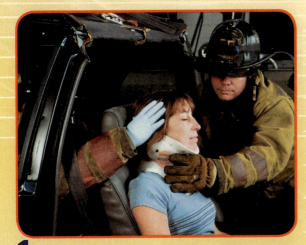

1 Check CMS. Move the patient's head to a neutral position and have another EMR apply a properly sized cervical collar.

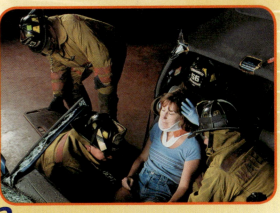

2 With an EMR on each side of the patient, the patient is gently lifted a couple of inches so a long spine board may be inserted under the patient's buttocks.

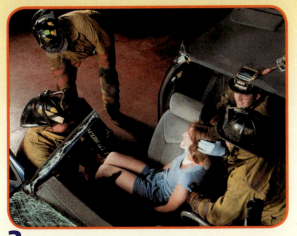

3 While an EMR continues to maintain manual stabilization of the spine, one EMR grasps the patient under the arms while another grasps the patient at the hips. Then, on command, the EMR rotates the patient to the side about 45 degrees. At this point, the EMRs may need to switch places if the car's B post becomes an obstruction. After two or three small turns to rotate the patient, the patient should be parallel to the long spine board.

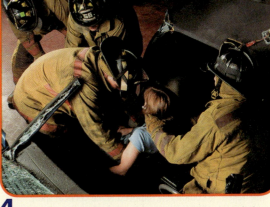

4 After the patient is parallel to the long spine board, the patient is lowered, as a rigid unit, to the long spine board while the EMRs maintain inline stabilization.

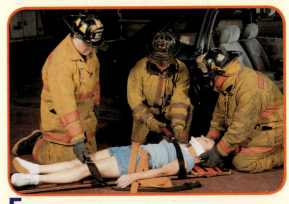

5 After the patient is on the long spine board, securely fasten the body and then the head and recheck the patient's CMS.

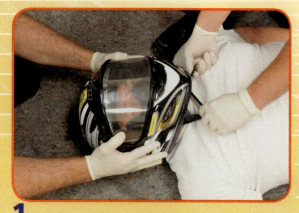

1 One EMR stabilizes the helmet while the other EMR cuts or unties the helmet strap. Check for CMS.

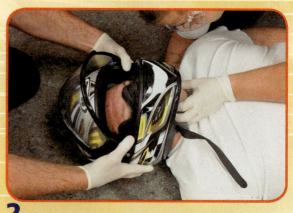

2 The EMR at the helmet slowly pulls the helmet back at a slight upward tilt while the second EMR stabilizes the cervical spine with one hand under the neck on the occiput and supports the chin with the other hand.

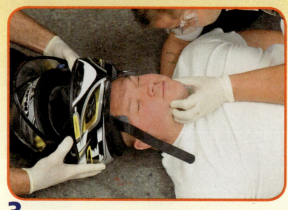

3 The helmet is completely removed while cervical spine stabilization is maintained.

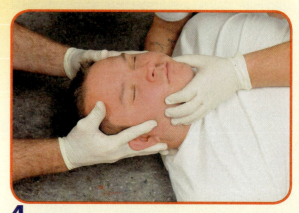

4 The second rescuer transfers spinal stabilization to the rescuer at the head. A cervical collar is placed on the patient. The patient is ready to be moved to a backboard and to have CMS rechecked.

SUMMARY

The EMR must understand the basics for applying various types of dressings, bandages, splints, and spinal immobilization devices. Practicing and mastering the skill sets in each area will prevent further injury to the patient.

REVIEW QUESTIONS

1. A bandage _____
   A. holds a dressing in place
   B. is placed directly over the wound
   C. must be sterile
   D. covers major wounds

2. Long bone fractures where no distal pulse or signs of circulation are found
   A. should never be straightened
   B. should be straightened by a trained responder
   C. must be splinted in position found by a trained responder
   D. is not a true emergency

3. What is "position of function?"
   A. The position the EMR finds the fracture
   B. The natural position of the hand or foot
   C. The manual repositioning of the fracture
   D. The manual reduction of an angulated fracture

4. When is a short backboard used?
   A. When a patient is lying supine
   B. When a patient is prone
   C. When a patient is sitting in a vehicle
   D. When a patient is in the water

5. The first thing you would do when finding a patient sitting in a vehicle after a collision would be to:
   A. place a cervical collar
   B. place the patient in a supine position
   C. place manual stabilization on the patient's head
   D. place the patient on a short backboard

6. An indication for removing a helmet from a possible spinal injury patient
   A. is the patient stable?
   B. does the patient insist on removing the helmet?
   C. does the patient have apnea?
   D. is the patient walking around?

7. What type of bandage would you use on a possible sprained ankle? _____

8. Bleeding is controlled on a forearm. To hold the dressing in place what bandage would you use? _____ _____

9. What are three methods used to stabilize an impaled object in the lower leg?
   _____,
   _____, _____

10. After a splint is applied, how would you provide support to a closed fracture of the upper arm? _____ _____ _____

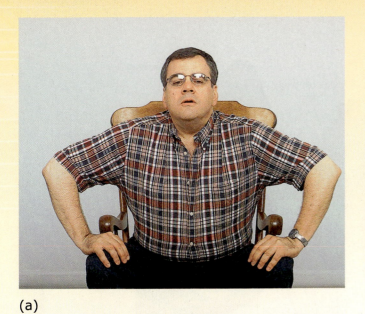

(a)

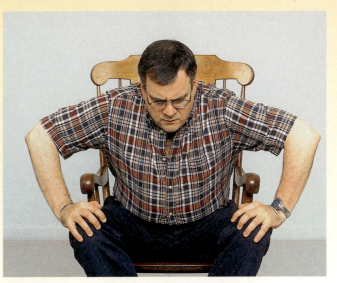

(b)

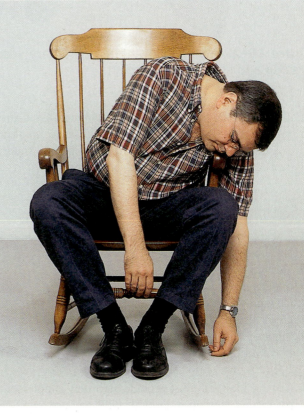

(c)

(d)

Figure 10-1 (a) The patient with respiratory distress will often be found sitting upright in a tripod position, using accessory muscles to assist in breathing. (b) As hypoxia worsens, the patient will often become anxious. (c) The patient with dyspnea may become tired because working to breathe is taxing. (d) The non-alert, cyanotic patient is extremely sick and in need of immediate oxygenation.

© Cengage Learning 2012

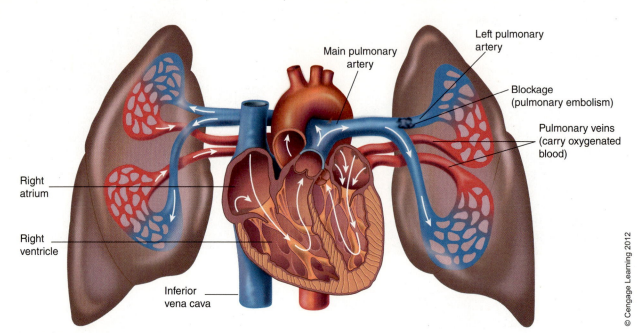

Figure 10-2 A blood clot in the pulmonary vessels will block oxygenation of the blood, resulting in hypoxia and shortness of breath.

usually show a sudden onset of difficulty breathing. Causes for pulmonary embolism include heart disease, smoking, major surgery, fractures, cancer, immobility, and trauma. Figure 10-2 illustrates this serious condition.

Signs and Symptoms of Pulmonary Embolism

- Unexplained shortness of breath with a sudden onset
- Difficulty breathing
- Tachypnea
- Sudden onset of chest pain
- Coughing up blood
- Cyanosis
- Signs of shock or cardiac arrest

Management of Pulmonary Embolism

- Critical interventions: provide high flow supplemental oxygen or ventilation, provide CPR and use an AED if indicated, treat for shock, and seek rapid transport.
- Allow a position of comfort or if supine prop upper body at approximately a 45-degree angle (Fowler's position).
- Keep the patient calm.
- Reassess every five minutes.

Asthma

Asthma is a chronic condition that causes narrowing of the airways. Airways can become narrowed by **bronchospasms** (a sudden contraction of the smooth muscle of the bronchi), and inflammation of the bronchial tubes. This narrowing may be complicated by the production of secretions. If the airway is completely obstructed, the condition may be life threatening.

Asthma can be caused by an **allergen** (a substance that causes an allergic reaction in certain people). Asthma emergencies may be triggered by cigarette smoke, pollen, pet dander, cold air, physical exertion, anxiety, or stress. Figure 10-3 illustrates the pathophysiology in the airways during an asthma attack.

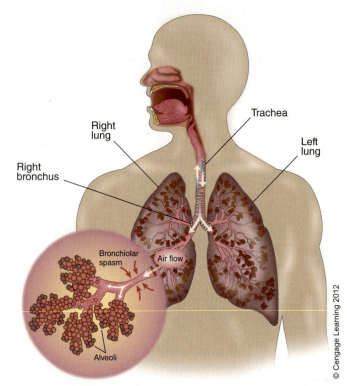

Figure 10-3 Asthma is a condition that involves bronchospasm and excessive airway secretions.

Signs and Symptoms of Asthma

- Shortness of breath, tachypnea
- Wheezing sounds
- Tightness or pain in the chest
- Bluish color of lips and face
- Anxiety

Management of Asthma

- Critical interventions: provide supplemental oxygen or ventilation and seek rapid transport.
- Allow a position of comfort.
- If the patient has a metered dose inhaler or dry powder inhaler, assist in administering medication. This medication can decrease bronchospasms and inflammation, as well as dilate the airway.
  - Check to be certain the inhaler belongs to the patient.
  - Shake a metered dose inhaler.
  - Have the patient exhale fully through her mouth, releasing as much air as possible. With the inhaler held upright, she should close her lip tightly on the mouth piece (Figure 10-4). And then while she inhales deeply through her mouth, have the patient discharge the medication and hold her breath for as long as possible up to approximately ten seconds. Repeat as prescribed.
  - The patient may use a spacer device with their inhaler, as shown in Figure 10-5.
  - The EMR only assists with the medication and does not administer it.
  - To prepare a dry powder disk inhaler, slide or twist a lever to expose the mouthpiece. Have the patient breathe in deeply and rapidly to discharge medication.
- Remove the patient from the irritant or the irritant from the patient.
- Try to calm the patient by allowing her to feel a fan or air on her, talking calmly, and providing a calm environment.
- Reassess every five minutes.

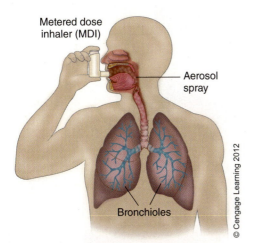

Figure 10-4 A metered-dose inhaler aerosolizes medication for inhalation directly into the airways. The Emergency Medical Responder should be familiar with the use of an inhaler so she may assist a patient with its use.

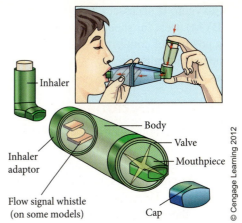

Figure 10-5 A spacer is a device that is commonly used in conjunction with an inhaler, especially by children, to effectively administer the medication.

Chronic Obstructive Pulmonary Disease

Chronic obstructive pulmonary disease (COPD) is a group of lung diseases that block airflow and make it increasingly difficult to breathe. COPD is chronic and can be caused by bronchospasm; inflammation; or irreversible causes of airway narrowing, such as scaring and destruction of air sacs. Two main types of COPD are chronic bronchitis and emphysema. A patient with **chronic bronchitis** produces excessive mucus and has swelling and thickening of the lining of the lower airways. The narrowed lower airway and thick mucus production prevent adequate airflow to the alveoli. The alveoli do not fully expand, causing respiratory distress and **hypoxia**, which is a deficiency in oxygen in the cells.

Emphysema, similar to chronic bronchitis, restricts air flow in the lower airways but also directly affects the elasticity of lung tissue. This irreversible loss of elasticity causes air to become trapped and the alveoli are chronically enlarged. Gas exchange is significantly disrupted. A patient works hard to exhale to rid the body of excess carbon dioxide. Cigarette smoking is one major cause of COPD. Respiratory infections, such as pneumonia, can exacerbate symptoms.

Signs and Symptoms of Chronic Bronchitis

- Difficulty breathing
- Use of accessory muscles while breathing
- Intense and productive cough with mucus

Signs and Symptoms of Emphysema

- Productive cough
- Barrel chest (large, rounded chest)
- Difficulty breathing, especially exhaling

Management of Chronic Bronchitis and Emphysema

- Critical interventions: provide supplemental oxygen initially with low-flow oxygen at 2 lpm via nasal cannula. If breathing continues to be compromised increase the flow of oxygen. If necessary, ventilate with a bag valve mask (BVM), treat for shock, and seek rapid transport.

- Allow a position of comfort.
- Keep the patient calm.
- Reassess every five minutes.

Respiratory Infections

Lower respiratory infections, such as pneumonia, can be caused by a virus or bacteria. The body's response creates inflammation and excess secretions in the lower airways of the lung. This results in narrowing the airways, making adequate ventilation difficult. Respiratory infections can exacerbate asthma and COPD. If severe, these infections can be life threatening, especially in a patient with a weakened immune system.

Signs and Symptoms of Respiratory Infection

- Fever or chills
- Nasal congestion
- Cough with green or yellow mucus
- Chest pain, especially with deep breathing or cough
- Fatigue
- Dyspnea
- Confusion, AMS
- Fever and chills

Management of Respiratory Infection

- Critical interventions: provide supplemental oxygen or ventilation.
- Allow a position of comfort.
- Reassess every five minutes.

Hyperventilation

Hyperventilation, overbreathing, is caused by a patient's breathing faster and deeper than normal. Hyperventilation can be caused by psychological reasons (such as anxiety and panic attacks) or by physiological reasons (such as in trauma or severe illness).

Signs and Symptoms of Hyperventilation

- Deep, rapid breathing
- Weakness
- Unsteadiness
- Lightheadedness
- Tingling or numbness around the mouth and fingertips
- Cramping of the fingers or toes

Management of Hyperventilation

- Critical interventions: provide supplemental oxygen or ventilation.
- Help the patient control breathing if it is caused by anxiety.
  - Instruct the patient to breathe only when you touch her hand.
  - Have the patient take a deep breath and then slowly exhale. Repeat.

- If the patient cannot slowly exhale, the problem may not be anxiety.
- Do not have the patient breathe into a paper bag. Hyperventilation may be associated with a more serious respiratory emergency. The patient then will need oxygenation, not exhaled carbon dioxide.
- Allow a position of comfort.

Cardiovascular Medical Emergencies

Cardiovascular emergencies involve the heart and blood vessels. Causes include narrowing of arteries, blood clots, and blood vessel spasms, which can all prevent adequate blood oxygenation. Because the circulatory system and the respiratory system are interrelated, cardiovascular and respiratory complications coexist. Early recognition and transport are critical.

Myocardial Infarction

Chest pain, also called **angina pectoris**, can occur when coronary (heart) arteries narrow or are blocked. With severe or total blockage, lack of oxygenated blood to the heart muscle causes an area or areas of the heart to die (Figure 10-6). This is called a heart attack or acute **myocardial infarction (MI).** Sudden-onset symptoms may be caused by physical exertion; emotional stress; extreme temperatures; cigarette smoking; eating a heavy meal; or use of stimulants, such as caffeine or cocaine. Chest pain and discomfort are classic symptoms, but other symptoms can indicate MI as well (Figure 10-7). Women's major symptoms are not usually the classic symptoms, and they include unusual fatigue, shortness of breath, feeling faint, and indigestion. Many patients do not recognize the symptoms and deny that they are experiencing a cardiovascular event (Figure 10-8).

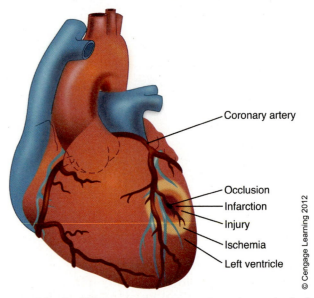

Coronary artery

Occlusion

Infarction

Injury

Ischemia

Left ventricle

© Cengage Learning 2012

Figure 10-6 When a coronary artery is occluded, the heart muscle, the myocardium can die.

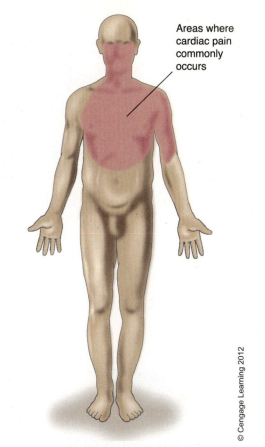

Areas where cardiac pain commonly occurs

© Cengage Learning 2012

Figure 10-7 Any pain from the "nose to the navel" is assumed to be cardiac until proven otherwise.

Assessment Tools for Chest Pain and Myocardial Infarction

After performing an initial assessment, providing critical interventions, and obtaining baseline vital signs, use the following assessment tools: SAMPLE, OPQRST, and pulse oximetry, if available. Obtaining the subjective information with SAMPLE is extremely important in regard to symptoms, pertinent past cardiac history, knowledge of use of medications such as nitroglycerin, and events leading up to the incident. Make sure that reassessment includes a trending of a pain rating. Look for medical identification jewelry on the neck, wrist, or ankle.

Signs and Symptoms of Myocardial Infarction

- Chest pain or discomfort described as pressure, squeezing, a vise grip, or a heavy weight on his chest
- Unexplained pain in the shoulder, back, jaw, or neck
- Pain radiating from the center of the chest to one or both arms
- Dyspnea, or a feeling of not having enough air
- Lightheadedness
- Indigestion or heartburn
- Nausea or vomiting
- Diaphoresis, or cold sweats

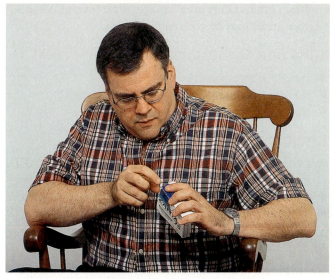

© Cengage Learning 2012

Figure 10-8 Many patients deny they are having a heart attack, thinking "it's only indigestion."

- Fast or irregular pulse, feels like the heart skips a beat or is racing
- Pale, grey, cyanotic skin color
- Weakness, unusual fatigue
- Feelings of impending doom, anxiety, irritability
- Altered mental status (AMS)

Management of MI

- Critical interventions: provide supplemental oxygen or ventilation, provide CPR and use an AED if indicated, treat for shock, and seek rapid transport.
- Have the patient stop activity.
- Allow a position of comfort or assist to a Fowler's position.
- Ask if the patient has taken any nitroglycerin or aspirin. If not, suggest and assist with a chewable regular aspirin and nitroglycerin, if local protocols dictate. An EMR can only assist in giving any medication. For nitroglycerin:
  - Identify that nitroglycerin belongs to the patient.
  - Assist with giving no more than three nitroglycerin tablets or sprays in 15 minutes, with each dose administered at 5 minute intervals.
  - Be aware that nitroglycerin can lower blood pressure.
  - Monitor vital signs and symptoms between each tablet. Many protocols state that if there is a systolic blood pressure below 100 mm Hg, additional nitroglycerin tablets should not be given. Also, ask the patient if he is feeling lightheaded, because this may be a sign of too low of a blood pressure for adequate perfusion.
- Keep the patient calm.
- Reassess every five minutes.

Cardiac Arrest

Cardiac arrest occurs when the heart stops beating. Causes can include MI, stroke, trauma, suffocation, severe allergic reaction, seizures, diabetic emergencies, drug overdose, poisoning, or choking. Respiratory arrest (cessation of breathing) often occurs after cardiac arrest or in children respiratory arrest may precede cardiac arrest.

Signs and Symptoms of Cardiac Arrest

- Patient is unresponsive
- No breathing or no normal breathing (gasping)
- No signs of perfusion

Management of Cardiac Arrest

- Critical interventions: provide CPR and use an AED. Provide ventilations with BVM at 100 percent oxygen.
- Follow the current American Heart Association guidelines.
- Seek rapid transport.

Heart Failure

Heart failure is a condition that affects one or both sides of the heart muscle resulting in an inability to pump a sufficient amount of oxygenated blood to meet the metabolic needs of the body, especially with activity. Blood backs up into the lungs and other areas of the body causing congestion. The accumulation of fluid is called edema and is often most evident visibly in the ankles and feet. Accumulation of fluid in the lungs is called **pulmonary edema**. Medications and fluid restrictions are used to decrease or eliminate the edema. Heart failure is often caused by a weakening of the heart from heart valve disease, heart attacks, hypertension, and diabetes.

Assessment Tools for Heart Failure

After performing an initial assessment providing critical interventions, and obtaining baseline vital signs, assessment tools used are SAMPLE, OPQRST, and a pulse oximeter reading, if available. When using SAMPLE, pay close attention to past pertinent history and medications used. When performing a survey on the legs, observe for swelling of the ankles and feet. Look for medical identification jewelry.

Signs and Symptoms of Heart Failure

- Dyspnea, tachypnea
- Use of accessory muscles such as pursed-lip breathing
- Assuming a tripod position
- Tachycardia or irregular pulse
- Coughing or spitting up of frothy, blood-tinged fluid
- Jugular vein distension (Figure 10-9)
- Crackling or wheezing sounds with respirations
- Extreme fatigue
- Recent weight gain
- Edema especially of the ankles and feet (Figure 10-9)
- Pale, grey, cyanotic skin color

Management of Heart Failure

- Critical interventions: provide supplemental high-flow oxygen or ventilation, provide CPR and use AED if indicated, and seek rapid transport.
- Keep the patient at rest.

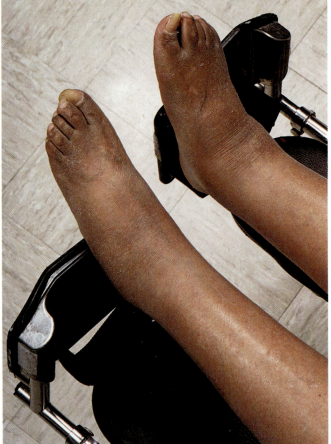

Figure 10-9 Edema is often seen in the ankles and legs of patients with heart failure.

- Allow a position of comfort or place supine in a Fowler's position.
- Reassess every five minutes.

Stroke

A **stroke** or **cerebrovascular accident (CVA)** occurs as a result of a disruption of blood flow to part of the brain. The brain does not receive adequate perfusion, and brain damage or death can result. There are two types of strokes: ischemic and hemorrhagic. An **ischemic stroke** is caused by a blocked blood vessel in the brain (Figure 10-10). A **hemorrhagic stroke** is the rupture of a blood vessel in the brain, which causes bleeding in the brain. Both types of strokes cause decreased blood flow to an area or areas of brain tissue resulting in potential brain damage or death (Figure 10-11). According to the National Stroke Center, approximately 85 percent of all strokes are ischemic, and 15 percent are hemorrhagic. Early recognition and rapid transport to a hospital stroke center are critical to the patient's outcome.

Assessment Tools for Stroke

After performing an initial assessment, providing critical interventions, and obtaining baseline vital signs use the assessment tools of SAMPLE, OPQRST, PERRL, visual changes,

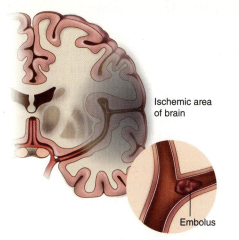

Ischemic area
of brain

Embolus

Figure 10-10 An embolus can lodge in a cerebral vessel, resulting in ischemia to the brain tissue supplied by that vessel.

and a pulse oximeter reading, if available. Look for medical identification jewelry. Perform the Cincinnati Prehospital Stroke Scale, also termed **FAST**. It is important to obtain information from the family or friends regarding the patient's baseline in regard to items on the FAST assessment.

F—*Face*: Ask the patient to smile. Look for drooping and lack of movement on one side of the face caused by facial weakness (Figure 10-12).

A—*Arms*: Have the patient close his eyes and raise both arms at shoulder level in front of his body with palms facing upward for approximately ten seconds. Note if pronator drift (one arm drifts downward) occurs, if there is weakness or no movement. See Figure 10-13 for an illustration.

S—*Speech*: Have the patient repeat a simple sentence. Determine if the patient can speak. Listen for slurring. Note if the patient is unable to speak, uses inappropriate words, or repeats the sentence incorrectly (Figure 10-14).

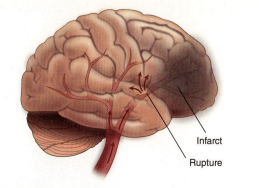

Infarct

Rupture

Figure 10-11 In hemorrhagic stroke, the rupture of a blood vessel results in decreased blood flow to an area of brain tissue.

T—*Time of the first sign*: Note the time when the patient's symptoms first appeared. Time is critical. You must get the patient to the hospital as soon as possible to prevent disability or death.

Signs and Symptoms of a Stroke

- Weakness or **hemiplegia**, paralysis on one side of the body
- Numbness or tingling, decrease in sensation
- Sudden severe headache
- AMS, confusion, disorientation
- Vision changes or abnormal PERRL
- Difficulty speaking or understanding others
- Difficulty swallowing
- Agitation or behavioral changes
- Lightheadedness
- Unsteadiness
- Difficulty breathing
- Seizures (in hemorrhagic stroke)

Management of Stroke

- Critical interventions: provide supplemental high-flow oxygen or ventilation, provide CPR and use an AED if

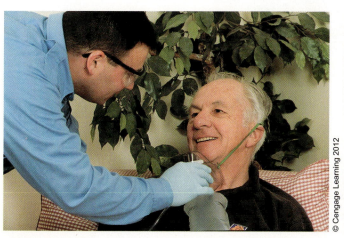

Figure 10-12 Asking the patient to smile helps demonstrate weakness of the facial muscles on one side of the face.

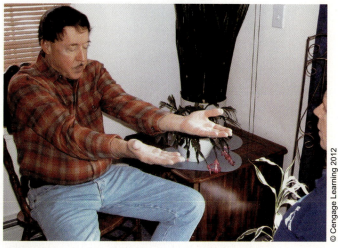

Figure 10-13 The presence of pronator drift indicates arm weakness, sometimes caused by a stroke.

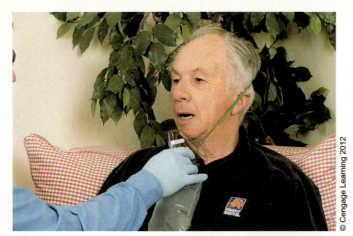

Figure 10-14 Garbled, slurred, inappropriate, or no speech can be indications of a stroke.

indicated, treat for shock, and seek rapid transport to a hospital stroke center.

- Do not have the patient take aspirin because bleeding in the brain may increase in a hemorrhagic stroke.
- Allow a position of comfort.
- Protect paralyzed extremities from injury.
- Do not give food or fluids.
- Document and report the approximate time of the event.
- Reassess every five minutes.

Allergic Reactions

An allergic reaction occurs when the patient's body is exposed to an allergen to which the body's immune system is sensitive, causing an exaggerated immune response. Common allergens include foods, insect stings or bites, plants, chemicals, new medications, and animal dander. Exposure to an allergen can cause a local reaction or a life-threatening, systemic reaction of anaphylaxis in which shock or death can occur within minutes. The severity of the reaction depends on the degree of airway swelling and dilation of the blood vessels throughout the body. Figure 10-15 illustrates the body systems that can be involved in an allergic reaction.

Assessment Tools for Allergic Reactions

After performing an initial assessment, providing critical interventions, and obtaining baseline vital signs, the EMR should use SAMPLE, making sure to obtain information on allergies, history regarding past reactions and interventions, medications, and events leading up to the reaction. Obtain an oxygen saturation reading with a pulse oximeter, if available. If indicated, use the OPQRST. Look for medical identification jewelry.

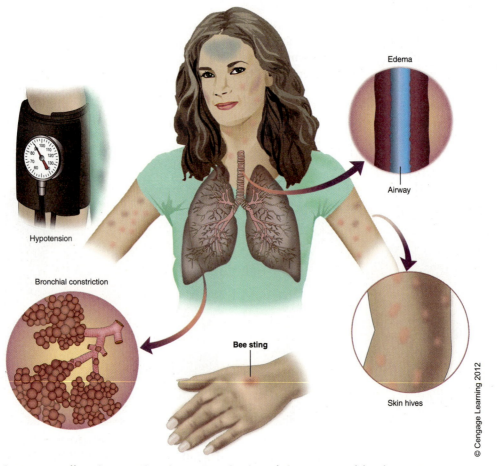

Edema

Airway

Hypotension

Bronchial constriction

Bee sting

Skin hives

Figure 10-15 A severe allergic reaction is systemic, involving several body systems.

Signs and Symptoms of a Mild Reaction

- Hives, usually itchy, swollen red bumps on the skin
- Swelling of the area
- Tenderness
- Sneezing, congestion
- Itching, watery eyes

Management of a Mild Reaction

- Monitor vital signs.
- If localized, use a cold compress at the site.
- Ask if the patient has taken an antihistamine.
- Remove the source of the allergen or the patient from the source. In the case of an insect stinger left in the skin, remove it by scraping the area with an edge of a credit card or dull side of a knife.
- Allow the patient to rest.

Signs and Symptoms of a Moderate to Severe Reaction

- Hives, itchy red bumps, either local or covering large body areas (Figure 10-16)

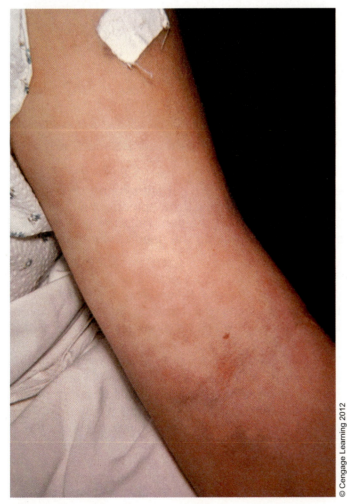

Figure 10-16 Hives are often the result of an allergic reaction.

- Difficulty breathing, talking, or swallowing or tightness in the throat
- Tachycardia
- Chest tightness or discomfort
- Wheezing
- Swelling of the face, eyes, lips, tongue, or throat
- Hypotension
- Dizziness, lightheadedness
- Nausea, vomiting
- AMS
- Anxiety, restlessness, feeling of impending doom

Management of a Moderate to Severe Reaction

- Critical interventions: provide supplemental high-flow oxygen or ventilation, provide CPR and use an AED if indicated, treat for shock, and seek rapid transport.
- If the patient is conscious, ask if she has taken an antihistamine.
- If agency protocols dictates, give epinephrine or assist the patient with an EpiPen or EpiPen Jr injection (according to weight) (Figure 10-17). Check for the patient's name on the pen label. Hold the autoinjector pen with a fist. Pull off the cap. Inject the epinephrine into the patient's upper, outer thigh by jabbing it into the area and not bouncing it. Hold it in place firmly for several seconds to fully inject the medication. After removing the needle, vigorously rub the area. Repeat epinephrine injection according to protocol. Figure 10-18 demonstrates how to give an epinephrine injection. Monitor vital signs because epinephrine will dilate the airway and constrict the blood vessels, causing an increased heart rate and blood pressure, tremulousness, and the pupils to dilate. Symptoms mimic the fight-or-flight response, as

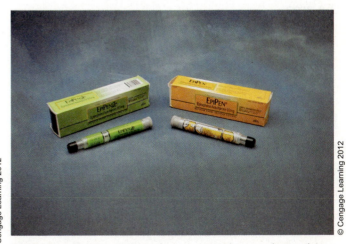

Figure 10-17 Epinephrine may be packaged in a preloaded syringe for ease of administration by adults and children.

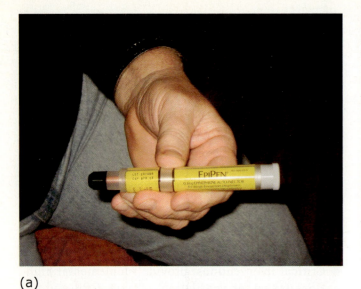

(a)

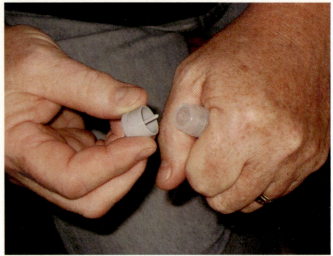

(b)

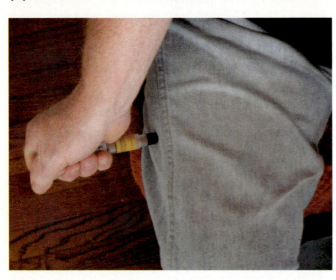

(c)

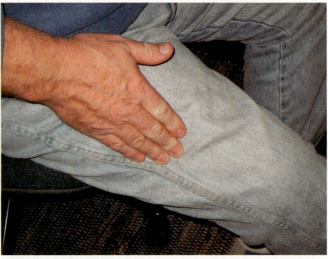

(d)

Figure 10-18   (a) The Emergency Medical Responder should check for the patient's name on the pen label. (b) Hold the autoinjector pen with a fist and pull off the cap. (c) Inject the epinephrine into the patient's upper, outer thigh by jabbing it into the area and not bouncing the pen. Hold the pen in place firmly for several seconds to fully inject the medication. (d) After removing the needle, vigorously rub the area.

illustrated in Figure 10-19. Be careful of the needle on the pen because it may not retract.

■ Reassess every 5 minutes.

Diabetes

The pancreas is responsible for the production of a hormone called insulin. Insulin absorbs glucose from the bloodstream into the cells and transports it to the brain and other body systems. The brain must have glucose. Without glucose, brain death could occur. **Diabetes mellitus** is a condition in which the pancreas no longer produces enough insulin or cells stop responding to the insulin that is produced. In these cases glucose in the blood cannot be absorbed into the cells of the body. Diabetes mellitus occurs in two different types. In type 1 diabetes, the pancreas either produces too little or no insulin. In type II diabetes, the pancreas may release some insulin, but the body does not effectively use the insulin.

A patient who does not produce adequate insulin needs insulin injections. A blood glucose or blood sugar reading is taken by a device called a glucometer. According to blood sugar readings, the patient may need insulin injections daily or even several times a day. Some people receive their insulin continuously through a small needle placed and secured in the abdomen and then delivered by an insulin pump. Monitoring and management of blood sugar levels as well as monitoring the type and amount of food intake are required for adequate control of diabetes.

© Cengage Learning 2012

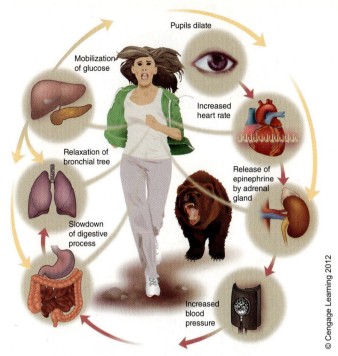

Figure 10-19 Epinephrine administration mimics the fight-or-flight response.

Labels in figure: Pupils dilate; Mobilization of glucose; Increased heart rate; Relaxation of bronchial tree; Release of epinephrine by adrenal gland; Slowdown of digestive process; Increased blood pressure

© Cengage Learning 2012

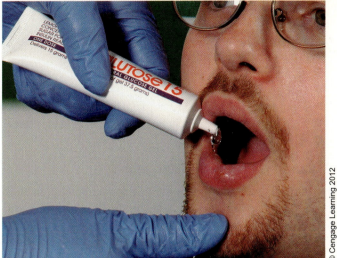

Figure 10-20 Oral glucose is given to a conscious patient with a diabetic emergency if agency protocol allows.

© Cengage Learning 2012

Assessment Tools for Hypoglycemia and Hyperglycemia

After performing an initial assessment, critical interventions, and baseline vital signs, the EMR should look for medical identification jewelry on the neck, wrist, or ankle. It is very important to obtain information from the SAMPLE assessment especially regarding diabetic medical history because symptoms of diabetes can mimic symptoms of stroke or intoxication. Obtain a blood sugar level with a glucometer if your agency allows or have the patient, family member, or caregiver obtain this reading.

Hypoglycemia

Hypoglycemia is a lower than normal blood sugar level. This is the most common type of diabetic emergency and can occur suddenly. Hypoglycemia can lead to brain damage or death if not corrected promptly. Severe hypoglycemia is called **insulin shock.** Blood sugar can become too low if the patient takes too much insulin, does not eat enough, or has significant physical or emotional stress.

Signs and Symptoms of Hypoglycemia

- Nervousness to unresponsiveness
- Low blood sugar level (patient or family data)
- Shaking, tremors
- Tachycardia, heart palpitations
- Headache
- AMS, confusion, disorientation
- Personality changes, agitation, restlessness, and possible combativeness

- Appears intoxicated by slurring of speech and staggering
- Pale-colored, cool, clammy skin
- Seizures

Management of Hypoglycemia

- Critical interventions: provide supplemental high-flow oxygen or ventilation, treat for shock, and seek rapid transport.
- If the patient is conscious and can swallow, give sugar, a sugar drink, or oral glucose *if your agency allows* (Figure 10-20). Do not give diet drinks.
- If the patient is unconscious and breathing, place him in the recovery position and follow your agency protocols.
- Reassess every five minutes.

Hyperglycemia

Hyperglycemia is a higher than normal glucose level. Onset is usually gradual and can take several days for life threatening symptoms. The patient may initially exhibit flu-like symptoms. Hyperglycemia can be caused by an insufficient dose of insulin, eating too much food, less than normal physical activity, illness, or emotional stress. In hyperglycemia, glucose levels become high, but glucose does not enter cells for use by the body. When glucose cannot be used, fats can be metabolized to provide energy. Ketones are acids created by the breakdown of fats and can be toxic to the body. In an effort by the body to rid itself of this excess acid, the patient will experience rapid, deep, labored breathing to blow off excess acid. This condition is called **diabetic ketoacidosis (DKA)** and is potentially life threatening.

Signs and Symptoms of Hyperglycemia

- Drowsiness to unresponsiveness
- Sweet or fruity breath

- **Kussmaul respirations:** deep, rapid, sighing
- Weakness
- Flu-like symptoms: aches, nausea, vomiting
- Abdominal aches or cramps
- Tachycardia, weak pulse
- Hot, flushed, dry skin
- Frequent urination
- Signs of dehydration, including dry skin and extreme thirst
- AMS, confusion

Management of Hyperglycemia

- Critical interventions: provide supplemental high-flow oxygen or ventilation, treat for shock, and seek rapid transport.
- Give sugar, sugar drinks, or oral glucose to a responsive diabetic patient who is able to swallow if you are unable to obtain an accurate glucometer reading. More sugar will not harm the victim, but a lack of sugar can cause serious problems in the brain. It is difficult to distinguish between hyperglycemia and hypoglycemia.
- Reassess every five minutes.

Seizures

A **seizure** is sudden, abnormal electrical activity in the brain. Seizures can be caused by a traumatic brain injury, brain tumor, high fever, alcohol or drug withdrawal, or hypoglycemia. There are basically two main types of seizures: partial and generalized (Figure 10-21). Symptoms of a seizure depend on what part of the brain is affected. A person with a history of seizures is said to have **epilepsy.**

Assessment Tools for a Seizure

Perform an initial assessment of PENMAN and LOC. For most cases wait until the seizure activity stops to perform critical interventions and obtain baseline vital signs. Assessment tools to be used by the EMR are SAMPLE, OPQRST, and a pulse oximeter reading, if available. It is important to obtain a pertinent past medical history and events leading up to the seizure. Look for medical identification jewelry.

Seizure Types and Phases

- A **partial seizure** is often brief and affects a limited area of the brain. Usually the patient has a sudden halt of consciousness. Additional symptoms can include, staring blankly, facial twitching, blinking, jerky movements, unusual emotions and sensations, and altered consciousness. The patient's symptoms depend on the part of the brain that is affected.
- A **generalized seizure** involves the entire brain. The patient will lose consciousness. Symptoms include a loss of muscle tone, rapid muscle contractions, or alternating symptoms of stiffening of limbs (**tonic phase**) followed by jerking (**clonic phase**). With a **tonic-clonic seizure**, breathing may be difficult or stop. During this phase, the patient may lose bowel and bladder control.

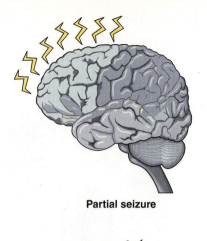

Partial seizure

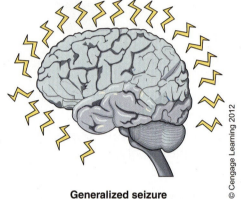

Generalized seizure

© Cengage Learning 2012

Figure 10-21 Abnormal electrical activity in a portion of the brain is a partial seizure. Chaotic firing all over the brain results in a generalized seizure.

- The **postictal phase** is the phase after seizure activity. The patient may be confused, sleepy, and exhausted. Breathing returns to normal.
- A generalized seizure usually lasts one to two minutes. If a seizure lasts longer than five minutes or if additonal seizures occur after the first without a lucid period between them, the patient is said to have **status epilepticus.** This is a potentially life-threatening situation.

Management of a Seizure

Management *during* a seizure:

- Protect the patient from further injury. Pad and protect body parts from striking hard surfaces.
- Never attempt to restrain an actively seizing patient.
- Do not place anything in the patient's mouth.
- Do not attempt to provide oxygen or positive-pressure ventilation to a patient who is actively seizing. Wait until the postictal phase.

Management *after* seizure:

- Critical interventions: give supplemental oxygen or ventilation, provide CPR and use an AED if indicated, control major bleeding, treat for shock, and seek rapid transport.
- Check the patient for a possible head or other injury.

- Place the post-seizure patient in the recovery position to allow secretions to drain from the mouth.
- Keep the patient calm and comfortable, provide privacy.
- In a handoff report give a complete description of the seizure, events leading up to the seizure, and the time and length of the seizure.

Abdominal Emergencies

Abdominal quadrants include the right upper quadrant, right lower quadrant, left upper quadrant, and left lower quadrant. These quadrants contain hollow and solid organs. An EMR does not need to identify the cause of abdominal pain but should treat abdominal pain as a potentially serious illness that can lead to shock from internal bleeding, infection, or dehydration.

Classifications of Abdominal Pain

If a patient is experiencing pain, it can be manifested in three different ways: visceral pain, parietal pain, and referred pain. Classifications and characteristics are as follows.

Visceral Pain

Visceral pain is pain that is poorly localized and more general in nature and is the result of an illness directly involving an organ. The patient will have difficulty pinpointing the exact location. The pain is constant or intermittent and often severe but can be dull or aching. Additional signs and symptoms may include nausea and vomiting.

Parietal Pain

Parietal pain usually occurs with an irritation of the outer lining of the abdominal cavity or peritoneum. This lining contains highly sensitive nerve endings; therefore, this pain is more severe, and the patient can pinpoint the exact location. Parietal pain is intense and localized and usually found on one side or the other of the abdomen. The patient may tell you the pain is sharp and constant. The patients will generally prefer lying on her back with her knees flexed toward the chest. This position may decrease pain in the abdominal muscles. The patient may breathe shallow and limit movement to reduce the pain.

Referred Pain

Referred pain is very similar to visceral pain and is located in an area of the body away from the point of origin. Referred pain occurs because an organ shares the same nerve pathway with a skin sensory nerve. This pain is dull and achy in nature and poorly localized, although it is usually constant. For example, if the spleen is injured, the referred pain may be in the left shoulder area or if the liver or gallbladder is affected, the referred pain may be in the right shoulder area or scapula.

Abdominal Medical Conditions

Many medical conditions can cause abdominal discomfort and pain. Following are some of the conditions that can result in medical emergencies.

Abdominal Aortic Aneurysm

An **abdominal aortic aneurysm** is caused by a weakness in the wall of the aorta, the largest artery in the body. The wall can balloon out (aneurysm) and leak or rupture. This causes massive bleeding and death.

Signs and Symptoms of Abdominal Aortic Aneurysm

- Abdominal or back pain with a sudden onset that may radiate to the pelvic area
- Lightheadedness
- Dyspnea
- Nausea and vomiting
- Signs of shock

Peptic Ulcer Disease

A **peptic ulcer** is an open sore in the lining of the stomach (gastric ulcer), duodenum (duodenal ulcer) (Figure 10-22), or esophagus (esophageal ulcer). If the ulcer involves a blood vessel, serious bleeding can occur and is called a bleeding ulcer.

Signs and Symptoms of Peptic Ulcer Disease

- Black, tarry stools
- Vomiting bright red blood
- Burning, cramping pain in the upper or mid abdomen
- Nausea, heartburn, belching
- Signs of shock

Esophageal Varices

Esophageal varices, dilated veins within the lining of the lower esophagus that may bleed profusely if they rupture. The most common cause is severe liver disease. The vessels become distended and rupture, causing uncontrolled bleeding.

Signs and Symptoms of Esophageal Varices

- Nausea, vomiting bright red blood
- Black, tarry stool
- Shortness of breath
- Signs of shock

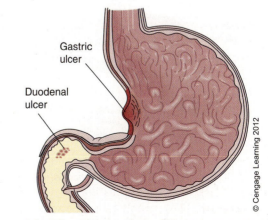

Gastric ulcer

Duodenal ulcer

© Cengage Learning 2012

Figure 10-22 Peptic ulcer disease can cause gastric or duodenal ulcers.

Gastroenteritis

Gastroenteritis is inflammation of the lining of the stomach and intestines from a bacteria, virus, or a parasite. Causes include contaminated food, unclean water, and handling of certain animals or reptiles. Illnesses such as stomach flu, travelers diarrhea, norovirus, giardia, dysentery, E. coli, and food poisoning can cause serious dehydration.

Signs and Symptoms of Gastroenteritis

- Nausea, vomiting
- Diarrhea
- Abdominal cramping
- Fever, chills
- Weakness
- Signs of hypovolemic shock

Bowel Obstruction

A **bowel obstruction** results from a narrowing or completely blocked bowel. If the blockage creates too much pressure, the bowel may rupture, and the contents of the bowel will enter the abdominal cavity resulting in serious infections leading to shock or death. Causes of bowel obstruction can result from surgical adhesions, hernias, loss of function, and tumors.

Signs and Symptoms of Bowel Obstruction

- Vomiting partially digested food
- Abdominal distension, rigidity
- Severe pain
- Fever, chills

Gallbladder Disease

Gallbladder disease can be caused by inflammation, infections, or stones in the gallbladder. Gallstones are created by a hardening of bile in the duct leading to the liver with resulting blockage (Figure 10-23). The constant, steady severe pain is called "a gallbladder attack."

Signs and Symptoms of Gallbladder Disease

- Fever
- Right upper quadrant or mid abdominal pain; referred pain to the right upper back, shoulder or flank (sides of back between the last rib and the hip); sometimes mistaken for a heart attack
- Nausea, vomiting, bloating, belching

Appendicitis

Appendicitis occurs when the appendix, a pouch attached to the beginning of the large intestine, becomes inflamed, distends, or ruptures causing a serious infection.

Signs and Symptoms of Appendicitis

- First symptom is usually a dull pain near the navel that becomes sharp as it moves to the right lower quadrant
- Fever, chills
- Rebound tenderness with palpation of the lower right quadrant
- Nausea, vomiting
- Signs of shock

Diverticulitis

Diverticulitis is an inflammation of a diverticulum. A diverticulum is a pouch in an area of the large intestinal wall. If the pouch wall weakens and becomes distended, a tear can result allowing spilling of intestinal contents into the abdominal cavity. The tearing and infection result in a medical emergency (Figure 10-24).

Signs and Symptoms of Diverticulitis

- Sudden and severe abdominal pain, usually in the left lower abdomen
- Fever, chills
- Nausea, vomiting, diarrhea

Pancreatitis

Pancreatitis occurs when the pancreas, a gland behind the stomach, becomes inflamed. Acute pancreatitis can be life threatening because of its role in insulin production.

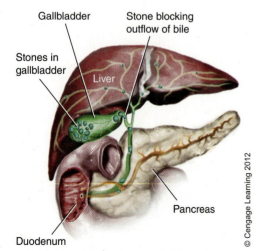

Figure 10-23 Gallstones can block the outflow of bile from the gallbladder.

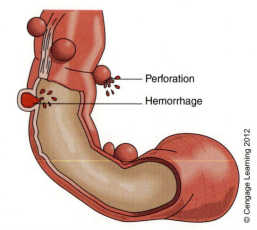

Figure 10-24 Diverticuli can become inflamed, perforate, or cause internal bleeding.

Signs and Symptoms of Pancreatitis

- Persistent, severe upper abdominal pain
- Abdominal tenderness and distension
- Nausea and vomiting
- Fever

Kidney Stones

Kidney stones are minerals that crystallize in the urine, become lodged in the ureter, and cause blockage to the bladder. Kidney stones are not usually a medical emergency, but the patient's severe pain makes this determination difficult.

Signs and Symptoms of Kidney Stones

- Severe flank pain radiating to the groin which may start and stop suddenly
- Nausea or vomiting
- Difficult getting into a position of comfort
- Difficulty or inability to urinate, blood in the urine
- Fever and chills

Assessment Tools of Abdominal Pain

After performing an initial assessment, providing critical interventions, and obtaining baseline vital signs use SAMPLE, OPQRST, and DRGERM. Check for distension, rigidity, guarding, evisceration, rebound tenderness, and pulsating masses. The EMR needs to use moderate palpation while assessing all quadrants of the abdomen.

Management of Abdominal Pain

- Critical interventions: provide supplemental oxygen or ventilation, provide CPR and use an AED if indicated, treat for shock, and seek rapid transport.
- Allow a position of comfort; patients often are in a supine position with the knees bent.
- Reassess every five minutes.

Poisoning

Each year, thousands of children and many adults become ill or die as a result of poisoning. Children investigate their environment with their mouths. Some substances they encounter can cause serious illness or death. Poisoning caused by an overdose of substances is discussed in Chapter 12.

Assessment Tools for Poison Emergencies

After performing an initial assessment, providing critical interventions, and obtaining baseline vital signs use SAMPLE and OPQSRT. It is important to check breath odor and for singe marks around the mouth and nose in case of ingested poison.

Types of Exposures

A person may be exposed to a poison by ingestion, inhalation, injection, or absorption.

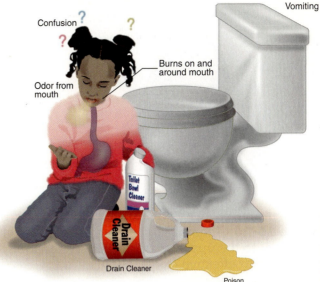

Figure 10-25 Ingested poisons can injure the mouth and throat when swallowed and are absorbed into the stomach and intestines and distributed throughout the body.

Ingested Poisons

This poisoning exposure involves a substance being swallowed and absorbed through the stomach and intestines. This is the most common poisoning exposure. Because of the slow absorption rate of the poison, the signs and symptoms may not appear for hours. Examples of ingested poisons are drugs, alcohol, insecticides, certain foods, and cleaning products. Ingested poisons can cause a variety of physical findings and symptoms (Figure 10-25).

Signs and Symptoms of Ingested Poisons

- Nausea, vomiting
- Difficulty breathing
- Signs of shock
- Airway compromise (with corrosive material)
- AMS
- Abdominal pain, diarrhea
- Chemical burns around the mouth
- Unusual odor on breath
- Signs of shock

Inhaled Poisons

Inhaled poison exposure occurs with gases, vapors, powders, or aerosols that are breathed or inhaled into the lungs. These inhaled substances rapidly absorb into the body and produce the signs and symptoms of the poisoning much sooner than ingested poisons. Inhaled poison may damage or destroy the respiratory tract (Figure 10-26). Common inhaled poisons include carbon monoxide, high levels of carbon dioxide, chlorine, ammonia, nitrous oxide, natural gas, and fumes from household or commercial cleaners.

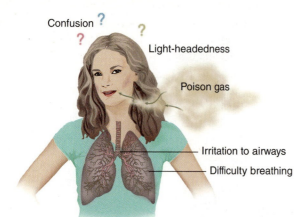

Figure 10-26 Inhaled poisons can cause irritation and injury to the upper and lower airways and may interfere with effective oxygenation.

Signs and Symptoms of Inhaled Poisons

- Difficulty breathing
- Chest pain
- Cough, hoarseness
- Headache, dizziness
- Seizures
- AMS
- Substance on face or hands
- Signs of shock

Injected Poisons

These poisons are injected into the bloodstream by a puncture through the skin. An immediate, or delayed, reaction occurs depending on the type of poison, speed of absorption, and distribution in the body. Reaction can be local or general (Figure 10-27). Injections may include drugs; stings from insects, spiders, or marine animals; and bites from ticks, scorpions, or snakes.

Signs and Symptoms of Injected Poisons

- Swelling, redness, irritation, and pain at an injection site
- Weakness, dizziness
- Fever, chills
- Nausea, vomiting
- Signs of anaphylactic shock

Absorbed Poisons

The absorption of poisonous substances can happen through the skin or mucous membranes. Some substances, such as liquids and dry powers, may cause a local reaction and lead to a more general-body reaction (Figure 10-28). Some examples include household chemicals; pesticides; fertilizers; and plants, such as poison ivy.

Signs and Symptoms of Absorbed Poisons

- Difficulty breathing
- Liquid or powder on the skin
- Burns
- Skin irritation, Itching
- Redness on area of exposure
- Signs of shock

Management of Poisoned Patients

- Critical interventions: provide supplemental oxygen or ventilation, provide CPR and use an AED if indicated, (extremely necessary to use a barrier device), treat for shock, and seek rapid transport.
- Notify the proper response teams for chemical or inhalation exposure. Special handling and personal protective equipment (PPE) may be required.
- If the patient is in anaphylaxis, assist with administering epinephrine if agency protocol allows.
- Look for signs of intentional poisoning, such as a suicide note.
- In an industrial setting, refer to Material Safety Data Sheets.

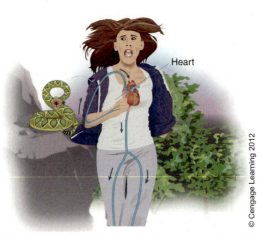

Figure 10-27 An injected poison will directly enter the bloodstream and be distributed around the body. Local blood vessel irritation may be seen.

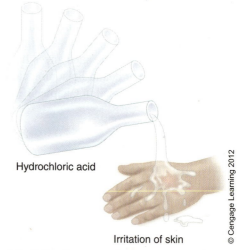

Figure 10-28 Some substances can be absorbed directly through the skin into surface blood vessels; others cause injury to the skin itself.

- If time allows, contact the Poison Control Center at 1-800-222-1222 for assistance.
- Be aware that vomiting caustic substances can seriously burn the gastrointestinal tract.
- For injection poisoning, look for the means of injection. Properly dispose of all sharps.
- For injection poisoning, keep the injected extremity lower than the heart.
- Carefully brush away dry chemicals, keeping in mind further exposure via air to patient, self, and others. Flush the affected area with copious amounts of clean water for at least 20 minutes or until handoff to Emergency Medical Services. If the chemical is in the patient's eye, remove contacts if necessary and tilt the head so the water does not run into the other eye.
- If the patient's clothing is involved, remove it with proper PPE and place it in a sealed bag.
- Reassess every five minutes.
- Send all containers and bottles observed at the scene with the transport unit.

SUMMARY

An EMR will routinely respond to medical emergencies and must perform critical interventions, obtain vital information, perform a secondary survey or rapid secondary survey incorporating objective and subjective information, and then focus on specific interventions. Using critical thinking skills and a basic knowledge of common medical conditions, an EMR can provide necessary care and determine if rapid transport is necessary.

MEDICAL EMERGENCY SCENARIOS

The following medical scenarios are designed to test the EMR student on the application of focused medical assessment, critical thinking skills, and management. To enhance application, use simulation to practice these scenarios.

Scenario 1

Your agency is called to a private residence at 0200 for a complaint of shortness of breath. Mrs. Jones, a 70-year-old woman, called 9-1-1. She meets you at the door and leads you to a room where you see an elderly male lying supine in bed using a nasal cannula at 4 lpm. The wife states that her husband has a history of heart failure, uses oxygen at home, and just woke up and said he couldn't breathe. Your initial assessment reveals a 72-year-old patient with A & O x 2. His breathing is labored, and he is using accessory muscles. A cyanotic skin color is noted around his lips. Your initial assessment reveals:

> Respiratory rate: 24 breaths/min
> Pulse: 120 beats/min and regular
> Blood pressure: 160/90 mm Hg
> Skin is warm to touch and diaphoretic

Critical Thinking Exercise

1. List your initial assessment.
2. What assessment tools would you use?
3. What signs or symptoms should be treated first? How?
4. Does this patient require rapid transport?
5. Write a patient care report (PCR) narrative for this patient using the principles of SOAP or CHART.

Scenario 2

Your agency arrives at 1900 to a private residence. Mr. Smith meets you at the door and states, "Twenty minutes ago my wife began complaining of a severe headache and started talking funny. She never gets headaches." When you enter the kitchen, you find Mrs. Smith sitting in a kitchen chair. She appears alert, but her speech is slurred. Upon assessment, she is unable to move her right arm. She has a facial droop and a dilated left pupil.

Critical Thinking Exercise

1. List your initial assessments.
2. What assessment tools would you use?
3. What are your priorities for managing this patient?
4. Does the patient require rapid transport? What assessment findings support your decision?
5. Write a PCR narrative for this patient.

Scenario 3

You are waiting for a friend to meet you at a coffee shop. When she arrives at 1030, she states that she just finished exercising at the gym. Ten minutes later, she becomes agitated and confused. She now appears nervous and is visibly shaking. Her skin is pale, cool, and clammy. She is unable to tell you what she ate this morning. Upon assessment, she has an A & O x 2 with baseline vital signs of:

> Respiratory rate: 24 breaths/min
> Pulse: 112 beats/min

Critical Thinking Exercise

1. What would you do first?
2. What assessment tools would you use?
3. What signs or symptoms should be treated first? How?
4. Does this patient require rapid transport? What assessment findings support your decision?
5. Write a PCR narrative.

REVIEW QUESTIONS

1. List three types of respiratory emergencies.
2. In what type of cardiovascular emergency does the heart stop beating?
3. What acronym is used to quickly assess a potential stroke victim?
4. What medication is used for patients in anaphylactic shock?
5. What diabetic complication is the result of a lower than normal blood glucose level?
6. Name three abdominal medical conditions that an EMR may encounter.
7. What type of poison exposure would most likely occur from household cleaner fumes?
8. What is meant by the term *myocardial infarction*?
9. What are two types of seizures?
10. What are the two types of strokes?

CHAPTER 11

ENVIRONMENTAL EMERGENCIES

LEARNING OBJECTIVES

By the end of this chapter, the reader should be able to

- Describe signs, symptoms, and management of cold exposure emergencies.
- Explain three types of heat exposure.
- Explain an Emergency Medical Responder's role during water-related emergencies.
- Explain lightning, altitude, and acute mountain sickness emergencies.
- Describe care for animal and insect bites and stings.

INTRODUCTION

The environments in which Emergency Medical Responders (EMRs) must work include excessive heat, cold, rain, snow, fog, and other potentially dangerous conditions. Exposure to environmental factors makes emergency responders susceptible to the same medical issues as the patients they treat. EMRs must protect themselves from the environment and effectively treat patients while keeping them safe. This chapter discusses classifications, assessment tools, signs and symptoms, and management of various environmental emergencies.

Principles of Environmental Assessment and Management

The EMR will assess environmental emergencies using PENMAN, spinal stabilization if the mechanism of injury (MOI) indicates, level of consciousness, and primary survey. Critical interventions will be performed and include providing supplemental oxygenation or ventilation, providing cardiopulmonary resuscitation and using an automated external defibrillator (AED), controlling major bleeding, and treating for shock. After performing critical interventions and if the patient has adequate perfusion to sustain life, the EMR will then obtain baseline vital signs and conduct a secondary or rapid survey. Using subjective and objective information along with critical thinking skills, the EMR will then manage the patient, provide a hand-off report and assist with transport if determined necessary.

Cold Exposure

Cold exposure occurs when a body part is exposed to a cold environment for an extended period of time. Wet clothing, consumption of depressants (such as alcohol or drugs), high altitude, prior cold exposure injury, dehydration, and large amounts of exposed skin create higher risks for complications with cold exposure injuries.

Assessment Tools for Cold Exposure

After performing an initial assessment, critical interventions, and obtaining baseline vital signs, the EMR will use the assessment tool of SAMPLE and OPQRST. Circulation, movement, and sensation (CMS) should be performed on any involved limb.

Frostbite

Frostbite is tissue damage resulting from exposure to freezing and subfreezing temperatures. Frostbite occurs when a body part is frozen and ice crystals form beneath the skin. Superficial frostbite is a local cold exposure involving the subcutaneous tissues. If frostbite is not treated it can progress to deep frostbite when blood supply to the tissue is halted, and the tissue begins to die.

Signs and Symptoms of Superficial Frostbite

- Soft and pliable skin texture
- Pale or white skin color
- Blisters
- Dulled, burning, or tingling skin sensation
- Pain and redness with rewarming when the circulation returns

Management of Superficial Frostbite

- Remove the patient from the cold environment.
- Provide active rewarming with warm packs in the armpits and groin. Rewarming should not be done if there is a chance of refreezing. Active rewarming may include immersing the part into body-temperature water for 20 to 30 minutes or using your warm hand contact.
- Provide passive rewarming by removing any cold or wet clothing and wrapping the patient in blankets.
- Have the patient move or perform light exercise, but not walk if their feet are affected.
- Do not rub the area.
- Do not put snow on the area.

Deep Frostbite

Deep frostbite occurs when unprotected skin is frozen and the tissues are permanently damaged (Figure 11-1). Deep frostbite tissue damage depends on the length of time exposed. Vessel damage occurs when blood leaks into the tissues causing blue to black skin appearance. Tissues damaged by a deep frostbite do not regain circulation or sensation after rewarming.

Signs and Symptoms of Deep Frostbite

- Skin texture is hard to the touch.
- Skin may be white or waxy yellow.
- Skin is pale or mottled.
- Skin has no sensation to touch.

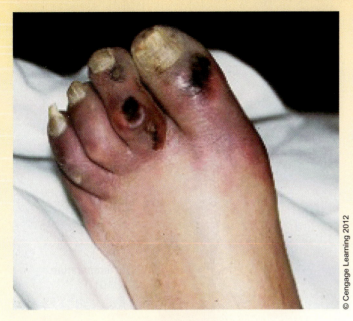

Figure 11-1 Deep frostbite results in permanent damage to tissue.

Management of Deep Frostbite

- Provide passive rewarming. Prevent further loss of body heat by removing wet or cold clothing, cover with a blanket, and provide shelter.
- Do not provide active rewarming if there is a chance of refreezing.
- Do not rub the area.
- Do not allow the patient to use the extremity.
- Carefully protect the affected area. Handle the area gently.
- Carefully bandage the area to prevent further injury.
- Elevate an extremity to reduce swelling.

Hypothermia

Hypothermia occurs when a person's core body temperature falls below 95°F. Hypothermia ranges in severity from mild to severe. A body temperature below 86°F is considered severe hypothermia. If the body's inner core temperature continues to drop, vital organs will stop working and the patient can die.

Hypothermia can occur even when the outside temperature is not below freezing. In fact, a temperature of 50°F with windy and wet conditions can start the process of hypothermia.

Factors Contributing to Heat Loss

- *Radiation:* The body is warmer than the environment. Heat transfers from the warmer body to the cooler environment. Figure 11-2 illustrates how heat is lost through radiation.

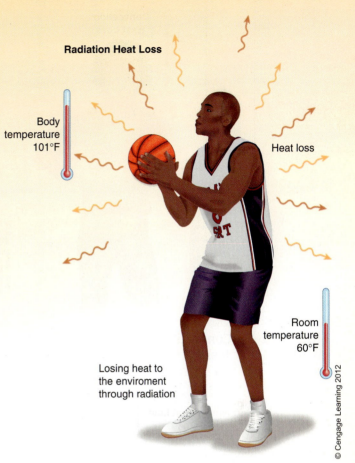

Figure 11-2 Radiation is an important means of heat loss.

- *Convection:* Air currents, such as wind or a fan, transfer heat away from the body, as depicted in Figure 11-3.
- *Conduction:* Direct contact with a cool object or substance cools the body. Figure 11-4 illustrates conduction.
- *Evaporation:* Sweating cools the body. Evaporation can account for up to 30% of the body's heat loss. Figure 11-5 illustrates evaporative heat loss from perspiration and from respiration.

Signs and Symptoms of Mild Hypothermia

- Core temperature between 90° and 95°F
- Shivering
- Poor coordination
- Dizziness
- Pale, cool skin (caused by vasoconstriction)
- Tachycardia, tachypnea
- Altered mental status (AMS)

Management of Mild Hypothermia

- Provide passive rewarming.
- Actively rewarm with hot packs in the armpits and groin.

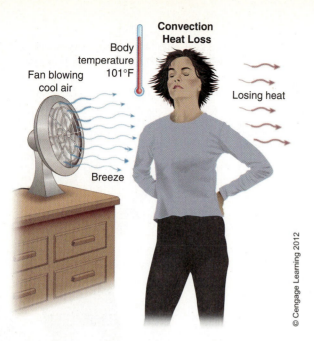

Figure 11-3 Convection is a mechanism that allows for heat loss.

Evaporation of sweat into environment

Losing heat

Body temperature 101°F

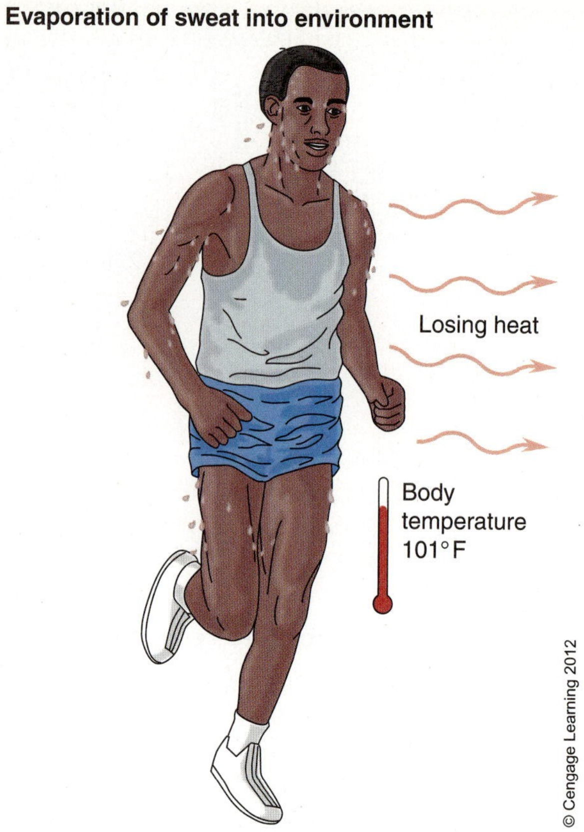

Figure 11-5 Humans use evaporation to disperse excess heat from the body.

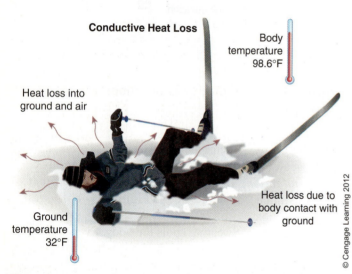

Figure 11-4 Conductive heat loss is a means of heat dispersal.

■ Do not allow walking or exertion.
■ Give the patient a warm drink (no alcohol).
■ Reassess every 15 minutes.

Signs and Symptoms of Severe Hypothermia

■ Core body temperature below 86°F
■ No shivering
■ Bradypnea, bradycardia
■ Hypotension
■ No fine motor muscle control, stiff joints
■ AMS, to coma
■ Inability to make logical decisions

■ Pupils no longer react
■ Unable to self-rescue
■ Paradoxical undressing; patient feels hot and removes clothing
■ Irregular heart rate

Management of Severe Hypothermia

■ Critical interventions: provide supplemental oxygen or ventilation, provide CPR and use an AED, if indicated, treat for shock, and seek rapid transport.
■ Provide passive rewarming. Do not use active rewarming unless you are far from medical care.
■ Avoid rough handling. Be gentle with the patient.
■ Reassess every five minutes.
■ Remember that you must make an effort to resuscitate the patient; survival chances may be increased because of the cold weather.

Heat Exposure

Heat-related emergencies frequently result from hot or humid weather, a lack of hydration, and improper clothing. Exercise and other physical exertion in these conditions cause the body to perspire more than 1 L of fluid per hour. If the body is not rehydrated, dehydration occurs. If the core body temperature is elevated above normal, the patient may have a condition called **hyperthermia**. Heat exposure can lead to hyperthermia, which usually begins with painful heat cramps that can quickly progress to heat exhaustion and then finally to heat stroke.

Assessment Tools for Heat Exposure

After performing an initial assessment, critical interventions, and obtaining baseline vital signs, the EMR should use the assessment tool of SAMPLE. With heat cramps, use OPQRST.

Heat Cramps

Heat cramps are brief and painful cramping or spasms that occur when significant amounts of fluids and electrolytes are lost through perspiration. These cramps are usually in the calf, thigh, or shoulder muscles.

Management of Heat Cramps

- Give water and electrolytes, if available. Electrolytes such as sodium, potassium, and chloride can be obtained from some energy and sports drinks.
- Get the patient into the shade or inside with air conditioning.
- Encourage rest.
- Gently massage the cramp to relieve the pain, starting distal to the cramp and progressing toward the heart.

Heat Exhaustion

Because the body has a decreased ability to compensate for heat and fluid loss, heat cramps can quickly progress to **heat exhaustion**, which is a form of generalized heat-related illnesses characterized by multiple symptoms and often by dehydration.

Signs and Symptoms of Heat Exhaustion

- Dizziness
- Nausea and vomiting
- Profuse sweating
- Pale, clammy skin
- Tachycardia, tachypnea
- Fatigue
- Muscle aches and cramps
- Dehydration

Management of Heat Exhaustion

- Stop all activity.
- Remove the patient from the hot environment.
- Remove excess clothing.
- Cool the patient with cool packs applied to the groin, armpits, and forehead or use a cool-water spray.
- Fan the patient.
- Give water and provide electrolytes, if available.

Heat Stroke

A **heat stroke** can be life threatening, especially when the victim has symptoms of an AMS and an increase in body temperature. During heat stroke, core body temperature may exceed 106°F. The patient's body temperature must be lowered as soon as possible.

Signs and Symptoms of Heat Stroke

- AMS
- Lack of coordination
- Headache
- Hot, dry, reddened skin, primarily
- Unresponsiveness, coma
- Tachycardia, tachypnea
- Possible seizure caused by elevated temperature

Management of Heat Stroke

- Critical interventions: provide supplemental oxygen or ventilation, provide CPR and use an AED, if indicated, treat for shock, and seek rapid transport.
- Passive cooling: remove the patient from the hot environment and remove clothing.
- Aggressive active cooling: place cool cloths or cold packs in areas where arteries are close to the skin, such as the neck, wrists, arm pits, groin, and behind the knees. Spray the patient with cool water. Use a fan if available.
- Reassess every five minutes.

Water-Related Emergencies

Drowning is suffocation and death resulting from filling the lungs with water, fluid, or other substances, so that gas exchange becomes impossible. Approximately 40 percent of drowning victims are children younger than 5 years of age. The bathtub is the most common location for an infant to drown. Incidences of drowning in teenagers and young adults usually occur in ponds, lakes, rivers, and oceans. Often, use of substances and medical conditions are associated with drowning incidents. Once the person is rescued CPR and using an AED may be needed. In cold water drowning, survival chances without oxygen are greater; therefore, the EMR must continue to provide resuscitative efforts until a higher level of provider is on the scene.

Near Drowning

A **near drowning** is survival after being submerged in water for any period of time. A near drowning can cause permanent disability depending on the length of time the brain is without oxygen. Even when submerged in water, the body forces the person to take a breath at some point, which allows water to enter the airway. Spasms may keep water from entering the lungs. However, the victim may swallow water, causing the stomach to become distended. As the oxygen level is reduced, the victim's heart rate and blood pressure decrease. After the person is rescued, CPR and AED may be initiated and immediate transport arranged. The victim's survival depends on the

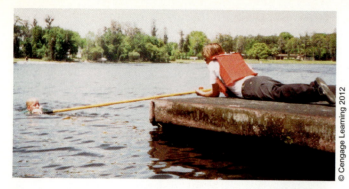

Figure 11-6   In any attempt to rescue a patient from a body of water, the first technique used is to reach out while securely holding on to a stable object.

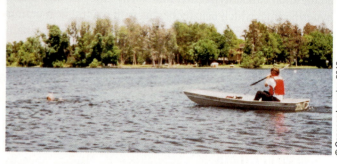

Figure 11-8   If the rescuer has been unable to reach the victim by reaching or throwing, he should use an appropriate watercraft to reach the patient if he is trained to do so.

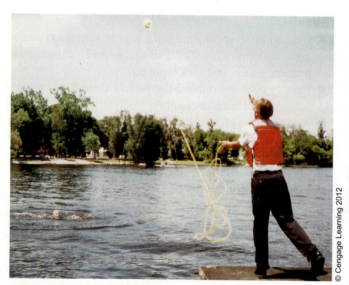

Figure 11-7   If the Emergency Medical Responder is unable to reach a victim in the water, the next step is to throw a rescue rope or flotation device for the patient to hold onto.

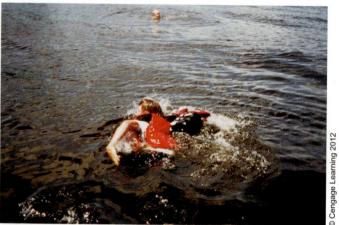

Figure 11-9   Only if all methods have failed or are not available should a rescuer enter the water to go after a water-bound victim and only if he is properly trained to do so.

length of time under water, clarity of the water, temperature of the water, chemicals in the water, and salt versus fresh water.

Seek rapid transport for all near drowning victims because of the high incidence of **secondary drowning**, which can take place within 24 to 48 hours. In secondary drowning, even a small amount of water can collect back into the lungs and cause hypoxia. The patient's neurological status should be evaluated for altered mental status.

Deep-water rescue needs to be done by trained water rescue professionals. Many rescuers with little or no training have died while attempting water rescues. If you are alone, you may reach or throw a rescue object to the victim (Figures 11-6 and 11-7). An EMR may attempt to rescue the victim by watercraft *only if trained to do so* (Figure 11-8). Then only if all other methods have failed or are not available should the EMR enter the water to go after a water-bound victim, and only if he is properly trained to do so (Figure 11-9).

Diving Emergencies

Diving into shallow water can result in striking the bottom of the pool or lake with the headfirst and may cause a neck injury. If a diving accident occurs, you will need to consider MOI and use spinal stabilization and place the patient on a long backboard. Treat for shock by covering the patient on the backboard with a wool blanket to maintain body heat. If the accident occurred in shallow water, you can safely enter and stabilize the patient's head in the supine position while standing in the water. If the patient is prone, acquire additional help and turn the patient while keeping the spine stabilized to prevent further injury. If the accident occurs in deep water, the EMR should not attempt a deep water rescue unless specifically trained to do so.

Deep Water Diving

In deep water diving, pulmonary, cardiac, and neurological complications can occur when descending or ascending too quickly. Divers can have problems with compression of air in the ears and sinuses during descent (squeeze). Symptoms of the squeeze include pain in the ears(s) and sinus cavities, and if the pressure increases, perforation of the ear drum can occur. Another problem is expansion of air during ascent (decompression sickness). If an ascent occurs too rapidly or if the diver does not exhale, the volume of air in the lungs increases and can cause the alveoli in the lungs to rupture. This process is illustrated in Figure 11-10.

The pressure with ascent may also cause problems in the joints, brain, and spinal cord.

Symptoms of decompression sickness include difficulty breathing, frothy blood coming from the mouth, joint pain, and mental status changes. Administer a high concentration of oxygen to the victim, treat for shock, and seek rapid transport. A medical center with a hyperbaric chamber might be necessary to treat the patient.

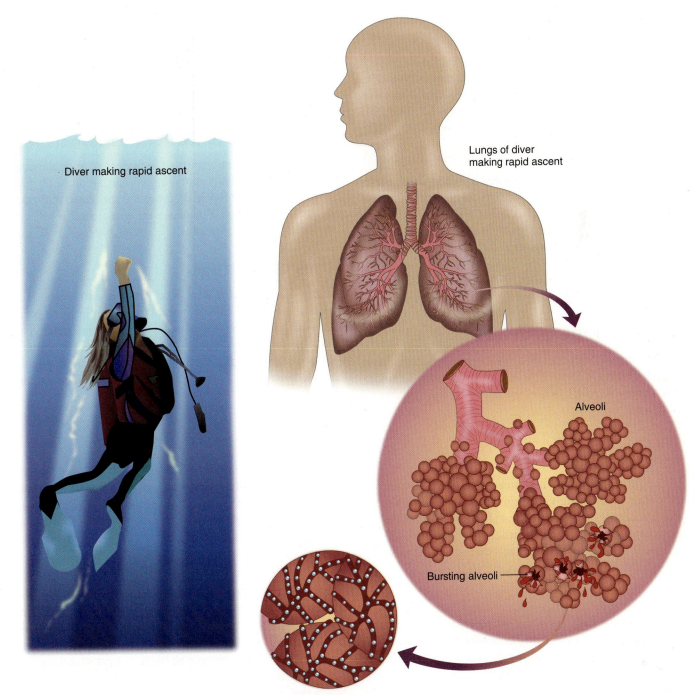

Diver making rapid ascent

Lungs of diver making rapid ascent

Alveoli

Bursting alveoli

Detail of alveoli

© Cengage Learning 2012

Figure 11-10 Expanding air can rupture a lung if not allowed to properly escape during ascent from a dive. Air can rupture into a pulmonary blood vessel during ascent from a dive.

Lightning Emergencies

A lightning strike is an electrical voltage that can stun the heart and lungs, causing hypoxia and ventricular fibrillation. Most deaths from lightning are caused by cardiac arrest. Survivors can sustain a complication or disability. Injuries from lightning that are not life threatening include rupture of the eardrum, fall-related injuries caused by the impact of the current, burns to the tissues, and entrance and exit wounds. Some other symptoms may include amnesia, headache, pain, numbness, and temporary visual or hearing problems.

Assessment Tools for Lightning Emergencies

After performing an initial assessment, critical interventions, and obtaining baseline vital signs, assessment tools used include SAMPLE, DOTS, TIC, and OPQRST. The EMR should look for entrance and exit open wounds.

Management of Lightning Emergencies

- Make sure the scene is safe. Keep in mind that the person struck by lightning does not carry an electrical shock.
- Critical interventions: provide CPR and use an AED (if indicated), provide high-flow oxygen or ventilation, control major bleeding, treat for shock, and seek rapid transport.
- Provide splinting, dressing, and bandaging as needed.
- Monitor AMS especially if a potential head injury.

Altitude Emergencies

Altitude emergencies include acute mountain sickness, high-altitude cerebral edema (HACE), and high-altitude pulmonary edema (HAPE). All of these can be life-threatening conditions.

Assessment Tools for Altitude Emergencies

After performing initial assessment, critical interventions, and obtaining baseline vital signs the EMR should use the assessment tool of SAMPLE, and OPQRST. For all altitude emergencies, patients must descend to a lower altitude immediately. Use the assessment tools during or after descending with the patient.

Acute Mountain Sickness

Acute mountain sickness is the body's reaction to changing elevation too quickly. This illness occurs when a person has not correctly acclimated to high altitudes. Symptoms include lightheadedness, difficulty breathing, headache, nausea, weakness, possible vomiting, and fatigue. The person with acute mountain sickness should be hydrated, rest, and descend to a lower altitude so the condition does not become more severe.

High-Altitude Cerebral Edema

If left untreated, acute mountain sickness can progress to HACE. Symptoms of HACE include AMS, lack of coordination, weakness, and if significant brain swelling, seizures, and coma. The patient should be given supplemental oxygen and moved to a lower altitude.

High-Altitude Pulmonary Edema

HAPE is another serious condition resulting from altitude sickness. Early symptoms of HAPE are a dry cough, dyspnea upon exertion, and tightness in the chest. If the illness progresses, the patient may have changes in mental status, lack of coordination, weakness, and dyspnea at rest. Fluid can build up in the lungs, causing crackles and there may be bloody secretions. This condition is managed by applying high-flow oxygen, immediately moving the patient to a lower altitude, and seeking rapid transport to a medical facility.

Management of Altitude Emergencies

- Critical interventions: provide high flow supplemental oxygen or ventilation, provide CPR and use an AED, if indicated, treat for shock, descend, and seek rapid transport.
- Provide hydration if the patient is conscious.
- Reassess every 5 minutes.

Bites and Stings

Various animals and insects pose environmental hazards to humans. An animal bite or insect sting can transmit a parasite, virus, or bacteria that causes a local reaction, anaphylactic shock, or long-term disease. Manifestation of symptoms may not be immediate, but a bite or sting can cause a medical emergency. Bite and sting emergencies are specific to the area of residence.

Assessment Tools for Bites and Stings

After performing initial assessment, critical interventions, and obtaining baseline vital signs, use the assessment tools of SAMPLE OPQRST, and CMS. CMS should be used with any swelling of an extremity. Also obtain subjective information regarding any travel the patient has recently completed.

Snake Bites

The severity of a snakebite injury depends on whether the snake is venomous. Even though there are several thousand reported venomous snake bites each year, the mortality rates are low. If the EMR practices in an area where venomous snakes can be found, she will be likely to treat snakebite.

There are two types of venomous snakes in the United States that can cause injury or death, pit vipers and the coral snake.

A pit viper is easily recognized by its two moveable fangs and the depression (pit) in front of each eye (Figure 11-11).

Pit vipers include rattlesnakes, water moccasins, and copperheads. These snakes emit hemotoxins that can break down the red blood cells and cause extensive edema, pain, nausea, and tachycardia (Figure 11-12). In very severe envenomization, the patient will appear acutely ill with hypotension, AMS, respiratory distress, and spontaneous bleeding.

Coral snakes, on the other hand, emit neurotoxins that affect the central nervous system. The coral snake can be recognized by the rhyme "red on yellow, kill a fellow; red on black, venom lack" (Figure 11-13). Venom from a coral snake has a toxic neurological decompensation on its victims. Tremor, salivation, respiratory paralysis, seizures, and other neurological problems can occur after a significant bite. The bite is usually on a hand or ankle because the coral snake has a very small mouth.

Management of a Snake Bite

- Critical interventions: provide supplemental oxygen or ventilation, provide CPR using an AED, if indicated, control major bleeding, treat for shock, and seek rapid transport.
- The part of the body bitten by the snake should be immobilized and positioned below the heart if possible.
- Keep the patient calm.
- Monitor the patient for AMS.
- Place a pressure immobilization bandage to slow absorption of the venom. Starting below the bite, begin using a figure of eight on the ankle or wrist and continue with a spiral bandage around the entire length of the bitten extremity (Figure 11-14). Keep the fingers or toes exposed. The bandage should not be too loose or tight, but it should be comfortably snug, allowing a finger to be slipped under it. Further immobilize the extremity with a splint for a leg or with a sling, and swathe for an arm. Remove jewelry and tight clothing. Do not use a tourniquet, cut the wound, suck out the blood, or apply heat or cold to the wound area.
- Do not attempt to catch the snake, but if you can describe the snake, medical personnel can determine the antidote to give the patient if necessary.

Spider Bites

The two most dangerous spiders in the United States are the brown recluse (commonly called the "fiddle back" because of the dark violin shape on its back) and the black widow.

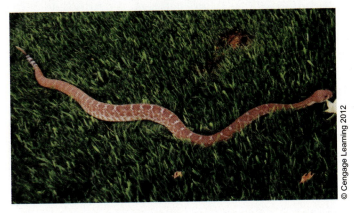

Figure 11-11 A pit viper can be recognized by the depression (pit) in front of each eye.

© Cengage Learning 2012

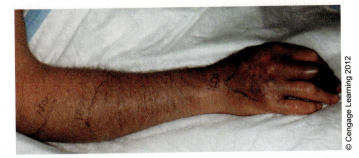

Figure 11-12 The bite of a pit viper can cause local pain and extensive edema.

© Cengage Learning 2012

Figure 11-13 Despite its beautiful coloring, the coral snake is quite venomous.

Source: Centers for Disease Control and Prevention

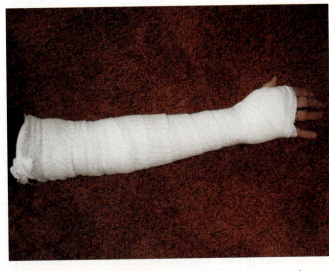

Figure 11-14 Pressure immobilization bandage for a snakebite. Splint the extremity after bandaging.

Joe Grafft, Stacy, MN

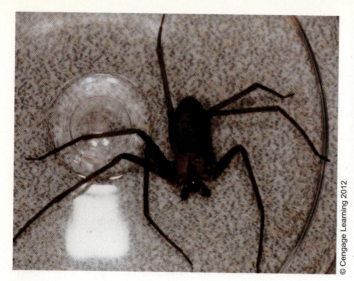

Figure 11-15 The brown recluse spider has a dark violin shape on its back.

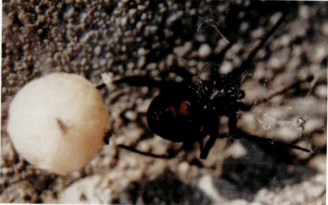

Figure 11-17 The black widow spider can be found in dark, dry, undisturbed areas.

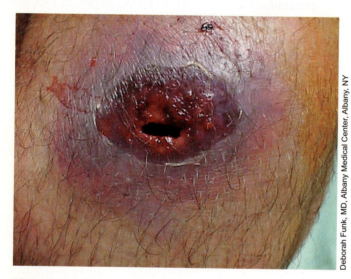

Figure 11-16 A distinctive wound from a brown recluse spider.

Bites from either of these two spiders can cause extensive damage and even death.

The venomous brown recluse (Figure 11-15) is found throughout the United States, but it is predominant in the southern and western sections. A brown recluse bite begins as a red lesion and progresses to a blister with a bluish discoloration (Figure 11-16). The tissue around and untreated bite can, with time, become necrotic (black in color due to cell death). Necrosis takes days or weeks to occur.

The black widow spider is a shiny black spider with a large abdomen that may have a bright red marking that resembles an hourglass. This spider is found throughout the United States in dark, dry, undisturbed areas (Figure 11-17). Only the female black widow spider is dangerous to humans. A black widow spider bite will look like tiny red fang marks at first. About an hour after the bite occurs, the victim will have redness and swelling at the site with progressive generalized muscle pain, abdominal cramping, and muscle weakness.

Animal Bites

If untreated, bites from both domestic and wild animals can be potentially life threatening. Bleeding, infection, and damage to muscle tissue, vessels, or bones can occur depending on the animal's size and the number of bite wounds. The threat of rabies must always be considered when the history of the animal's vaccinations is unknown. While on the scene, an EMR needs to obtain subjective and objective information about the animal, control bleeding, irrigate the wound with copious amounts of water, and dress and bandage the wound area. Advise the patient to seek medical care.

Human Bites

Make sure the scene is safe from violence before entering. Human bites can cause serious infections. Stop bleeding from the wound by applying a sterile dressing and bandage. When bleeding is controlled, irrigate the wound with copious amounts of water. Have the patient seek medical care.

Marine Animal Bites and Stings

A wide variety of injuries can be caused by marine animals ranging from shark bites to jellyfish stings. Symptoms can include bleeding, infection, headache, nausea, fever, chills, tissue and bone damage as well as the possibility of an allergic reaction. Jellyfish stings are managed by pouring vinegar over the affected area to inactivate the venom load and then immersing the area in hot water to relieve the pain but not hot enough to cause a burn. The EMR must be familiar with the marine life in the geographic area and be prepared to provide treatment based on local protocol.

Additional Bites and Stings

Stings or bites from bees, fire ants, and scorpions can cause a local reaction or a life-threatening anaphylactic reaction. The stinger of a bee should be removed by scraping a credit card, knife, or other rigid object over the stinger to release it from the skin. Fire ants get their name from the intense burning pain caused by the fluid-filled vesicles on the skin. A local skin reaction may include swelling, redness, and pain. Scorpions very rarely cause fatal injury in adults, but their sting can cause a slightly reddened area and a stinging or burning feeling on the skin (Figure 11-18).

Management of Bites and Stings

- Make sure the scene is safe and that the source of the bite or sting will not harm you.
- Critical interventions: provide supplemental oxygen or ventilation, provide CPR using an AED, if indicated, control major bleeding, treat for shock, and seek rapid transport.
- Ask if the patient has taken any antihistamines or has an EpiPen.
- Allow a position of comfort.
- Remove any jewelry from an affected extremity caused by swelling.
- Clean the area and cover with a dressing and bandage.

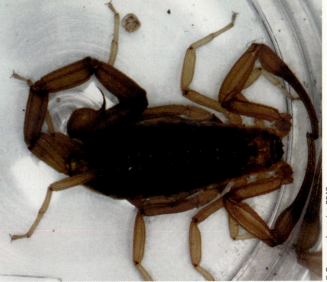

© Cengage Learning 2012

Figure 11-18 Scorpion bites rarely cause significant illness.

- Ask the patient if he has recent vaccinations (tetanus).
- Obtain information from the patient or bystanders regarding the description of the source of bite or sting.
- Use ice for pain and swelling.

SUMMARY

EMRs need to be prepared for various types of environmental emergencies. To provide the best possible care for patients, EMRs must have a basic knowledge of heat and cold exposure emergencies; water-related emergencies; lightning emergencies; and animal, human, or insect bites and stings. Environmental emergencies can be life threatening, and EMRs must be prepared when encountering any of these situations.

▶ ENVIRONMENTAL EMERGENCY SCENARIOS

The following environmental scenarios are designed to test the EMR student on the application of focused medical assessment, critical thinking skills, management, and documentation. To enhance application, use simulation to practice these scenarios.

Scenario 1

You are providing care at a first aid station at the local county fair. At 1400, a woman approaches and tells you that she was stung on the lip by a bee. The bee was in her soda can. Her lip is swollen, and she states, "I'm having trouble breathing." She tells you that she has an allergy to bees and carries an EpiPen. She is alert and anxious. Your initial assessment reveals:

Vital Signs

First Set	*Second set at 14:05*
Pulse: 100 beats /min	A & O × 2
Respiratory rate: 22 breaths /min	RR: 28 breaths /min and struggling to breathe
Blood pressure: 100/70 mm Hg	Pulse 120 beats /min
A & O × 3	Blood pressure: 92/60 mm Hg

Swelling is noted on the right side of her face and neck.

Assessment

1. List the findings of your initial primary assessment.
2. What are your first actions?
3. What do the second set of vital signs and patient symptoms indicate?
4. What are your two main priorities with the change in status?
5. Write a patient care report (PCR) narrative for this patient using the principles of SOAP or CHART.

Scenario 2

Your agency is called to a local park, where you encounter a 28-year-old man who was cross-country skiing with some friends. The outside temperature is 5°F. One of the friends explains to you that he noticed his friend is confused, disoriented, not shivering, complained of being "too hot" and began removing his jacket, and has refused to eat or drink. Your initial assessment indicates A & O × 2 and reveals:

Vital Signs

Pulse: 52 beats /min
Respiratory rate: 10 breaths /min
Blood pressure: 96/68 mm Hg
Skin is cool and pale. There is a lack of fine motor control and inability to make logical decisions.

Assessment

1. What do you think the patient is experiencing? Why?
2. What would be your critical interventions?
3. How would you warm this patient?
4. Does this patient require rapid transport? Why?
5. Write a PCR narrative for this patient.

Scenario 3

It is a very hot day with a temperature of 98°F and 80 percent humidity. Your agency receives a 9-1-1 call to an apartment complex, where at 1730 you find a 68-year-old woman lying on the floor. You note there is no air conditioning in the apartment. The husband, who is extremely anxious, tells you that after returning from the store, he found his wife not moving. Your initial assessment reveals:

Vital Signs

Respiratory rate: 8 breaths /min
Pulse: 110 beats/min
Blood pressure: 132/84 mm Hg
Responds only to painful stimuli
Skin is hot and dry

Assessment

1. What do you think the patient is experiencing? Why?
2. What would be your critical interventions?
3. How would you cool this patient?
4. Does this patient require rapid transport? Why?
5. Write a PCR narrative for this patient.

REVIEW QUESTIONS

1. What are the signs and symptoms of deep frostbite?
2. Define *hypothermia*.
3. List the four factors contributing to heat loss.
4. What type of warming technique would you use with a patient in severe hypothermia?
5. What causes heat cramps?
6. Define *near drowning*.
7. What are the symptoms of acute mountain sickness?
8. What are the two types of venomous snakes in the United States that can cause injury or death?
9. In the United States, bites from what two spiders are the most dangerous to humans?
10. What assessment tools would you use for a person struck by lightning?

CHAPTER 12

SPECIAL POPULATIONS

LEARNING OBJECTIVES

By the end of this chapter, the reader should be able to

- Explain obstetrics and related medical emergencies.
- Name and explain the stages of labor.
- Describe the assessment and management of neonates.
- Explain the pediatric assessment triangle.
- Describe the assessment and management of a pediatric patient.
- Describe the assessment and management of a geriatric patient.
- Identify assessment and management challenges for specially challenged patients.
- Explain different types of abuse and neglect and methods for managing victims.
- Describe seven categories of mental health disorders.
- List signs and symptoms of stimulant, hallucinogen, and depressant use.
- Describe methods for managing crisis situations.

INTRODUCTION

Emergency Medical Responders (EMRs) work with many different populations, including obstetric, neonatal, pediatric, geriatric, and the specially challenged. EMRs also encounter patients with mental health disorders and substance abuse problems. This chapter gives an overview of these special populations and the methods for assessing and managing these patients.

Obstetric Patients

Obstetrics (OB) is a medical specialty involving pregnancy and childbirth. Most OB patient emergency calls involve complications with pregnancy or labor and delivery. Many of these complications can be life threatening.

Ectopic Pregnancy

In an **ectopic pregnancy**, a fertilized egg implants somewhere outside the uterus, usually in a fallopian tube. This type of pregnancy is commonly referred to as a tubal pregnancy. Ectopic pregnancy complications occur as the **embryo**, the developing human from the fourth day after fertilization to the end of the eighth week, grows and expands in the fallopian tube, causing the tube to rupture. Symptoms include abdominal pain; pelvic pain; vaginal bleeding; and symptoms of shock, such as lightheadedness or dizziness. An ectopic pregnancy is potentially life threatening. Seek rapid transport and manage the mother as you would a potential shock patient with positioning and oxygen. Observe and note the amount of vaginal bleeding as scant, light, moderate, or profuse. Ask a woman of childbearing age who has abdominal pain when her last menstrual cycle occurred. If her last cycle was 4 to 6 weeks prior, suspect an ectopic pregnancy.

Miscarriage

Another condition that can occur during a pregnancy is a **miscarriage**, or spontaneous, unintentional termination of a pregnancy. The embryo or nonviable **fetus** (developing human from nine weeks after fertilization until birth) is prematurely expelled, usually during the first six to 12 weeks of pregnancy. Symptoms of a miscarriage include uterine contractions, uterine bleeding, dilation of the cervix, and presentation or expulsion of all or part of the embryo or fetus. Manage the patient as you would a patient with an ectopic pregnancy.

Gestational Diabetes Mellitus

Sometimes women develop a form of diabetes called **gestational diabetes mellitus** during pregnancy. This type of diabetes is similar to type II diabetes and usually disappears after the birth of the baby. Prenatal complications for mothers with gestational diabetes include elevated blood sugars, preeclampsia, early labor, and an increased risk for kidney and bladder infections. Complications for the fetus may include high birth weight, stillbirth, cesarean section birth, and possible delivery problems. Manage a patient with a gestational diabetes emergency like any diabetic emergency.

Preeclampsia and Eclampsia

Preeclampsia is a condition of pregnancy marked by high blood pressure and excess protein in the urine after 20 weeks of pregnancy. Cases can be mild to severe. Symptoms may include high blood pressure and swelling of the face, hands, and feet. Some patients have visual changes and complain of severe headaches. If left untreated, symptoms may progress to include nausea, vomiting, and seizures. Preeclampsia with seizures is called **eclampsia**, which is a life-threatening complication. Without treatment, the mother may lapse into a coma. Provide oxygen and seek rapid transport.

Blunt-Force Abdominal Trauma

A developing fetus is well protected by the pelvis during early pregnancy. After approximately the 12th week of pregnancy, the uterus expands outside the pelvis and is more susceptible to injury. Subjecting the uterus to blunt force trauma may cause a rupture that could quickly lead to a life-threatening internal bleed. Remember that you are really treating two patients. The fetus's survival depends on the mother's survival.

Because of a pregnant woman's 35 percent increase in blood volume, her baseline respiratory rate and pulse are higher than normal, and her blood pressure is lower than normal. When the patient is supine, place padding under one hip for slight rotation to take the weight of the baby off the mother's major vessels (Figure 12-1). If placing the mother on a backboard, slightly tilt the board, as little as 15 degrees, to aid in circulation and prevent hypotension (Figure 12-2).

Obstructed Airway

If an obviously pregnant woman is conscious and experiencing an obstructed airway, do not use traditional abdominal thrusts to clear her airway. Follow the American Heart Association (AHA) guidelines for clearing the airway of a pregnant woman.

Motor Vehicle Crash

A motor vehicle crash is particularly dangerous if the pregnant woman is not wearing her seat belt properly. If the woman is properly restrained with lap and shoulder restraints

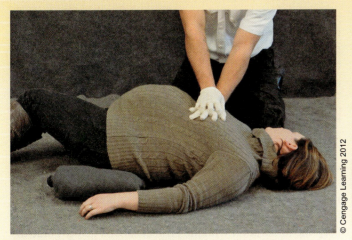

Figure 12-1 When providing care for a pregnant woman, place padding under one hip for slight rotation to aid in circulation.

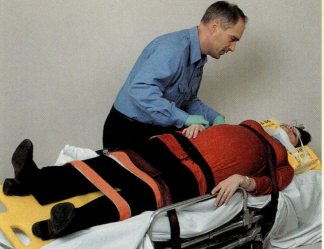

Figure 12-2 Tilting the backboard as little as 15 degrees can aid in circulation and prevent hypotension.

and the vehicle deploys an airbag, the chance for abdominal injury is greatly reduced. If the seat belt is not properly placed across the pelvis (Figure 12-3), the woman may experience serious abdominal trauma.

Childbirth

The EMR's job is to assist the woman in having a successful delivery, if necessary, while waiting for the Emergency Medical Services (EMS) agency. If time allows, do an initial assessment and history of the mother. If the mother has an obstructed airway, follow the current AHA guidelines.

Assessment of Labor

Assess for signs of **labor**, the process by which the uterus expels the fetus and placenta. Signs of labor may include losing the mucus plug, contractions or cramps with a consistent pattern, and leaking amniotic fluid. Labor contractions get progressively stronger and last longer with shorter intervals of time between contractions. **Braxton Hicks contractions** (false labor) can occur sporadically for several weeks before true labor. Braxton Hicks contractions are generally irregular and nonprogressive and may stop with a change in activity, eating, drinking, or emptying the bladder. Generally, an EMR cannot distinguish between Braxton Hicks contractions and true labor.

Obtain an OB history. Ask if the mother has a medical condition that may complicate her delivery and whether she is on medications. Ask the expected due date and if she has had other pregnancies. If she has had prior pregnancies, ask how many were live births. Look for a **bloody show** (expulsion of a small amount of thick, bloody mucus from the cervix as the cervix begins to thin and starts to dilate in preparation for childbirth) and signs that the bag of waters (amniotic sac) has ruptured. Assess whether contractions are regular and three minutes or less apart. If you observe a bloody show followed by a rupture of the bag of waters, remain calm, and prepare the mother for delivery. Most deliveries occur without any complications; however, it is essential for EMRs to have an understanding of the stages of labor.

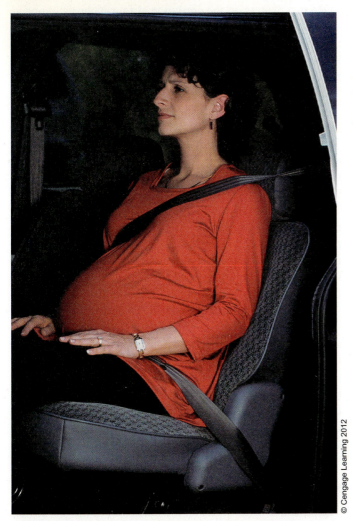

Figure 12-3 A properly worn seat belt can decrease injuries sustained by a pregnant woman in a motor vehicle crash.

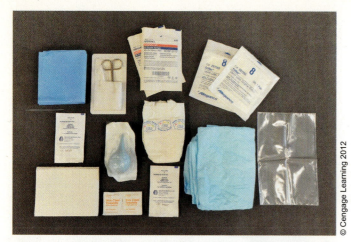

Figure 12-4 The obstetrics kit contains items to be used for an emergency delivery.

© Cengage Learning 2012

Labor

Labor for a first pregnancy usually takes 12 to 16 hours but can take up to 30 hours. Subsequent labor time can be much shorter, so you need to know if the patient has had a previous pregnancy. The EMR must decide whether to await transport of the patient or to deliver the baby on site. This decision may be influenced by the response time of EMS. If transport to a medical facility is delayed, put the patient in a private area (if possible), positioned on her back with towels beneath her and a blanket draped over her legs. Lay out the OB kit, which includes towels, sheets, a bulb syringe, a baby blanket, gloves, a gown, eye protection, cord clamps, gauze sponges, sterile scissors or a scalpel, dressings, sanitary napkins, and a plastic bag (Figure 12-4).

Stage One: Dilation

A bloody show is often the first sign of impending labor. Although it does not actually indicate the beginning of labor, it indicates the thinning and effacement of the cervix. In the first stage of labor, contractions begin and become increasingly more frequent and intense as the cervix dilates. Amniotic fluid may leak with every contraction or the amniotic sac may rupture with a gush of clear fluid. Wear goggles, gloves, mask, and a gown for protection. Stage one is completed when the cervix dilates to 10 cm.

Stage Two: Delivery

Uterine contractions force the baby's head through the uterine opening and into the vaginal canal. As the baby moves down and pushes against the rectum, the mother may have the urge to move her bowels. This feeling is followed by increasing vaginal pressure as the baby continues to move. The baby's head forms a bulge at the vaginal opening and becomes visible, which is called **crowning**. Encourage the patient to hold her breath and bear down to push the baby through the birth canal during her contractions. If you see the amniotic sac still intact, use a gloved hand to tear the sac as the baby's head is delivered. The sac should be removed from

the baby's nose and mouth. If the amniotic fluid is green or has an odor, infection or **meconium** (newborn feces) may be present in the sac. Document this finding in the report for the receiving facility. At this point, the infant makes a series of movements to work his way out through the birth canal. Place three fingers on the head to support the head and to prevent an explosive birth, which could tear the perineum.

As soon as the baby's head is delivered, use the bulb syringe to suction the baby's mouth and nose. Check to see if the umbilical cord is wrapped around the baby's neck. If the cord is around the baby's neck, encourage the mother to stop pushing. Then use two fingers to carefully remove the cord from the infant's head and shoulders. Next, holding the baby's head, keep the infant level with the birth canal and gently guide the baby downward to deliver the shoulder. The remaining shoulder as well as the rest of the baby will be delivered quickly. Remember that the baby will be very slippery, and you must have a good hold on her. Lower the baby's head and suction the mouth again. Note and record the time of birth. For multiple births, record the time of each birth and identify babies to indicate birth order, such as Baby A, Baby B, and so on.

Clamp the umbilical cord immediately after delivery. Place two clamps on the cord: one at four inches and one at six inches from the naval of the baby. Cut the cord between the clamps. If you have no clamps or cutting device in the OB kit, use shoe strings soaked in alcohol and scissors soaked in alcohol. If you do not have scissors, clamp or tie off the cord and leave it uncut.

Quickly dry and wrap the baby in a blanket, towel, or thermal covering to prevent heat loss. Place the baby on the mother's abdomen to initiate mother–baby bonding and to keep the baby warm. Encourage the mother to breastfeed the baby. Nipple stimulation slows or even stops uterine bleeding.

Assess the baby and assign an Apgar score within one minute after the birth. The **Apgar score** is a numerical expression of the color (appearance), heart rate (pulse), reflex irritability (grimace), muscle tone (activity), and respiratory effort (respiration) of a newborn, usually determined at 60 seconds after birth. Table 12-1 details the point assignments of the Apgar scoring system. To determine the Apgar score, uncover the infant, stimulate his feet, and attempt to straighten his legs to check for active kicking (Figure 12-5). Use the bulb syringe and suction the infant's nose again to test whether the baby will cough, sneeze, or only grimace (Figure 12-6). Next assess the strength of the baby's cry (Figure 12-7). The quality of circulation is determined by checking pulses and skin color (Figure 12-8). The soles of the feet can be checked for a pink color (Figure 12-9). Conduct a second Apgar scoring assessment five minutes after birth.

Stage Three: Placenta

The **placenta** is the organ on the inner wall of the uterus that provides a blood supply via the umbilical cord to the baby. Within an hour after the baby is delivered, the placenta is expelled and is often called the afterbirth. Place the placenta in

Table 12-1 Apgar Scoring System

A = Appearance
2—Completely pink
1—Cyanotic extremities
0—Central cyanosis
P = Pulse
2—Greater than 100 beats/min
1—Less than 100 beats/min
0—No pulse
G = Grimace
2—Cough or sneeze
1—Grimace
0—Unresponsive
A = Activity
2—Active
1—Flexion
0—No motion
R = Respiration
2—Good respiration, strong cry
1— Slow or irregular respiration, weak cry
0—Apneic

© Cengage Learning 2012

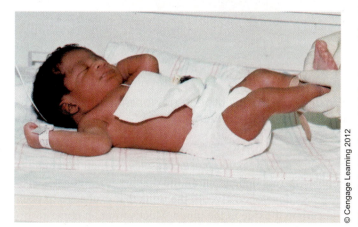

Figure 12-5 An active, kicking newborn is awarded 2 points on the Apgar score.

a plastic bag and transport it to the hospital with the mother and baby. The hospital will determine if the placenta is complete. If it is not complete, the mother could have excessive uterine bleeding.

EMRs do not deliver babies very frequently. With that in mind, it is helpful for EMRs to review the delivery process in a step-by-step manner. **Skill 12-1** at the end of this chapter presents the steps involved in an emergency delivery.

Delivery Complications

Most deliveries occur without a problem, but EMRs need to be aware of potential childbirth complications and how to manage them.

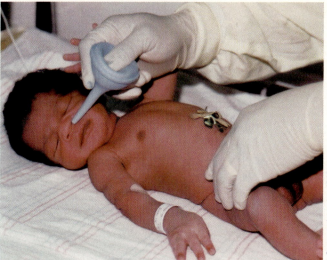

Figure 12-6 If a newborn sneezes when his nostrils are suctioned, he is awarded 2 points on the Apgar score.

Breech Delivery

Most babies are delivered head first, but sometimes a baby will have a **breech presentation**. This means that the baby's buttocks or a limb delivers first (Figure 12-10). This delivery is much more difficult, and the mother will need to be transported to the hospital as soon as possible.

Prolapsed Umbilical Cord

When the umbilical cord precedes the baby's head through the birth canal, the cord gets compressed, which is called a **prolapsed umbilical cord**. The baby's head puts pressure on the cord and stops blood flow from the mother to the baby, which compromises the oxygen flow to the baby. Place the mother in a head-down buttocks-raised position to relieve the pressure on the umbilical cord (Figure 12-11). The mother must be given high-concentration oxygen via a non-rebreather mask.

Newborn Resuscitation

If the baby's color is not pink, oxygen may be needed. Provide blow-by oxygen near the baby's mouth and nose. If the baby is unresponsive, not breathing or has no normal breathing (gasping), check a brachial pulse. If the pulse is absent or less than 60 beats/min, start compressions. To ventilate, use a bag valve mask (BVM) to deliver 40 to 60 breaths/min. Follow current AHA guidelines.

Postdelivery Care of the Mother

After the baby is born and placed with the mother, concentrate on the mother's bleeding. Postbirth vaginal bleeding can be reduced by externally massaging the uterus and allowing the baby to breastfeed. The uterus will feel spongy but contracts and becomes hard when massaged, thus slowing or stopping the bleeding. Use sanitary napkins to contain external bleeding not controlled by massaging the uterus or

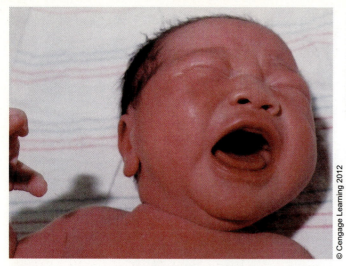

Figure 12-7 A newborn with a strong cry is awarded 2 points on the Apgar score.

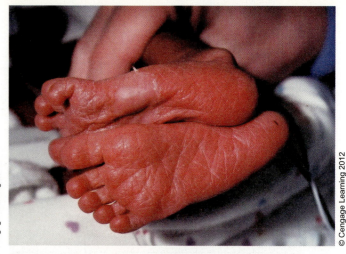

Figure 12-9 If the soles of the feet and the palms of the hands are pink, the newborn is awarded 2 points on the Apgar score.

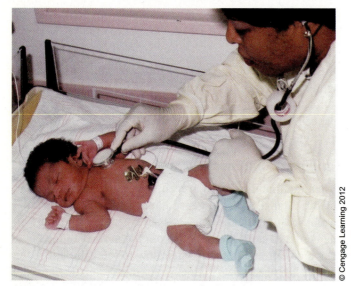

Figure 12-8 A newborn with a heart rate greater than 100 beats/min is awarded 2 points on the Apgar score.

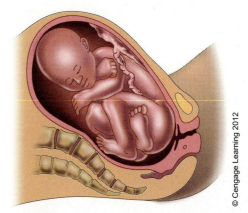

Figure 12-10 A breech newborn is at great risk of injury during delivery.

breastfeeding. Also, the mother may need oxygen because of the stress of delivery and loss of blood. Provide supplemental oxygen with a nasal cannula.

Neonates

A **neonate** is a newborn infant from birth up to one month of age. Neonates younger than 30 days old may have trouble with body temperature and respirations, called problems of transition. In the mother's body, the fetus lives in an incubator with a regulated temperature of approximately 98.6°F. After birth, a neonate must produce her own body heat. The newborn uses special energy stores called brown fat to keep her temperature between 98° and 100°F. If the neonate is premature, she will have little or no brown fat and cannot produce heat well.

Neonates are nose breathers except when in pain or experiencing air hunger from a lack of oxygen (hypoxia).

Neonates have weak intercostal muscles, so their breathing is almost entirely dependent on the diaphragm. Neonates also have less developed alveoli, the units that exchange oxygen and carbon dioxide in the lungs. Mucus from an upper respiratory infection can obstruct the airway, causing the neonate to breathe through his mouth. Mouth breathing increases heat loss and moisture loss and causes increased respirations. Neonates may lose 5 to 10 percent of body weight in the first week of life by merely working to maintain body temperature and breathing.

Neonatal Assessment and Management Considerations

Assess airway, breathing, and circulation (**ABCs)** and manage them if needed. When opening an infant's airway, the neck is to be hyperextended *only* to the point that chest movement can be seen during ventilations. Hyperextending the neck too far can block the airway and injure the neck. If an obstruction is suspected or there is no breathing or no normal breath, refer to the AHA guidelines for an infant's

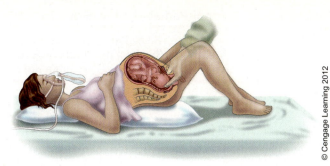

Figure 12-11 The Emergency Medical Responder can help to prevent complete compression of the umbilical cord and the vessels within it by holding the infant's head away from it during contractions.

obstructed airway and cardiopulmonary resuscitation (CPR). When providing supplemental oxygen, use blow-by oxygen. Use the infant section of the Pediatric Glasgow Coma Scale (discussed in Chapter 8) to assess the neonate. Keep the neonate warm and reassess her frequently.

Pediatrics

Pediatrics is a specialty dealing with children, the development and care of children, and the nature and treatment of diseases of children. The AHA classifies pediatric patients in two categories for CPR and obstructed airway management:

- **Infant:** Age ranging from birth to one year
- **Child:** Age ranging from one year to puberty

Pediatric patients have a good ability to compensate. They may look stable up until the time they present with life-threatening symptoms; therefore, it is important to constantly monitor them. It is also important to keep the parents or caregiver close by at all times.

Pediatric Assessment Triangle

After PENMAN, use the **pediatric assessment triangle (PAT)**, an observational tool for assessing the patient's appearance, work of breathing, and circulation to the skin. PAT helps an EMR form a general impression of the patient's condition. Use PAT, illustrated in Figure 12-12, for a child who is too young to communicate. PAT takes no more than 30 seconds to perform.

Appearance

Use the acronym TICLS to assess a child's appearance.

- **T:** Muscle tone. Note whether the child's muscles are limp, rigid, or move effortlessly.
- **I:** Interactivity. Observe if the child is alert, easily distracted, paying attention to her surroundings, making eye contact, reaching for objects, wanting to play, or interacting with her parent or caregiver.
- **C:** Comforting level. Observe whether the parent or caregiver is able to console or comfort the child.
- **L:** Look or gaze. Observe whether the child's eyes appear alert and clear or appear dull and have a blank stare.

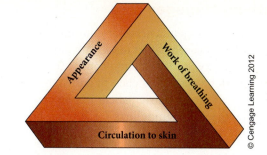

Figure 12-12 Pediatric assessment triangle.

Note whether the child keeps eye contact with and tracks (follows) a person or an object.
- **S:** Speech or cry. Observe whether the child's cry is strong, weak, or high pitched and if the speech is hoarse, slurred, and age appropriate.

Work of Breathing Assessment

Determine whether the child's airway and breathing appear to be normal or compromised. Look and listen for signs of respiratory difficulty, such as unusual breathing sounds and abnormal rate. Observe whether the child is using accessory muscles or leaning forward in a tripod position to breathe. Investigate the possibility of an obstructed airway.

Circulation Assessment

Assess the color of the child's skin. Determine if the skin color is pale, cyanotic, or mottled. Be aware that sometimes when crying, an infant may appear cyanotic around the mouth, hands, and feet. Check the peripheral pulses and capillary refill, which can indicate circulatory adequacy or perfusion. Check capillary refill by squeezing and releasing the child's thumbnail. The nail should blanch (go pale) and then return to pink within two seconds of release. If it takes longer than two second for the nail color to return to pink, the child may be hypoperfused.

Pediatric Assessment and Management Considerations

After obtaining a general impression from PAT, conduct a primary survey, critical interventions, obtain baseline vital signs, and then perform a secondary or rapid survey. Additional considerations in regard to the pediatric patient are addressed below.

Altered Mental Status Assessment

A hypoxic child may have an altered mental status (AMS), usually evidenced by cognitive and behavioral changes. Common conditions that can cause hypoxia are a traumatic brain injury (TBI), seizure, diabetes, and poisonings. Other causes of AMS in pediatric patients include alcohol ingestion, hypoglycemia, dehydration, and infection. The Pediatric Glasgow Coma Scale or AVPU (see Chapter 5) can be used to assess for AMS. If the child is not responding appropriately and AMS is suspected, manage the child's ABCs. Seek rapid transport.

Breathing Management

If supplemental oxygen is necessary during the primary assessment, use a non-rebreather mask with high-flow oxygen. Give blow-by oxygen if the child cannot tolerate a mask. Place the mask on the child's chest to enrich the atmosphere with oxygen. If the pediatric patient has an obstructed airway, follow the AHA guidelines for foreign body airway obstruction.

Circulatory Emergency Management

If the pediatric patient is unresponsive, not breathing, or showing no normal signs of breathing (gasping), follow the current AHA guidelines for CPR for the pediatric patients. If the patient has life-threatening bleeding, control the bleeding and seek rapid transport.

Vital Signs

When obtaining vital signs in a pediatric patient, use the brachial artery (Figure 12-13) in an infant and the radial pulse in a conscious child. In an unconscious child, use the carotid pulse. Pediatric blood pressure cuffs come in various sizes, and the correct size must be used to take the blood pressure. Follow the range markings on the inside of the cuff and read manufactures' comments on the cuff. The ranges of normal for vital signs of infants and children are different than for adults. See Table 12-2 for a list of normal pediatric vital signs by age.

Trauma Emergencies

Trauma causes more deaths in children than all other causes combined. The majority of these deaths are in motor vehicle crashes in which the child was not properly restrained in a car seat. Other trauma emergencies include drowning, burns, and falls, as listed in Table 12-3. Use PENMAN, PAT, spinal stabilization, AVPU or the Pediatric Glasgow Coma Scale, and the ABCs to assess a pediatric trauma patient. Assessing a conscious child can be challenging. You will have to look for increased or decreased pulse and respirations as well as changes in mental

Table 12-2 Normal Pediatric Vital Signs by Age

Age	Respiratory Rate (breaths/min)	Heart Rate (beats/min)	Systolic Blood Pressure (mm Hg)
Newborn	30–60	100–160	50–70
1–6 weeks	30–60	100–160	70–95
6 months	25–40	90–120	80–100
1 year	20–30	90–120	80–100
3 years	20–30	80–120	80–110
6 years	18–25	70–110	80–100
10 years	15–20	60–90	90–120

© Cengage Learning 2012

status. Look for facial grimacing, guarding, or crying as you palpate during the secondary survey. Look for signs of bleeding, bruising, burns, and deformity. A child's bones are more flexible and require a greater force to cause them to fracture. Do not rule out internal injuries or damage to tissue by blunt trauma even if you do not see evidence of injury. A pediatric patient has a smaller amount of blood volume than an adult and a good compensatory mechanism, so a pediatric patient may become unstable more quickly. Therefore, you must act rapidly with any changes in condition.

Medical Emergencies

When performing an assessment in a conscious child or infant, calmly approach the patient and position yourself at the child's eye level. Engage the child whenever possible, such as allowing the child to touch the equipment you will be using. Begin interaction with an infant by playing with the patient's feet and then working your way up to the head. If one is available, use a toy or stuffed animal to distract the child. A penlight or flashlight also works very well. Have a parent or caregiver stay with the child or hold and comfort a young child during the assessment. In pediatric medical emergencies, use SAMPLE (see Chapter 5) to get information about the child from the parent or caregiver.

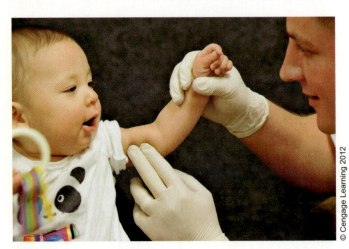

Figure 12-13 The brachial artery is used to take the pulse in an infant.

Table 12-3 Pediatric Trauma by Age Category

Age Category	Types of Trauma	Examples
Toddlers	Blunt trauma	Motor vehicle crash
	Drowning	Pool and bucket
	Burn trauma	Scalding
	Poisoning	Household cleaners or pills
School age	Blunt trauma	Motor vehicle collision
	Falls	Bicycle
	Burn trauma	Intentional fire
Adolescents	Blunt trauma	Motor vehicle crash
	Penetrating trauma	Suicide or homicide
	Poisoning	Overdose

© Cengage Learning 2012

Airway Emergencies

Foreign objects, spasms, and inflammation are common airway emergencies in children. These can be life-threatening emergencies. Inflammation can be caused by viral, bacterial, or fungal infections. Some pathogen causes for inflammatory airway obstruction are croup, bacterial tracheitis, epiglottitis, and pneumonia.

Croup

Croup is swelling and inflammation of the larynx, trachea, and bronchi (to some extent), usually caused by a viral infection. A child who has inflammation in these areas often presents with a cough, sore throat, and runny nose. As the symptoms progress, the patient may have breathing difficultly because the swelling narrows the upper airway. A defining symptom of croup is a loud barking cough.

Bacterial Tracheitis

Bacterial tracheitis is an acute croup-like bacterial infection of the upper airway in children. It is characterized by coughing and high fever and may occur after a viral upper respiratory infection. Young children's tracheas are small and easily become blocked by swelling. Signs and symptoms of tracheitis may include high fever, a barking cough, high-pitched breathing sounds with inspiration, and increasing difficulty in breathing. The child will use accessory muscles to breath.

Epiglottitis

Epiglottitis is a bacterial infection characterized by a swollen, inflamed epiglottis that can cause upper airway obstruction. It usually has a rapid onset but may range from a few hours to a few days. Symptoms include high fever, a brassy cough, difficulty speaking and swallowing (drooling). Patients use accessory muscles to breathe and can often be found sitting in a "sniffing position" (leaning forward with the nose tipping upward). Breathing will be high pitched and will make a whistling noise.

Pneumonia

Pneumonia can be caused by a bacterial, viral, or fungal infection of the lungs with symptoms that can include fever, chills, lethargy, irritability, dehydration, and chest discomfort. A cough may produce mucus that is green, rusty, or blood tinged in color. Shortness of breath, an increased respiratory rate, and shallow breathing are evident.

Asthma

Pediatric asthma involves reversible spasms of the smaller airways in the lungs. Some of the common triggers of asthma include respiratory infections, exercise, animal dander, dust, smoke, airborne irritants, and cold. Ask specific questions about the child's medication use. Find out if the child has an inhaler and if the child can use the inhaler unassisted. If the child cannot administer her own medication, have the parent or caregiver administer it. If a parent or caregiver is not available assist the child in using the inhaler. Remember to verify that the medication is prescribed for the child by checking the name on the inhaler and follow your agencies protocol. See Chapter 10 on assisting a patient to use an inhaler.

Management of Airway Emergencies

When giving supplemental oxygen during any airway emergency, use blow-by oxygen if the child cannot tolerate a nasal cannula or mask. If the child shows increasing signs of respiratory distress, a BVM may be used to ventilate the airway. Allow the child to assume a position of comfort and try to maintain a calm environment. If the child has a high fever, be aware of possible dehydration. Allow the parent or caregiver to stay as close to the child as possible to provide comfort. Seek rapid transport.

Poisonings

Children explore with their mouths, so accidental ingestion is a common pediatric medical emergency. Some poisons children find in the home include alcohol, drugs, poisonous plants, cleaning supplies, gasoline, and other petroleum-based products.

When you encounter a pediatric poisoning, secure the ABCs. Seek rapid transport and monitor the child's ABCs. Call the National Poison Control Center at 1-800-222-1212 to get information concerning the suspected poison and treatment advice. Give a container of suspected poison to EMS.

Dehydration

Dehydration is a medical condition that can occur very quickly in an infant or child. Dehydration can be caused by inadequate fluid intake, vomiting, or diarrhea. Signs and symptoms of dehydration in a child are AMS, fever, absence of wet diapers, diarrhea, vomiting, inadequate drinking, and lethargy. Loss of consciousness can happen quickly. Seek rapid transport.

Seizures

The most common seizures in children are caused by high fever and are usually referred to as febrile seizures. When a child is found having seizure activity, protect him from injury, manage his airway, and seek transport immediately. Provide supplemental oxygen or ventilate after the seizure, if needed, as described in Chapter 10.

Type I Diabetes

Children can be diagnosed with Type 1 diabetes, a condition in which the pancreas secretes little or no insulin. Complications from Type 1 diabetes can result in a medical emergency. Look for signs of hypoglycemia or hyperglycemia and manage accordingly, as addressed in Chapter 10.

Sudden Infant Death Syndrome

Sudden infant death syndrome (SIDS) is the sudden and unexplainable death of a healthy-looking infant during the first year of life. The infant will stop breathing, usually while sleeping. As a result, the infant's heart stops. Show compassion and aggressively attempt to resuscitate the infant. Make sure law enforcement is notified in case of potential child abuse.

Geriatrics

Geriatrics is the medical specialty that focuses on problems specific to adults age 65 years and older. The majority of the calls for this age group are medical emergencies. Common emergencies include heart attack, heart failure, stroke, hypertension, chronic obstructive pulmonary disease (COPD), kidney failure, pneumonia, complications of diabetes, falls and fractures (Figure 12-14), hypovolemia, infection, and poor nutrition. Geriatric patients have a decreased physical and physiological ability to compensate for medical and trauma issues.

Aging Factors

Approximately 85 percent of geriatric patients have a chronic disease, and 30 percent have three or more chronic diseases. Geriatric patients often have vague and poorly defined complaints. Patient may have diminished or absent senses, AMS, depressed temperature regulation, depressed thirst

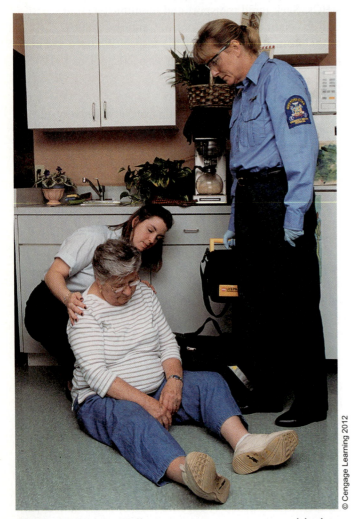

Figure 12-14 Falls are common among elderly adults. A detailed assessment should be done to ensure no bones are broken.

mechanisms, osteoporosis, and limited mobility because of a decreased flexibility of the bones and joints. The physiological systems of the body decrease functioning as aging occurs. See Figure 12-15 for a summary of these changes.

Assessment and Management

Begin assessment with PENMAN and provide spinal stabilization if needed. Perform a primary survey, critical interventions, obtain baseline vital signs, and conduct secondary or rapid survey. Before taking baseline vital signs, look and feel for possible internal or external medical devices such as an intravenous line or dialysis access. Do not take a blood pressure in an arm with these devices.

Communication

When responding to a call involving a geriatric patient, approach respectfully and speak directly to the patient first. Do not let someone else speak for the patient unless the patient is unable to communicate. Speak to the patient alone if necessary. Ask for the patient's chief complaint and then ask more specific questions to find what other signs and symptoms the patient may have. Note the patient's answers, even ones that seem trivial and not pertinent.

When communicating, position yourself near the center of the patient's visual field, stay at eye level, and make eye contact. Look for eyeglasses that might be close at hand. Do not shout. Speak slowly and enunciate clearly. Find out if the patient hears better with one ear than the other. If so, speak toward that ear (Figure 12-16). If you see hearing aids, ask if they are turned on or if the battery needs to be changed.

Geriatric Interventions

It is important to be familiar with some of the illnesses that occur more commonly or require unique considerations in elderly adults. During geriatric assessment and interventions, always consider specific age-related differences and needs.

Altered Mental Status and Dementia

Trauma and some medical conditions can cause an AMS in geriatric patients. These conditions include head injury with a cerebral hematoma, brain tumor, alcohol or drug intoxication, infection of the central nervous system (CNS), heart failure, hypoglycemia, hypoxia, and medication side effects. You may have difficulty, without additional information, distinguishing between AMS caused by a specific event or from dementia. Dementia is a group of symptoms caused by many disorders and can affect cognition, movement, and emotions different from the normal aging process. Similarly, depression and anxiety often present with AMS. Talk with family members or caregiver regarding the patient's baseline orientation and cognition.

Depression

The EMR needs to be aware that depression is the number one mental health problem in the geriatric population. Symptoms of depression often lead elderly adults to neglect their

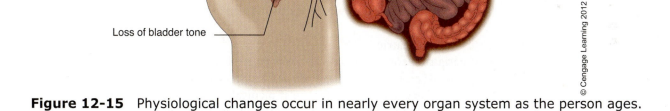

CNS

Sensory changes

Less blood flow to brain

Respiratory

Decreased lung volumes

Decreased cough reflex

Greater secretion buildup

Cardiovascular

Decreased cardiac output

Decreased heart rate

Thickening of left ventricle

Increased coronary artery occlusion

Increased blood pressure

Gastrointestinal

Decreased gastrointestinal motility

Inefficient nutrient absorption

Renal

Decreased kidney function

Less blood flow to the kidneys

Loss of bladder tone

© Cengage Learning 2012

Figure 12-15 Physiological changes occur in nearly every organ system as the person ages.

physical health. If evidence of depression and loneliness is noted, do not overlook the possibility of substance abuse, suicidal thoughts, and gestures.

Skin

By the time an adult is classified as geriatric, her skin has thinned by 20 percent. In addition, the sweat gland function is reduced, and sweating decreases. These changes in the skin can affect the severity of burn injuries, frostbite, wound healing, and cold and heat tolerance. In geriatric emergencies, the patient's body temperature needs to be maintained to prevent shock. Two blankets can be placed under the patient, and one or more can be placed on top of the patient to maintain body heat. Burns, frostbite areas, and external injuries should be covered with sterile dressings to prevent infection and reduce pain. Handle and move the patient gently to prevent bruising or tearing the skin. To reduce skin injury, use minimal amounts of tape on the skin when applying dressings.

Hypovolemia

Geriatric patients have a decreased ability to compensate for hypovolemia, commonly caused by blood loss, lack of fluid intake, side effects of medications, diarrhea, and vomiting. Hypovolemia can very rapidly progress to decompensated shock. Geriatric patients have difficulty tolerating hypoperfusion, even for short periods of time. If not treated quickly, the patient's organs can be permanently damaged and death can occur.

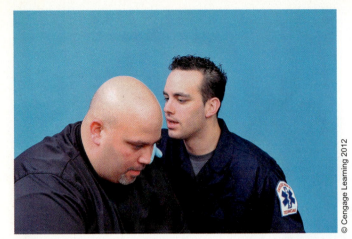

Figure 12-16 Speak into the ear that has the hearing aid or better hearing.

Diabetes

Many geriatric patients have diabetes. Whether caused by improper communication or lack of understanding about their medical condition, they may have hypoglycemic or hyperglycemic complications. Consider a change in mental status or behavior as a possible diabetic emergency.

Trauma

Geriatric patients are likely to incur head injuries even with minor trauma. These patients have an increased risk of bleeding with an internal or external injury especially when taking blood-thinning medications. In assessing a head injury, watch for a possible bleed by looking for signs of increased intracranial pressure such as an AMS. The patient may have no memory of the injury, and his symptoms may be mistaken for a stroke. Additionally, a possible head injury may also indicate a possible cervical spine injury.

Falls are a very common occurrence in the geriatric population. Approximately 33 percent of geriatric people fall each year. One in four patients will be hospitalized from an injury caused by a fall. **Osteoporosis** (a loss of bone density in which bones become weak and brittle) as well as a narrowing of the vertebral canal can lead to fractures, even with minimal trauma. When splinting or back boarding an elderly patient, pad bony prominences and any open areas or voids.

Medications

The average geriatric patient takes several prescription medications in addition to multiple over-the-counter vitamins and herbal supplements. Sometimes medical problems are caused by a lack of compliance with medication or lack of understanding how to take the medication. Geriatric patients are more susceptible to developing adverse effects to medications. If the patient's medications are available, ask permission to gather all of the drug containers or a list of medications to send with EMS when the patient is transported.

Specially Challenged Patients

Specially challenged children and adults may have physical, cognitive, sensory, emotional, or **developmental challenges** or some combination of these. The degree of involvement can vary significantly. Challenges may be acquired (occurring during a person's lifetime) or congenital (present at birth). Conditions such as cerebral palsy, Down syndrome, and visual impairment may be congenital. Acquired challenges may be caused by trauma resulting in a TBI or spinal cord injury or caused by a medical emergency such as a stroke. In both of these incidences, there is CNS involvement leading to a challenge or a combination of challenges.

Because specially challenged adults and children have varying levels of physical, cognitive, and behavioral impairments, you may not initially notice some challenges. Rely on a parent or caregiver to provide baseline information regarding the patient's specific challenges or impairments. Ask the caregiver how the patient usually behaves, communicates, or is best handled. Encourage the transporting agency to allow the parent or caregiver to accompany the patient.

Legal Issues

Patients with special challenges are often considered to be vulnerable. **Vulnerable patients** are individuals with disabilities who are susceptible to injury or illness or at risk for abuse and neglect because of their existing health conditions, impairments, age, or dementia. Look for signs and symptoms of abuse or neglect during assessments. Some specially challenged patients often have advance directives or Do Not Resuscitate (DNR) orders, dictating the scope of medical care to be provided. Many adults with special needs have guardians or may be wards of the state. Guardianship papers must be viewed to determine who can make decisions for the patient.

Considerations Before an Emergency

People with special challenges or their caregivers can contact the 9-1-1 dispatch system and provide valuable information for later use if medical care is needed. The dispatcher can gather information and make notations next to the person's address regarding his special circumstance.

Physically Challenged

Physical challenges range from being hearing impaired to being paralyzed. Causes include trauma, congenital, or physiological impairments. Some physically challenged patients, such as those with cerebral palsy, have spasticity, which is an unusual increase of muscle tone often with reflexive and involuntary movement of the arms and legs (Figure 12-17). A patient with muscular dystrophy might have flaccid muscles resulting in a weakness or lack of muscle tone and coordination. The muscles of a patient who has had a stroke or spinal cord injury might be atrophied with loss of movement and muscle mass. Some patients who have neurological conditions such as Parkinson's disease have ataxia, or tremors, resulting in a loss of ability to control their movements.

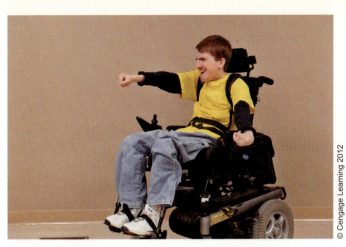

Figure 12-17 Spasticity or involuntary movement can occur at any time in a physically challenged person.

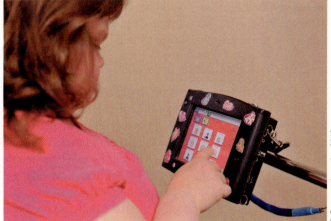

Figure 12-18 An electronic communication board being used.

Medical Complications

Children and adults with physical challenges have frequent and often recurrent complications from health conditions, including dehydration, bowel obstruction, urinary tract infections, hypothermia, upper respiratory infection, seizures, and congenital heart defects. Because of other existing medical conditions, many of these patients have medical equipment and devices with or on them. You may encounter tubes to assist in feeding such as a gastric tube, tracheostomies, insulin pumps, breathing machines (ventilators), urinary catheters, colostomy or urostomy bags, oxygen equipment, customized wheelchairs, seating devices, or braces.

Assessment and Management

- Do not assume that a patient with a physical challenge will also have a cognitive or behavioral challenge.
- Do not assume that a person has good balance and perception as he walks. Provide support or standby assistance. When assisting a visually impaired person to walk, extend your elbow for the person to hold on to as you guide her.
- Patients with physical challenges may also have osteoporosis. To prevent fractures, be careful when lifting and moving them.
- Patients with spasticity may have reflexive or involuntary movements caused by emotion or a change in position.
- A spastic or contracted limb often cannot be relaxed or extended. The patient may not be able to tolerate some positions.
- Patients with scoliosis or kyphosis (curvatures of the spine) are often more comfortable lying on one side rather than the other. Find out from the caregiver or parent which side is better.
- A flaccid patient seems heavier when lifted because of the lack of muscle tone.
- Do not take a temperature orally because some patients could involuntary bite the thermometer. Take a temperature under the arm, noting this location or use a tympanic (ear) thermometer if available.
- Keep a severely disabled patient's head elevated at a greater than 45 degree angle to prevent food, liquid, and secretions from being aspirated into the airway.
- Communicating with a patient who has hearing or language impairment can be challenging. Remain calm and be gentle when working with patients with hearing impairments. Seeing alarm on your face may frighten the patient. Using eye contact, speak clearly, and slowly so the person can read your lips. Ask if the patient uses alternative communication devices or techniques to communicate. Figure 12-18 demonstrates a communication board being used. If possible, use gestures or demonstrations to communicate with the patient before physical contact. For patients who are unable to communicate intelligibly, ask the caregiver about using alternative forms of communication such as gestures or facial expressions. For example, a patient may communicate with his eyes. Looking up could mean "yes" and looking down, "no."
- Remain calm and use a calm voice while working with visually impaired patients. Explain in detail everything you are doing and when and where you will be touching the person.

Wheelchair Considerations

Many of the patients with special challenges remain in their wheelchairs and are unable to assist with position changes. As an EMR, you will need to consider alternative techniques to perform lifesaving measures. You will need to know when to keep a patient in his wheelchair and when to remove him. Performing a conscious obstructed airway technique is a procedure that can be done with the person in a wheelchair. To perform obstructed airway technique for a conscious patient in a wheelchair, push the wheelchair up to a hard surface (wall, car, or tree) and lock the brakes. The brake on a wheelchair can be found at the side or back of the chair. If the patient is wearing an orthosis (brace), you may have to remove it. Most braces have Velcro fasteners so they can be removed quickly if necessary. Kneel in front of the patient and perform abdominal thrusts. **Skill 12-2** at the end of the chapter illustrates the process for performing an obstructed airway technique on a physically challenged patient in a wheelchair.

Removing Patients from Wheelchairs

If the patient is unconscious with an obstructed airway, needs CPR, has major bleeding, or is exhibiting signs of shock, take the patient out of the wheelchair. If using an automated external defibrillator (AED), remove the patient's braces or sitting devices because they may contain metal rivets. Three people are optimal for removing a larger patient from a wheelchair. Lock the brakes and unfasten the belts. Have two people stand on each side of the wheelchair. Have both use one hand to hold the seat frame and place the other hand on the wheelchair handle. Gently lower the wheelchair backward toward the ground. Have the third person hold the patient's head. Gently but quickly slide the patient out of the chair onto the floor. At the end of the chapter, **Skill 12-3** illustrates three people lifting an unconscious patient out of a wheelchair.

A two-person method can be used if three people are not available. Lock the brakes of the wheelchair and, if possible, remove the arm rest on the side you will be moving toward. While maintaining proper body mechanics, one person stands behind the wheelchair and places his arms under the arms of the patient while another person, positioned in front of the wheelchair, cradles both legs with her arms. Bend your knees before lifting and do not use your back. On the count of three, slide or lift the patient sideways out of the wheelchair. **Skill 12-4** at the end of the chapter demonstrates this lift. For a light child, use proper body mechanics to cradle and lift the patient from the chair. Remember to anticipate possible uncontrollable movements.

Cognitive and Behaviorally Challenged

Patients with cognitive challenges have varying levels of comprehension, judgment, memory, and reasoning. These patients may also have behavioral challenges from physiological, psychological and emotional conditions that cause inappropriate thoughts, verbalizations, and actions (Figure 12-19).

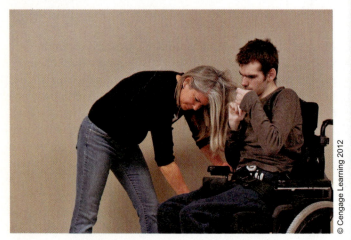

Figure 12-19 Cognitively challenged patients may have inappropriate behavior at times.

Cognitive and behavioral challenges can range from mild to severe and temporary to chronic. Some causes of cognitive or behavioral challenges include:

- **Congenital:** genetic causes or in utero events
- **Trauma:** hypoxia at birth or from a TBI
- **Physiological factors:** diabetic coma, seizures, stroke
- **Psychological:** traumatic life event, inability to cope
- **Substance abuse:** alcohol, drugs both prescription and illegal

Patients with cognitive and behavioral challenges may have physical impairments as well. For example, patients with Down syndrome (Figure 12-20), a genetic condition, have decreased muscle tone and may also have congenital heart defects that can lead to cardiac and respiratory compromise.

Assessment and Management

After initial assessment, performing critical interventions, and obtaining baseline vital signs ask the caregiver about the patient's baseline abilities, cognition, and behavior if the patient is unable to accurately describe symptoms or provide accurate information when questioned. Communicate with direct short phrases and allow time for delayed responses. Requests should be repeated calmly and gently. If necessary, rephrase questions. Give simple explanations and demonstrate care to be given to the patient. If necessary, use alternative forms of communication, such as sign language, picture cards, or computer devices.

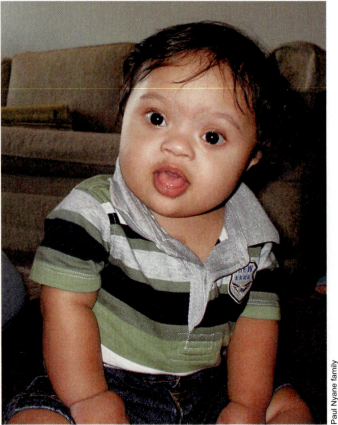

Figure 12-20 A child with Down syndrome.

Some patients may be insensitive to pain. In these cases, the patients may not be aware of their medical symptoms or physical trauma. In other cases, the opposite may be true. The patient may perceive a minor scrape or cut as a major injury. Remember that for some patients, a gentle touch may be perceived as painful. A patient with cognitive or psychological problems may become hyperactive and want to run away. Others might become limp. Do not take away items held by the patient unless the item could be used as a weapon. A parent or caregiver should be at the scene and encouraged to go with the patient during the transport.

Self-Stimulating Versus Self-Injurious Behaviors

Many adults and children with special challenges may exhibit self-stimulating behaviors. These behaviors can include hand flapping, finger moving and playing, head tapping, head or body rocking, and spinning. The patient may visually fix, for extended periods of time, on objects such as falling leaves, snowflakes, or even grains of sand. They may stare trancelike at flashing lights or ceiling fans. You may observe repetitive behavior, such as constantly spinning a ball or switching a ball from hand to hand. The patient may laugh or cry inappropriately for no apparent reason may repeat what you say. The patient may get stuck on a topic for long periods of time. Do not attempt to stop this self-stimulatory behavior.

However, do stop self-injurious behavior, such as head butting or banging, self-biting, or scratching. The patient's condition could be worsened or the patient could be harmed by self-injurious behavior.

Fire Rescue of a Challenged Adult or Child

Remember that people with cognitive or behavioral challenges often gravitate to places of comfort or quiet during times of stress or danger. These places may include a bedroom, an attic, a crawl space, a closet, a corner, or under a bed. They may put themselves at risk during a fire because they frequently hide in a comfortable place even if the location is close to the fire. A special challenged adult or child with limited understanding may unexpectedly move away from you to seek comfort despite heat, fire, or noise. The person may block out or fail to comprehend the danger of situation and try to hide from the fire or go to his comfort zones. If a special challenged adult or child gets away or cannot be found during a fire, immediately get information on the person's favorite locations. If the individual is spotted in a rescue setting, grab the person and go. Prepare for possible resistance or lack of cooperation because of the person's inability to understand the gravity of the situation.

Abuse and Neglect

Abuse and neglect is a national health care problem that can have long-term physical and psychological effects. Abuse and neglect involves all age groups, from newborn to geriatric

patients, and all types of relationships. **Abuse** is intentional physical, emotional, sexual, or economic injury to a dependent person that may lead to serious injury or permanent disability. **Neglect** is failure to provide for the basic needs of a dependent person. EMRs need to contact law enforcement if they suspect abuse or neglect.

Pregnant Women

Pregnant women may become the target of anger from a spouse, boyfriend, or biological father of the infant. They and the unborn child can become victims of abuse. Obtain a focused assessment in regard to trauma. If the perpetrator is present, you may have to leave and request law enforcement. Do not confront the perpetrator and make sure the scene is safe before providing assistance.

Child Abuse and Neglect

Federal law defines **child abuse** as "any act, or failure to act, on the part of responsible adults which results in death, serious physical or emotional harm, sexual abuse or exploitation, or an act or failure to act that presents an imminent risk of serious harm." Child neglect is defined as the failure to provide for a child's basic physical, emotional, or educational needs or failure to protect a child from harm or potential harm. You must look for signs of child neglect or abuse as a possible reason for illness, injury, or death. Signs include fear of the child to return to the parent or caregiver or to return home, sexual gestures or speech by a child, the incident of the illness or injury related by the parent or caregiver differs from the child's description, malnutrition, begging for food, dirty clothes and body, or an excoriated buttocks or perineum from diapers not being changed. A child might exhibit signs of trauma from being burned, hit, kicked, shoved, or shaken or say that he was left unattended. Look for signs of pattern bruises or burns that suggest abuse (Figures 12-21). Look for bruises or injuries that do not fit the story of the injury. Look for bruises on uncommon parts of the body such as the chest or genital area. Look for signs of substance abuse in the caregiver or parent and observe for indifference in regard to the child condition. Table 12-4 lists some of the physical signs that suggest child abuse.

Geriatric Abuse and Neglect

The needs of elderly adults may exceed the abilities of the caregiver, causing frustration and anger. This applies to both domestic and institutional settings. A caregiver may be physically and mentally stressed. Many caregivers experience a loss of financial resources by taking time off from work, loss of social relationships, and loss of time for themselves and other family members. This stress or sense of loss is compounded by the emotional strain of dealing with the loved one's loss of ability or impending death.

Abuse or neglect most often occurs in dysfunctional families, and the abusers are relatives. Some patients do not report neglect or abuse, which is most likely to be from an adult child. They may believe they have no choice but to stay

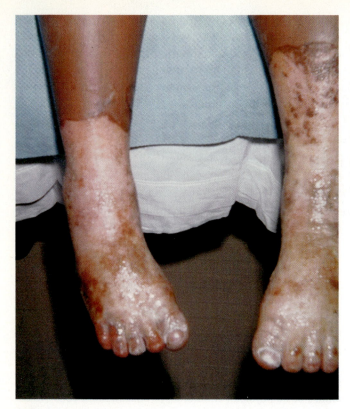

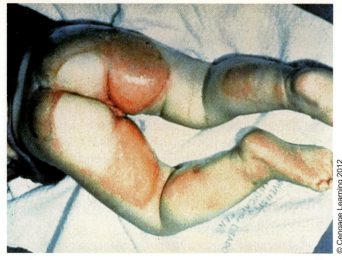

(b)

(a)

Figure 12-21 Burns in a pattern suggest child abuse.

Table 12-4 Physical Examination Findings Suggesting Child Abuse

1. Bruising
   a. Bruising inconsistent with mechanism of injury
   b. Atypical locations for bruise
   c. Bruises in multiple stages of healing
2. Bite
   a. Back
   b. Arms
   c. Thighs
   d. Genitals
3. Burns
   a. Cigarette
      i. Palms of hands
      ii. Soles of feet
   b. Hot water immersion
      i. Stocking burn
      ii. Glove burn
      iii. Donut burn
   c. Stoves
      i. Grill marks
4. Broken bones
   a. Multiple fractures
   b. Spiral fractures

© Cengage Learning 2012

in the abusive environment. Signs or symptoms of abuse include fear of speaking in front of the caregiver, malnutrition, begging for food, bedsores, need for medical or dental care, and concern about money or missing valuables.

Sexual Abuse

Sexual assault refers to physical and psychological trauma of a sexual nature. A victim of sexual assault may exhibit fear, shame, guilt, embarrassment, humiliation, anger, revenge, and a feeling of loss of control. Do not be judgmental. If the victim is undressed, cover the victim and begin caring for the injuries. If the victim requests a provider of the same gender, honor the request. Ask the patient who you can contact and what else you can do to help.

Notify law enforcement. Gather clothing and bag it. Do not let the victim shower, eat or drink, clean her fingernails or hair, or go to the bathroom because doing so may destroy valuable evidence. A sexual assault evidence collection kit is shown in Figure 12-22. The victim may show signs of memory loss if she was given a date rape drug. Arrange to transport the victim to a hospital as soon as possible so a complete physical examination can be done.

Assessment of Abuse and Neglect

Look for the mechanism of injury (MOI) such as weapons or items that might have caused the harm. Look at the injuries to see if they match what the patient is telling you. Check for signs of physical trauma, such as bites, contusions, burns, various stages of bruising, and untreated sores or injuries in

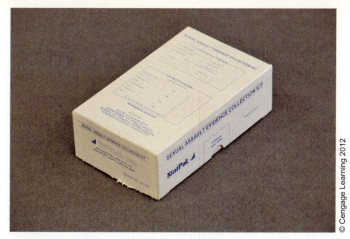

Figure 12-22 A sexual assault evidence collection kit.

various stages of healing. Look for internal injuries, concussions, and fractures. Look for unexplained injuries. Check for evidence of medication abuse, such as overmedicating to keep a patient sedated. Look for evidence of restraints or isolation. Note the patient's statements, signs of emotion, or body language that exhibits fear, agitation, or anxiety. Additionally, note if the patient does not agree to being touched by medical responders. If so, do not touch the patient and be aware of your legal responsibility to always ask for permission first.

While assessing the patient, take the opportunity to observe whether the spouse, partner, caregiver, or parent is cooperative. Look for signs of substance abuse by the people with the patient.

Note also the living conditions, even if the patient lives in a nursing home, foster home, or group home.

Management of Abused and Neglected Patients

Evidence of abuse or neglect could be a possible crime scene. If neglect or abuse is suspected, notify and report your findings to law enforcement. Your legal duty is to contact law enforcement as soon as possible. Do not confront a caregiver, partner, or family member at the scene.

Approach the patient in a nonjudgmental way and be empathetic. If possible, communicate with the patient without the abuser present and ask if he feels safe. Ask the patient to describe what happened and identify the victim's support system. Obtain assistance from another EMR with a secondary survey and ask permission to touch the patient to do an assessment. Do not press for answers. Encourage the patient to be transported to a medical facility.

Mental Health Disorders

A mental health disorder is a pronounced emotional or behavior impairment which affects a person's ability to function comfortably and effectively in their environment. Some mental health disorders can be attributed to physical conditions,

such as a medical illness or the effects of a TBI. Examples of mental health disorders are depression, anxiety disorders, personality disorders, schizophrenia, dissociative disorders, somatoform disorders, and eating disorders.

Depression

Depression is a mood disorder characterized by persistent sadness and lack of interest in usual life pleasures. A depressed person may have feelings of worthlessness, hopelessness, difficulty concentrating, social withdrawal, avoidance of eye contact, verbalization of inability to cope, or suicidal thoughts or plans.

Anxiety Disorders

Anxiety disorders are chronic conditions characterized by an excessive and persistent sense of apprehension often with physical symptoms such as sweating, palpitations, and hyperventilation. A person with an anxiety disorder may exhibit mild symptoms of anxiety to severe symptoms of panic to perceived threats. Patients with an anxiety disorders can have generalized anxiety, phobias, panic attacks, and posttraumatic stress disorder.

Personality Disorders

A person with a personality disorder is unable to follow mainstream social cues. These individuals have socially inappropriate thinking or behavior and tend to unknowingly respond inappropriately to others. These thoughts and behaviors may include paranoia and antisocial or obsessive-compulsive behavior.

Schizophrenia

Schizophrenia is a chronic disorder characterized by symptoms of being completely out of touch with reality. Behaviors may be exhibited only intermittently. A person with schizophrenia may have hallucinations or hear voices. The patient may also have paranoid delusions making her believe she is in danger with no basis in reality.

Dissociative Disorder

A person with a dissociative disorder has a sudden, temporary disruption in identity, memory, perception, or awareness. This disorder causes the person to cope by segregating themselves from a situation. Amnesia, post traumatic stress disorder, and multiple personality disorder are some familiar types.

Somatoform Disorders

A patient who has a somatoform disorder will describe physical symptoms that cannot be attributed to any real physical cause and appear to be psychiatric in origin. The patient may be preoccupied with these unfounded physical symptoms. These complaints and symptoms were formerly classified as psychosomatic symptoms.

Eating Disorders

Anorexia and bulimia are two types of eating disorders. Anorexia is lack of adequate nutrition caused by a refusal to eat. Bulimia is characterized by binging on food and then purging the food by self-induced vomiting or use of laxatives. People with eating disorders have low self-esteem and body image issues. Depression and denial are common. Eating disorders can lead to medical problems such as bradycardia, hypotension, loss of cardiac muscle, and seizures. Severe weight loss can have life-threatening consequences of dehydration or sudden death from cardiac arrest.

Substance Abuse and Misuse

A substance is an illegal or legal drug or chemical that affects the processes of the mind, body, or both. Substances include those ingested, inhaled or injected such as alcohol, sedatives, cocaine, methamphetamines, over the counter (OTC) medications gasoline, propellants, and **narcotics**. **Substance abuse** is the use of chemical substances that are not prescribed for a medical or psychological condition. **Substance misuse** is taking a substance that was prescribed but not for the purpose intended. This can include taking too much of a dosage or using a substance that was intended for another person.

Substance Abuse Considerations

- **Tolerance** happens with repeated, constant use of a substance, when more quantity is needed to achieve the desired effect.
- **Synergy** occurs when the patient takes a combination of substances. An example is drinking a beer and smoking marijuana. Both are depressants, so the effect of the combined drugs is intensified.

- **Addiction** is a physical or psychological dependency of a substance despite the negative side effects.
- **Withdrawal symptoms** are the unpleasant physical and psychological effects experienced by a physically addicted patient who stops use of the drug.

Types of Substances

The three basic categories of substances are stimulants, hallucinogens, and depressants. Patients using these substances exhibit varying signs and symptoms based on the amount of the substance taken, the length of time since the substance was taken, and the combinations of chemicals used. Symptoms and behaviors can change at any point depending on the amount of drug taken and its effects. A list of commonly abused drugs can be found in Table 12-5.

Stimulants

Substances classified as **stimulants** are psychoactive drugs that induce temporary changes in mental, emotional, and physical function. Stimulants can be found in cigarettes (nicotine), drinks (caffeine), prescription medications, and illegal substances used for recreation. Stimulants speed up the CNS.

Signs and Symptoms of Stimulant Use

Many people use some forms of legal stimulants such as caffeine or nicotine on a daily basis. If the person does not get the caffeine or nicotine, mild symptoms of withdrawal such as headache and nervousness occur. When the person gets more caffeine or nicotine than usual, he may experience a rapid heart rate, elevated blood pressure, nervousness, and sleeplessness. Illegal stimulants such as cocaine, amphetamines, methamphetamine, ecstasy, lysergic acid diethylamide (LSD), and phencyclidine (PCP) are stimulants.

Table 12-5

Commonly Abused Drugs Name	Street Names	Source	Effect
Amphetamines	Uppers, speed	Manufactured	Stimulant
Caffeine	N/A	Coffee, chocolate	Stimulant
Cocaine	Coke, crack	Coca plant	Stimulant or euphoria
Ecstasy	E, Adam, E-bomb 2C-E, Bath Salts	Manufactured	Hallucinogen or stimulant
Hashish	Tar	Resin of cannabis	Euphoria
Heroin	H, smack, horse	Opium plant	Depressant or euphoria
Inhalants	Huffing, bagging	Lighter fluid, gas	Depressant or euphoria
Lysergic acid diethylamide (LSD)	Acid	Chemistry laboratory	Euphoria
Marijuana	Pot, grass, weed K2 – Spice Drug	Cannabis plant	Euphoria
Methamphetamine	Crank, ice, stove top	Manufactured	Stimulant or euphoria
Nicotine	N/A	Cigarettes, tobacco	Stimulant
Sedatives	Downers, barbs	Manufactured	Sedative

N/A, not applicable.

© Cengage Learning 2012

Depending on the stimulant used and the length of time it is abused, signs and symptoms range from mild to very serious. Symptoms include tachycardia, elevated blood pressure, increased energy, staying awake for extended periods of time, dilated pupils, respiratory or cardiac distress, aggressiveness, agitation, malnutrition, and paranoia.

You may see injection marks, "track marks," along the length of veins in the arms, between the toes, behind the knees, in the groin, or under the tongue. You may find marks well hidden in a tattoo. In a patient who abuses methamphetamines, you may notice crank bug scars that are formed by the abuser's scratching and picking at nonexistent bugs. The drug releases toxins through the skin, making the user feel as if bugs are crawling on his skin. Picking and scratching at the skin results in sores and eventually scars. You may also encounter patients who snort drugs, resulting in the destruction of the septum (wall between the nostrils).

Hallucinogens

A patient abusing a **hallucinogen**, a substance that induces hallucinations in any of the five senses, may be out of touch with reality. Hallucinations make the patient see or hear things that are not real. The patient may also be delusional. Do not agree with any of the hallucinations or delusions that a person on drugs might have. This patient may act appropriately and be compliant but then very quickly change and act inappropriately and be noncompliant or violent. Be on guard at all times in case the patient perceives you as a threat. Examples of hallucinogens are LSD, Ecstasy, and PCP.

Signs and Symptoms of Hallucinogen Use

Commons signs and symptoms include dilated pupils, tachycardia, diaphoresis, tremors, and acute hearing. You may find the abuser in the fetal position. A patient using PCP may be extremely strong and have a very high pain tolerance. Do not agitate the person. Stay away until law enforcement arrives and makes the scene safe.

Depressants

Depressants decrease the mental, emotional, and physical function of a person. Abuse or misuse of depressants can be life threatening whether it is voluntary or involuntarily. Prescription sedatives and narcotic pain medications (morphine, codeine, OxyContin) are often abused or misused by the person for which the prescription was written or by someone who obtains the drug illegally. Opiates, such as heroin and methadone, are also depressants. Date rape drugs, such as Rohypnol, ketamine, and gamma-hydroxybutyric acid (GHB or GBH) are also depressants. Alcohol is a depressant that affects the CNS. A person dependent on alcohol will develop symptoms of withdrawal or **delirium tremens** (DT's) if he suddenly stops drinking. Signs and symptoms of alcohol withdrawal include irritability, agitation, uncontrollable body tremors, sweating, increased heart rate, decreased blood pressure and respirations, AMS, hallucinations, seizures, or

suicidal thoughts and actions. Alcohol withdrawal can start within 24 hours of the last drink and can be life threatening. An overdose of alcohol may result in death.

Signs and Symptoms of Depressant Use

Signs and symptoms of depressant use include slurred speech, dilated pupils, coordination problems, and difficulty walking. The patient may show signs of impaired judgment, sleepiness, or irritability. Progressive symptoms may include decreased blood pressure and respiratory depression followed by convulsions and coma. Opiates such as heroin have depressant side effects but have specific differences of which the EMR should be aware. In the early stages, the user experiences euphoria followed by pinpoint pupils and impairment in attention, judgment, and memory. You may see needle tracks. During the later stages of opiate use, the victim's pupils may become dilated when the patient becomes hypoxic. Respiratory arrest and coma are possible.

Substance Abuse Patient Management

Remain alert with substance abuse patients. They are at risk for breathing difficulties. If possible, raise the patient's head to a 45-degree angle and use high-flow oxygen. This position will decrease the possibility of aspiration and further airway problems. Monitor the level of consciousness (LOC) and ABCs every five minutes. Manage bleeding from wounds. Stay alert for contaminated sharp objects on the patient during your assessment and management. Abusers of stimulants, hallucinogenics, and depressants can be aggressive, agitated, depressed, or suicidal. Crisis management of these behaviors is essential to patient treatment and EMR safety.

Crisis Management

You may need to deal with crises regarding mental health disorders or substance abuse. Safety is paramount. You must always have law enforcement on scene before you enter a residence of or provide care for a suspected drug user.

Agitated or Aggressive Patients

An agitated patient may have varying reactions in a crisis situation. This patient may have a fight-or-flight, sympathetic nervous system response.

Signs and Symptoms of Agitated or Aggressive Patients

The patient will have physiological changes, such as increased pulse, rapid heartbeat, chest pain, palpitations, increased blood pressure and respirations, and seizures. The patient may sweat, feel short of breath, hyperventilate, feel dizzy, and be nauseous. The patient may also have tremors in the extremities, restlessness, irritability, muscle tension, vocal tremors, feelings of impending doom, and an inability to focus. Reasoning and communication may be impaired.

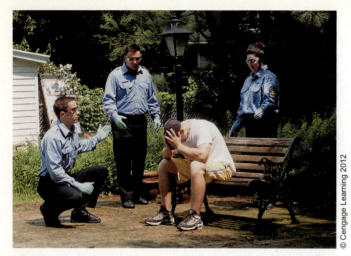

Figure 12-23 A show of force is sometimes all that is necessary to obtain a patient's cooperation.

Management of Agitated or Aggressive Patients

First make sure the scene is safe and law enforcement is present. The patient may be dangerous to herself or others. Scene safety is the most important intervention. Never enter the scene alone. Determine if the patient presents a continuous threat to herself or others. At times, patients may try to harm those who are trying to help. Never kneel or sit directly in front of the patient. Never let the patient get between you and an exit. A show of force from law enforcement is sometimes all that is necessary to obtain a patient's cooperation (Figure 12-23).

After the scene is safe, approach the patient slowly. Speak slowly in a gentle, calm tone. Listen to the patient. Do not say or imply that the patient's experiences or thoughts are not real. Show concern. Determine and note for EMS if the patient needs psychological assistance. If allowed by the patient, monitor medical issues and provide interventions. Try to determine if the patient has taken medications or abused substances. Use caution because the scene can become unsafe at any time. Be prepared to retreat.

You may need to restrain the patient but only if you have been trained to do so by your agency or if you are assisting another agency. Do not restrain the patient too tightly in the chest or abdominal area and monitor for breathing. If the patient is hallucinating, do not under any circumstances agree with what the patient is saying. Reassure the patient that you will get him help and that you will not leave him alone unless your safety is threatened. Seek transport to a medical facility.

Management of Depressed and Suicidal Patients

Suicide threats or attempts must be taken seriously. Suicidal thoughts and gestures are pleas for help from people who still wish to live. An example of a suicidal gesture can be when someone cuts her wrist superficially. Contact law enforcement immediately as well as EMS. Suicidal thoughts or attempts may result from depression, anxiety disorder, schizophrenia, personality disorders, and substance abuse.

Signs and Symptoms of Suicidal Behavior

- Signs of depression
- Self-inflicted wounds with minor bleeding
- Telling others of plans to take one's own life
- Statements such as "I can't take it anymore," "Life isn't worth living," "I wish I were dead," or "Everyone would be better off if I died"
- Leaving a note
- Giving away private possessions and getting affairs in order
- Not taking care of themselves
- Unusual improvement in mood after being depressed

Management for Attempted Suicide

After the scene is safe and law enforcement has been notified, directly and gently ask the patient if she intends to harm herself. Ask if she has a plan. Speak in a calm, supportive, nonjudgmental manner. Try to determine if the patient has a medication issue, either abuse or absence of necessary medication. Look for evidence of suicidal plans such as a gun or sharp objects lying nearby. Look for a suicide note. Ask the patient if you can contact a spouse, relative, counselor, or caregiver. Document all objective and subjective information and give the information to EMS who will transport the patient to the proper facility. Be aware that the patient may have difficulty making decisions.

Potential medical emergencies in the depressed patient can result from an attempted suicide, substance abuse, or overdose of medications. Look for airway problems, decreased respirations, heart rate changes, low blood pressure, AMS, lethargy, extreme fatigue, slurred speech, confusion, an inability to answer questions, lack of coordination, and despondency.

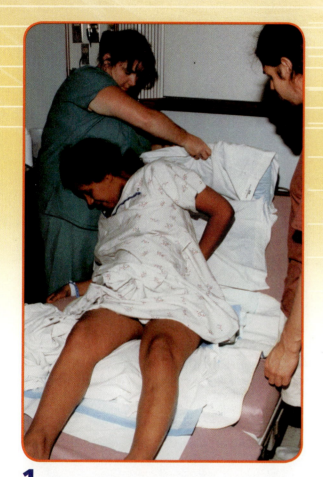

1 Position the mother supine with knees drawn up and spread apart. Assist the mother by helping her to elevate her buttocks on a pillow or blankets.

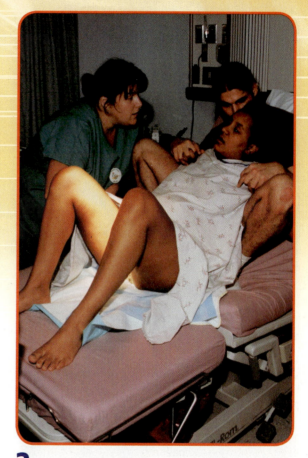

2 Create a clean area around the vaginal opening with clean towels or paper barriers.

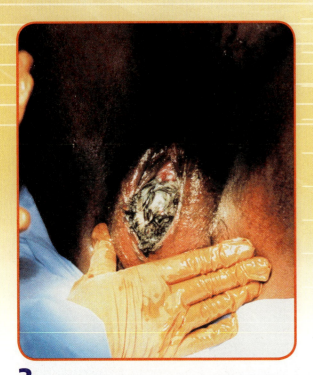

3 As the infant's head appears during crowning, place your fingers gently on the skull and exert very gentle pressure to prevent an explosive delivery.

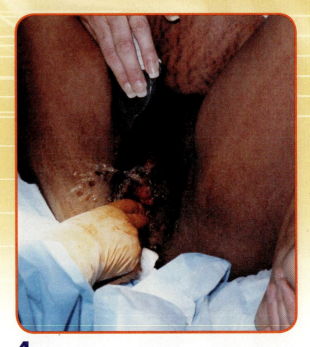

4 If the amniotic sac has not broken, use your thumb and forefinger or a clamp to puncture the sac and push it away from the infant's head and face.

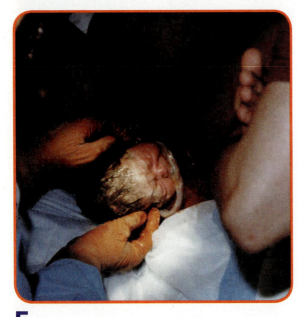

5 As the infant's head is delivered, determine whether the umbilical cord is around the neck and, if it is, slip it over the infant's head or shoulder. If it is not possible to slip the cord, clamp the cord in two places, cut the cord between the clamps, and unwrap the cord from the infant's neck.

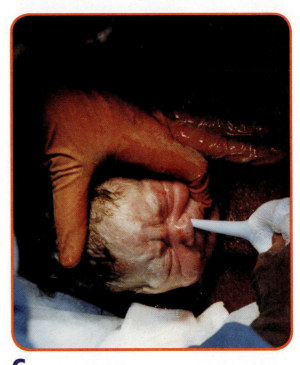

6 After the infant's head is born, support the head and suctions the newborn's mouth and then the nose several times with the bulb suction device.

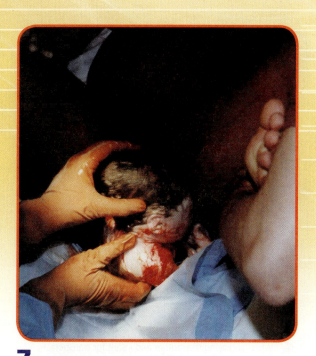

7 As the torso and full body are born, support the infant with both hands. As the feet are born, grasp them firmly.

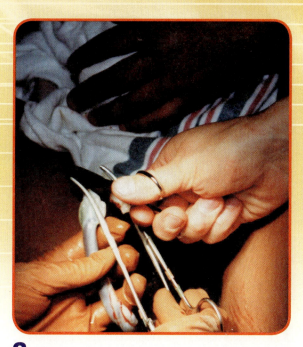

8 After pulsations cease in the umbilical cord, clamp the cord in two places with the closest clamp about four fingers' width away from the infant and then cut the cord between the clamps.

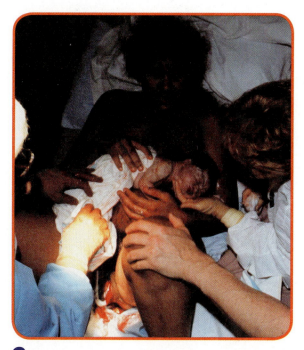

9 Gently dry the infant with towels and wrap the infant in a warm blanket. The infant should be placed on the infant's side, preferably with the head slightly lower than the trunk.

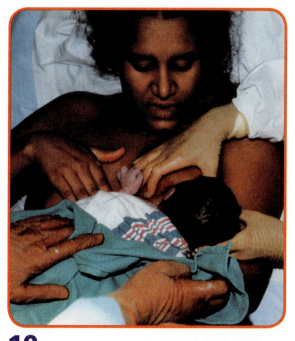

10 Another EMR should monitor the infant and complete initial care of the newborn.

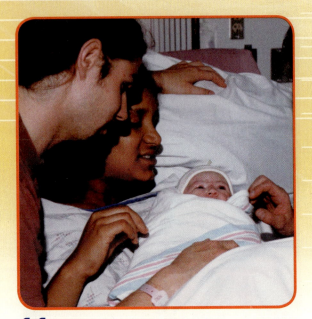

11 Place a sterile sanitary napkin between the mother's legs and have her close her legs. Comfort the mother and monitor vital signs.

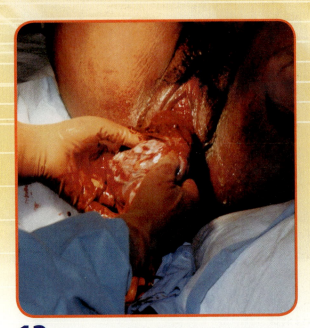

12 While preparing the mother and infant for transport, watch for delivery of the placenta. When the placenta is delivered, wrap the placenta in a towel, place it in a plastic bag or container, and transports it to the hospital with the mother.

Skill 12-2 Performing Obstructed Airway Technique on a Conscious Person who Uses a Wheelchair

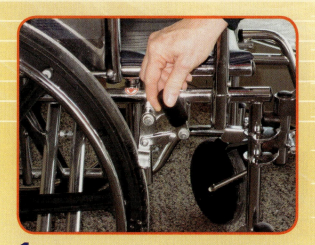

1 Back up the wheelchair to a wall and lock the brake. Most wheelchairs have the brake at the side of the chair.

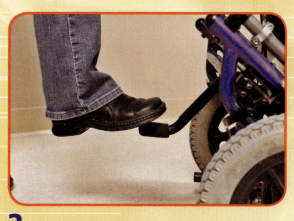

2 On some wheelchairs, the brake is located at the back.

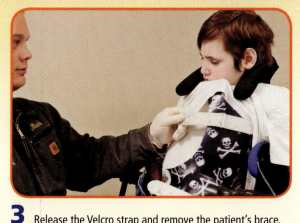

3 Release the Velcro strap and remove the patient's brace.

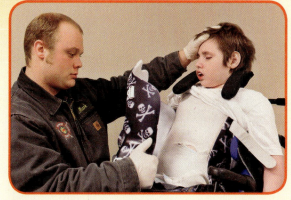

4 Remove the anterior portion of the brace.

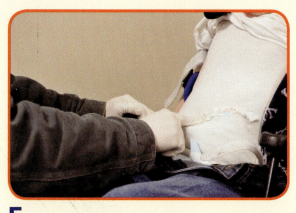

5 Locate the landmark on the patient.

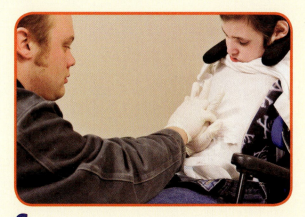

6 Use the abdominal thrust hand position following American Heart Association guidelines.

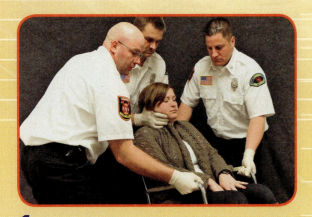

1 Lock the brakes and remove any fastening belts and support the patient

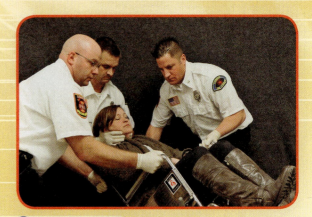

2 Two people stand on each side of the wheelchair, with one hand holding the seat frame and the other hand holding the chair handle. The third EMR, positioned at the back, supports the patient's head. Simultaneously, lower the wheelchair backward toward the floor. Then carefully slide the patient out of the wheelchair onto the floor.

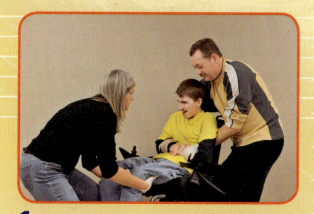

1 After locking the brakes and removing the arm rest from the side the patient is being moved toward, release any fastening straps. The person behind the wheelchair then places his arms under the arms of the patient while the person in front cradles the legs of the patient.

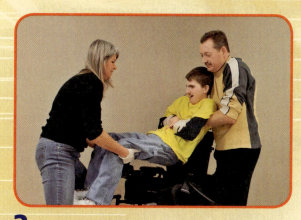

2 Simultaneously, bending at the knees, slide or lift the patient sideways out of the wheelchair.

The EMR must be knowledgeable of basic physical, cognitive, and behavioral conditions that may be present in special populations of all ages. An EMR needs to be aware of medical conditions that frequently occur in OB patients, neonates, pediatric patients, and geriatric patients and the care that should be provided as well as medical problems that frequently affect specially challenged populations. The EMR will also respond to emergency calls involving abused children and adults and substance abuse or overdoses. Ensuring scene safety and activating law enforcement are common threads in the care of all behavioral and mental health disorders.

REVIEW QUESTIONS

1. Preeclampsia is a condition of pregnancy marked by
   a. Elevated blood pressure
   b. Tachycardia
   c. Bradypnea
   d. Cardiogenic shock
2. Braxton Hicks contractions are referred to as
   a. False labor
   b. Stage one dilation
   c. Dilation
   d. Delivery
3. Neonates are newborn infants from birth to _____ days old.
   a. 50
   b. 40
   c. 30
   d. 60
4. Which tool gives a quick observation of the severity of a child's condition and helps the EMR form a general impression?
   a. AVPU
   b. LOC
   c. LLF
   d. PAT
5. The acronym AMS refers to
   a. Alert motor sensory
   b. Acute mental sickness
   c. Altered mental status
   d. Acute motor sensation
6. Croup is
   a. Swelling and inflammation of the larynx, trachea, and bronchi
   b. A bacterial infection of the upper airway
   c. A swollen epiglottis
   d. An infection of the lungs
7. Seizures in children are often caused by
   a. Dehydration
   b. High fever

c. Poisoning
d. Diabetes

8. Dementia is defined as
   a. A specific event causing a loss of cognitive ability
   b. Several disorders causing a loss of cognitive ability
   c. A central nervous system disease causing a loss of cognitive ability
   d. AMS caused by blunt trauma
9. The number one mental health problem in the geriatric population is
   a. Substance abuse
   b. Alzheimer's disease
   c. Depression
   d. Dementia
10. Individuals with disabilities who are susceptible to injury or illness or at risk for abuse are referred to as:
    a. Vulnerable
    b. Geriatric
    c. Pediatric
    d. Adolescent
11. Which of the following is classified as a stimulant?
    a. Crack cocaine
    b. Marijuana
    c. Opiates
    d. LSD
12. Which of the following is a hallucinogen?
    a. Cocaine
    b. Seconal
    c. Hashish
    d. Angel dust
13. Which of the following is a depressant?
    a. MDA
    b. Shrooms
    c. Phenobarbital
    d. Dexedrine

CHAPTER 13

OPERATIONS AND EXTENDED CARE

LEARNING OBJECTIVES

At the end of this chapter, the reader should be able to

- List and explain the three phases of emergency operations.
- Define FADE.
- Explain NIMS and ICS.
- Describe HAZMAT and MCI concerns during incident response.
- Explain the four steps of a CDC Field Triage Decision Scheme.
- Describe START and JumpSTART Triage Systems.
- Differentiate among the four levels of trauma centers.
- Describe air transport and landing zones.
- List examples of special response conditions.

INTRODUCTION

Emergency Medical Responders (EMRs) need to be familiar with field operations while keeping safety at the forefront. EMRs also need a basic understanding of incident evaluation tools, situational awareness strategies, and all-hazard incident management structures. While maintaining personal and personnel safety, EMRs need to be able to assess patients for transport to a higher level of care, decide where to send patients, and determine the best method of transport. Even though effective patient care is important, public and emergency responder safety in field operations is critical for the best possible outcome for all involved in the incident.

Emergency Operations

All incidents follow a three-phase resolution pattern. This pattern consists of mobilization and then an on-scene phase followed by demobilization.

First Phase

The first phase is mobilization. This phase has the least amount of on-scene activity. Emergency vehicles mobilize and drive to the scene. Often emergency personnel mobilize using a **Code 3** response (emergency response requiring lights and sirens), and safety precautions must be taken. Many responders die needlessly each year in Code 3–related accidents. Remember that using Code 3 does not automatically give responders the right of way on the road. Extreme care must always be used when passing through intersections. When going against a red traffic light, the emergency vehicle should come to a complete or near-complete stop depending on state laws (Figure 13-1). Civilian vehicles may, or may not, pull to the side and yield the right of way to an emergency vehicle. The emergency vehicle operator should look both ways for oncoming traffic and attempt to make eye contact with drivers or other vehicles before proceeding through the intersection.

As resources arrive on the scene, safety hazards must be identified and incident strategies determined to stabilize and mitigate the incident.

Second Phase

The second phase is the on-scene phase. During this phase, on-scene activity increases as incident strategies are put into action. With an increase in activity comes an increased risk to casual observers. Also, responders may become **task fixated** and lose situational awareness. Task fixated means being focused or engaged on an observed object or the accomplishment of a task that awareness of other obstacles or hazards can diminish. An example is an EMR so focused on bandaging a child's open wound that he does not hear the horn honking, does not hear the others at the scene yelling, and does not see the large truck that is driving directly toward him. EMRs must be able to focus on the tasks while being aware of the scene around them.

Third Phase

This third and last phase is demobilization. As the incident is resolved, resources are released. Scene activity is reduced. Roles change as scene priorities shift. By this phase, most hazards have been mitigated or eliminated. Although scene activity may ebb and flow, personal and personnel safety must remain paramount in everything an EMR does.

Incident Evaluation

Operations are the creation of strategies, development of tactics necessary to fulfill those strategies and use of resources to execute the identified tactics. Safe operations have ongoing, methodical evaluations of incident conditions. An incident can begin with PENMAN and can continue with FADE, a critical thinking acronym that can be used during the management of the incident.

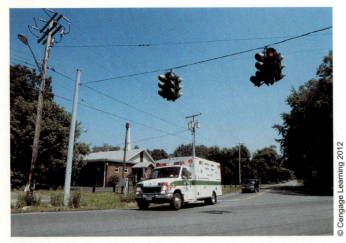

© Cengage Learning 2012

Figure 13-1 A complete stop at an intersection gives the emergency vehicle operator time to be sure that drivers of other vehicles in the intersection know of her intent to go through it.

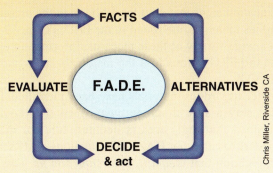

Figure 13-2 FADE (facts, address the facts, decide and act, and evaluate).

FADE

FADE (facts, address the facts, decide and act, and evaluate) is an acronym for a circular decision-making tool that responders can use during an incident. A responder, possibly under tremendous stress, can use FADE to help make decisions for patient care or incident organization (Figure 13-2).

F—Facts

"F" represents the need to collect the facts. The EMR must learn the facts about the patient or the incident. The EMR may have to do a reconnaissance lap of the incident first to gather the facts.

A—Address the Facts

"A" represents addressing the facts. After the facts are known, determine alternatives for what must be done to treat the patients, mitigate and resolve the incident, and get resources to fulfill EMR and incident requirements.

D—Decide and Act

"D" represents deciding and acting. After collecting facts and considering alternatives, the EMR must make decisions and act on those decisions, thus carrying out the plan of action.

E—Evaluate

"E" represents evaluation. The EMR must evaluate the facts, which may be constantly changing; consider new alternatives; and decide and act on possible new information. One way to remember this circular decision-making tool acronym is "FADE the incident away."

Situational Awareness

Situational awareness refers to an EMR continually looking for hazards at the scene. An EMR must be aware of exposure to already-identified hazards and other potential hazards. Therefore, an EMR must know where she is geographically within the perimeter of the incident and watch for hazards using a 360-degree prospective. A **360-degree perspective** means that the EMR is aware of potential hazards in front, behind, to the sides, and even above and beneath her. This perspective is illustrated in Figure 13-3. There is no distance

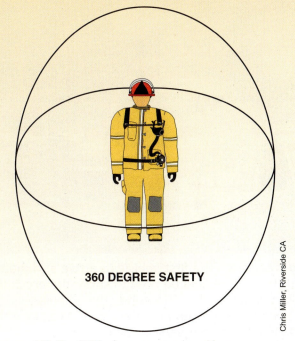

360 DEGREE SAFETY

Figure 13-3 360-degree perspective.

limitation to the safety sphere around the EMR. Safety concerns for the victims, patients, and bystanders should also be part of the EMR's safety considerations.

Situational awareness also includes personnel accountability. When a **personal accountability report (PAR)** is requested, all personnel on the scene must verbally or physically check in with their scene supervisors. An EMR should stay with his team or know where his partner is.

Traffic Collisions

Traffic is the number one killer of emergency responders. EMRs working near moving motor vehicles must practice 360-degree perspective for safety. This safety practice applies to roadways and parking lots. If necessary, you must request additional resources to control traffic flow and direction. Although traffic control may not happen immediately, it must be immediately initiated. The first public safety or agency vehicles to arrive on the scene can be used to block traffic from the incident scene; however, situational awareness should be maintained when taking this action (Figure 13-4).

Other possible on-scene safety concerns at a traffic collision may include vehicle stabilization, which must occur before safe extrication can begin; leaking fluids, which may produce a flammable or slippery environment; the possibility of down power lines, which may energize the vehicle(s) involved; and vehicle supplemental restraint systems, which may not have deployed or have the capability of deploying twice. To stabilize a vehicle shift to park, turn off the ignition, set the parking brake, and disengage the battery if possible. Do not stand in front of a vehicle; stand off to the side because a collapsed bumper can spring back. With electric cars even when the battery

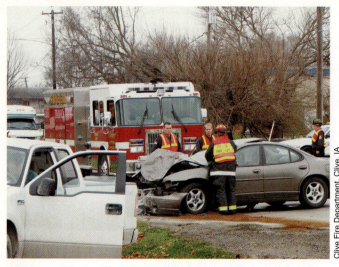

Figure 13-4 The first vehicle to arrive at a motor vehicle crash should be used to shield the accident from passing traffic. If possible, the ambulance should never be used in this manner. Fire apparatus or law enforcement vehicles are preferred.

in back is disconnected a charge can exist. Follow your agency protocols.

As previously mentioned, after equipment is deployed and action at the scene increases, even more hazards are present. Hoses from extrication tools can create a tripping hazard. Sometimes a vehicle needs to be cut and spread apart to extricate the patient. To remain with the patient throughout the extrication process, EMRs must wear the same level of personal protective equipment (PPE) as those working on the vehicle. If PPE is not available, EMRs should wait outside the perimeter of the collision until the area is safe enough to enter.

Incident Management

Incident management provides the best possible outcome for the responders, the victims, the bystanders, and the public in general. Good incident management begins when the first responder arrives on the scene.

Types of Incidences

An EMR must be prepared for various types of incident responses. Types of incidents include hazardous material (HAZMAT) and multiple casualty incidents.

Hazardous Materials

Hazardous materials are substances—biological, chemical, or physical—that have the potential to cause harm to animals, the environment, or humans, either by themselves or through interaction with other agents. Hazardous materials cause damage by exposure to skin, the respiratory tract, the digestive tract, or the eyes. The *Emergency Response Guide* (ERG) is the best resource to assist EMRs in identifying hazardous materials on vehicles or in storage areas. Placards, or

identification signs that alert the EMR as to the presence of hazardous materials, are found in the ERG. Figure 13-5 displays a wide variety of these placards. Information on how to use the ERG is found on the inside cover, as shown in Figure 13-6.

After hazardous materials have been identified, EMRs should stay a safe distance away until the HAZMAT (hazardous material) area is deemed safe for medical responders to enter. For HAZMAT situations, EMRs should find a location that is *uphill*, *upstream*, and *up wind* from the hazardous material. To maintain a safe distance, EMRs should stay at least 2,000 feet from the hazardous materials. EMRs must keep safety a top priority. Only responders with specialized training should handle the HAZMAT component of the incident.

Three zones are set up by HAZMAT Response Teams, the hot zone, warm zone, and the cold zone. Specially trained responders from an emergency response team (ERT) wearing proper PPE enter the hot zone, the actual incident scene, and rescue patients. A designated warm zone, where trained decontamination teams wearing proper PPE usually dilute the chemical with large amounts of water and decontaminate the patient, lies outside the warm zone. The EMR needs to stay in the cold zone, where no special training is required and only standard PPE should be worn. In this zone the EMR assists the Emergency Medical Services (EMS) responding agency with managing and packaging the patient for transport. Figure 13-7 illustrates the zones.

HAZMAT scenes may become **victim generators**, a dynamic incident component that continues to produce victims. As already mentioned, exposure to the hazardous materials may continue to create victims. In some circumstances, the area may need to be evacuated, which is typically a law enforcement responsibility. In large areas of contamination, individuals may have to be sheltered in place, meaning that people in the affected area are asked to close their windows, turn off their heating and cooling systems, and remain indoors for the duration of the event.

Patients exposed to the hazardous material may need to be decontaminated before being medically assessed, treated, and transported. The decontamination process removes contaminates from the person. The twofold goal of decontamination is: (1) Determine the decontamination zones and the way in which patients will be decontaminated and (2) Clean the patient(s) and keep the hazardous material restricted to the decontamination zone. The decontamination team oversees this process. When complete, the decontaminated patient can be transferred to the on-scene medical team, which consist of EMR's and EMS agencies (Figure 13-8).

The Federal Emergency Management Agency (FEMA) also offers *IS5, an Introduction to Hazardous Materials*, online for free through the Emergency Management Institute's (EMI's) Independent Study Program. It is also located at http://training.fema.gov/IS/.

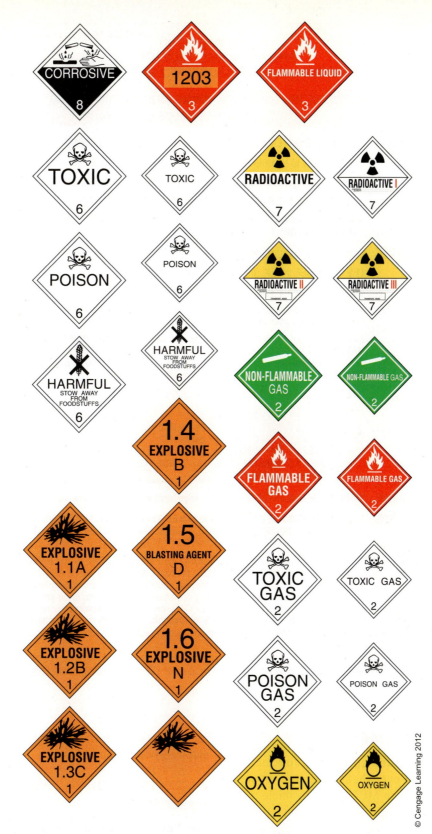

Figure 13-5 A wide variety of placards are used to mark different types and quantities of hazardous materials.

© Cengage Learning 2012

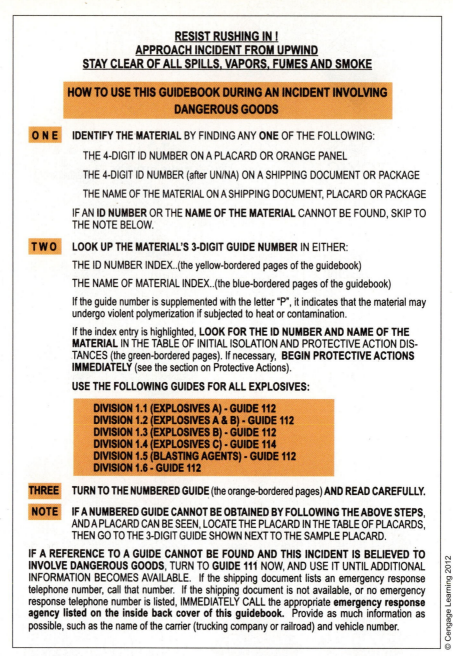

RESIST RUSHING IN !
APPROACH INCIDENT FROM UPWIND
STAY CLEAR OF ALL SPILLS, VAPORS, FUMES AND SMOKE

HOW TO USE THIS GUIDEBOOK DURING AN INCIDENT INVOLVING DANGEROUS GOODS

ONE **IDENTIFY THE MATERIAL** BY FINDING ANY **ONE** OF THE FOLLOWING:

THE 4-DIGIT ID NUMBER ON A PLACARD OR ORANGE PANEL

THE 4-DIGIT ID NUMBER (after UN/NA) ON A SHIPPING DOCUMENT OR PACKAGE

THE NAME OF THE MATERIAL ON A SHIPPING DOCUMENT, PLACARD OR PACKAGE

IF AN **ID NUMBER** OR THE **NAME OF THE MATERIAL** CANNOT BE FOUND, SKIP TO THE NOTE BELOW.

TWO **LOOK UP THE MATERIAL'S 3-DIGIT GUIDE NUMBER** IN EITHER:

THE ID NUMBER INDEX..(the yellow-bordered pages of the guidebook)

THE NAME OF MATERIAL INDEX..(the blue-bordered pages of the guidebook)

If the guide number is supplemented with the letter "P", it indicates that the material may undergo violent polymerization if subjected to heat or contamination.

If the index entry is highlighted, **LOOK FOR THE ID NUMBER AND NAME OF THE MATERIAL** IN THE TABLE OF INITIAL ISOLATION AND PROTECTIVE ACTION DISTANCES (the green-bordered pages). If necessary, **BEGIN PROTECTIVE ACTIONS IMMEDIATELY** (see the section on Protective Actions).

USE THE FOLLOWING GUIDES FOR ALL EXPLOSIVES:

DIVISION 1.1 (EXPLOSIVES A) - GUIDE 112
DIVISION 1.2 (EXPLOSIVES A & B) - GUIDE 112
DIVISION 1.3 (EXPLOSIVES B) - GUIDE 112
DIVISION 1.4 (EXPLOSIVES C) - GUIDE 114
DIVISION 1.5 (BLASTING AGENTS) - GUIDE 112
DIVISION 1.6 - GUIDE 112

THREE TURN TO THE NUMBERED GUIDE (the orange-bordered pages) AND READ CAREFULLY.

NOTE IF A NUMBERED GUIDE CANNOT BE OBTAINED BY FOLLOWING THE ABOVE STEPS, AND A PLACARD CAN BE SEEN, LOCATE THE PLACARD IN THE TABLE OF PLACARDS, THEN GO TO THE 3-DIGIT GUIDE SHOWN NEXT TO THE SAMPLE PLACARD.

IF A REFERENCE TO A GUIDE CANNOT BE FOUND AND THIS INCIDENT IS BELIEVED TO INVOLVE DANGEROUS GOODS, TURN TO **GUIDE 111** NOW, AND USE IT UNTIL ADDITIONAL INFORMATION BECOMES AVAILABLE. If the shipping document lists an emergency response telephone number, call that number. If the shipping document is not available, or no emergency response telephone number is listed, IMMEDIATELY CALL the appropriate **emergency response agency listed on the inside back cover of this guidebook.** Provide as much information as possible, such as the name of the carrier (trucking company or railroad) and vehicle number.

© Cengage Learning 2012

Figure 13-6 The inside cover of the *Emergency Response Guidebook* provides information on how to use this book.

Multiple Casualty Incidents

A **multiple-casualty incident (MCI)** is any incident in which the patient load overwhelms the first on-scene responders. An example of an MCI is a two-vehicle traffic collision with four critically injured patients and only three responders on the scene. Another example is an auto versus pedestrian incident in which the pedestrian and three persons in the car need care but only two EMRs are on the scene. In each example, the on-scene presentation of victims overwhelms the first arriving EMS responders' abilities to assess, treat, and transport all patients. MCIs require more resources than a typical medical incident. Because of the ratio of the injured versus the available resources, MCIs require victims to be rapidly and efficiently assessed, treated, and transported appropriately.

National Incident Management System

The **National Incident Management System (NIMS)** is a structured but flexible framework used nationwide by agencies to work together to respond to disasters, natural or manmade. NIMS is designed to be used at the national, state, regional, and local levels.

The FEMA offers *ICS-100* (ICS is the Incident Command System), *Introduction to ICS*, and *NIMS: An Introduction* as well as several other free ICS and NIMS courses online

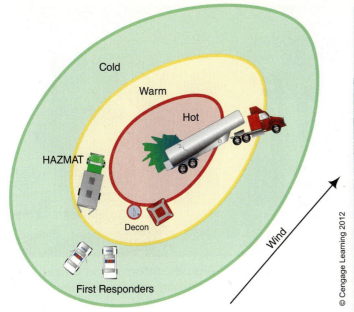

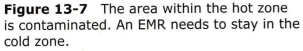

Figure 13-7 The area within the hot zone is contaminated. An EMR needs to stay in the cold zone.

through the EMI's Independent Study Program. This program is located at http://training.fema.gov/IS/. The purpose of this training is to ensure that all responders understand and use the same terminology and incident command structure.

Components of NIMS include preparedness, communications, and information management; resource management, command and management, and ongoing management and maintenance. The ICS is a part of the command and management component.

Incident Command System

The **Incident Command System (ICS)** is a standardized, on-scene, all-hazard incident management structure that is designed for emergency scene management. ICS is based on a flexible response configuration that provides a common framework within which responders can work together effectively. It provides a coordinated response that allows for integration of facilities, equipment, personnel, procedures, and communication and establishes common processes for planning and managing resources.

Public and private emergency response agencies are federally mandated to use and adhere to ICS. The first arriving responder should activate ICS. After it is in place, ICS can be expanded as additional resources arrive.

The ICS command structure optimizes communication and coordination. The command section of ICS consists of an incident commander (IC), command staff, and general staff. In some small events, the IC may handle all of these functions. In large events, the IC assigns ICS components to other responders. The IC assigns these ICS components as they are needed. ICS positions and incident resources are then released as the incident gets smaller and comes to an end.

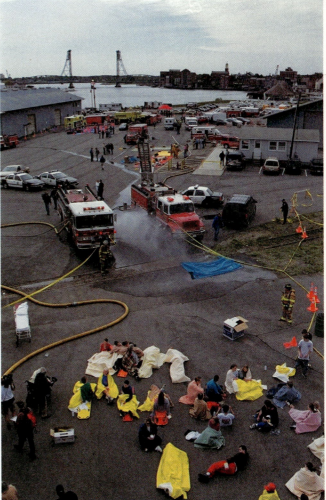

Figure 13-8 EMS usually awaits arrival of patients at the end of the decontamination corridor in the cold zone.

Minimally, all incidents have an IC (Figure 13-9). The IC is usually the highest-ranking responder to arrive on the scene, who may be a fire, police, or EMS chief. This IC position can be transferred as more experienced personnel arrive on the scene. Transfer of command should be a formal face-to-face turnover followed by a radio announcement of the IC change. The IC is located in the command post, a centralized location that is often off site where information is gathered and on-scene operations are regulated.

The IC delegates responsibilities according to incident needs. Every ICS position has a fully developed job description. Most positions can be immediately filled as resources arrive; however, some ICS positions require specialized training and experience. Additionally, the number of personnel that any position can supervise is defined as the **span of control**, which is defined as one officer for a maximum of five personnel. All people delegated responsibilities ultimately report directly to their supervisors, who in turn report to the IC. This reporting mechanism is called the chain of command. Branches of responsibilities include a safety officer, public information officer (PIO), staging officer,

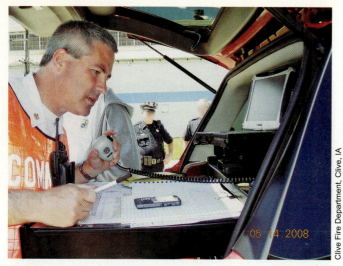

Figure 13-9 The incident commander establishes an incident command post.

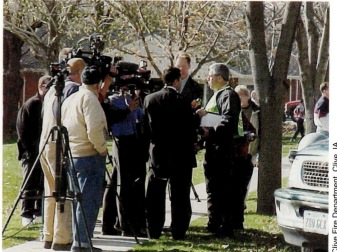

Figure 13-11 The public information officer designee is the only person who interfaces with the media.

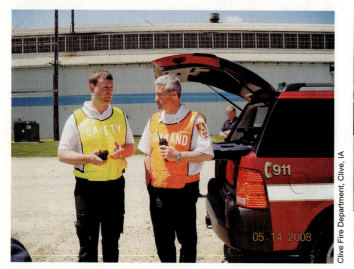

Figure 13-10 The safety officer has the responsibility for the safety of all personnel.

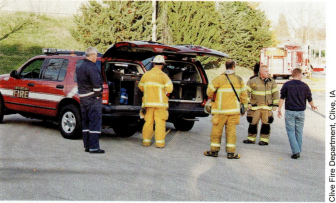

Figure 13-12 The staging officer assembles needed vehicles, personnel, and equipment.

triage officer, treatment officer, and transportation officer. An EMR functions under one or more of these officers depending on their specialty.

A safety officer should be a person who understands the common hazards that are present and is trained in ways to mitigate them (Figure 13-10). The PIO meets with the media to report on the incident. All information that is given to the public should only be provided by the designated PIO (Figure 13-11). The staging officer is a manager of the staging area, an off-scene location where personnel and vehicles assemble and await assignment (Figure 13-12). The treatment officer manages the field hospital, a temporary onsite treatment facility. The transportation officer is responsible for the overall movement of patients from the scene to the appropriate hospital. The triage officer is the manager who helps decide priorities for treatment and transportation of the patients involved. The duties of a triage officer are listed in Table 13-1.

Table 13-1 Triage Officer Duties

1. Performs the first evacuation triage
2. Appoints assistants as needed
3. Performs second treatment or transportation triage as needed
4. Coordinates EMS activities on scene
5. Coordinates patient movement to triage or transportation
Personnel
Extrication officer
Triage support personnel
Patient handlers
Equipment
Radio
Multiple-casualty incident plan
Identifier or vest
Long backboards
Triage tags

© Cengage Learning 2012

Triage Systems

Rapid patient assessment is called **triage**, which is a French word meaning "to sort." Triage is a system that sorts patients into treatment classifications according to their severity of injury. An evacuation triage is frequently the fist triage performed. Several triage systems are available. You will need to check with your agency as to which system it uses to identify priority patients. Two triage systems, the Centers for Disease Control and Prevention (CDC) Field Triage Decision Scheme and the START triage system, are described below.

CDC Field Triage Decision Scheme

The national standard for triage is the method developed in 2006 by a group of EMS experts working with the Centers for Disease Control and Prevention (CDC). This system, known as the **CDC Field Triage Decision Scheme**, looks at four different areas: physiological criteria, anatomic criteria, mechanism of injury (MOI), and special considerations to set priority for treatment and transportation. Figure 13-13 illustrates the triage system.

Step 1: Physiological Criteria

This first step rapidly identifies critically injured patients by measuring vital signs and assessing level of consciousness.

If any of the following are identified, the patient should be transported to a trauma center:

- Glasgow Coma Scale score <14 (see Chapter 5)
- Systolic blood Pressure <90 mm Hg
- Respiratory rate <10 breaths/min or >29 breaths/min in an adult; <20 breaths/min in an infant younger than one year old

Step 2: Anatomic Criteria

This step identifies patients who need care at a high-level trauma center but have physiological parameters that do not meet the criteria of Step 1.

If any of the following are identified, transport to a trauma center is recommended:

- All penetrating injuries to head, neck, torso, and extremities proximal to the elbow and knee
- Two or more proximal long bone fractures
- Crushed, degloved, or mangled extremity
- Amputation proximal to the wrist or ankle
- Pelvic fracture
- Open and depressed skull fracture
- Paralysis

Step 3: Mechanism of Injury

If a patient does not meet the criteria in Step 1 or 2 but has a severe injury, transport might still be indicated. The MOI should be evaluated next.

If any of the following have occurred, transport to a trauma center is recommended:

- Falls: An adult who has fallen from higher than 20 feet (approximately two stories); a child who has fallen from higher than 10 feet
- High-risk auto crash
  - Vehicle body intrusion greater than 12 inches into the victim's space or vehicle body intrusion greater than 18 inches
  - Ejection (partial or complete) from automobile
  - Death in the same passenger compartment
- Automobile versus a pedestrian or bicyclist thrown, run over, or with significant impact (greater than 20 mph)
- Motorcycle crash traveling greater than 20 mph

Step 4: Special Conditions

Step 4 identifies patients who may require a high-level of trauma care because of a co morbid (additional but not the primary) condition despite appearing to have no substantial injury after evaluation using physiological, anatomical, and MOI criteria.

If any of the following are identified, transport to a trauma center or specific resource hospital should be considered:

- All penetrating injuries to head, neck, torso, and extremities proximal (closer to the body) to the knee and elbow
- Flail chest (three ribs broken in two or more places to create a floating segment and paradoxical motion)
- Two or more broken proximal long bones
- Crushed, degloved, or mangled extremity
- Amputation proximal to the wrist or ankle
- Pelvic fractures
- Open or depressed skull fractures
- Paralysis

The CDC has much more information available regarding the Field Triage Decision Scheme at http://www.cdc.gov/fieldtriage/.

START Triage System

START is another triage system that has been developed to manage victims. START stands for simple triage and rapid treatment. JumpSTART is a term describing specific assessment techniques used for infants and children. Patients in both systems are quickly evaluated on their ability to walk (except infants), respirations, perfusion, and mental status (Figures 13-14 and 13-15). Color tags are placed on the wrist (most common) or foot to designate different levels of response. Four colors are used to designate patient status: green for those who can walk and are in no immediate need of transportation, yellow for those who can have treatment delayed, red for those who need intervention and immediate transport, and black for a patient who is considered deceased or for whom death is likely (Figure 13-16). Remember that color assignment can be subject to change because a patient who is stable can become unstable at any point.

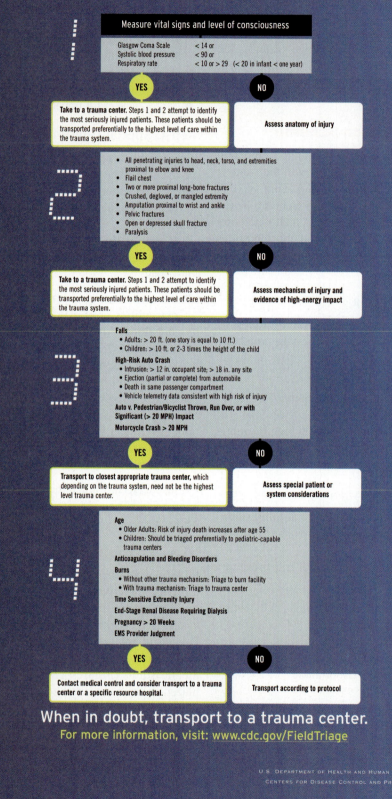

FIELD TRIAGE DECISION SCHEME: THE NATIONAL TRAUMA TRIAGE PROTOCOL

Measure vital signs and level of consciousness

Glasgow Coma Scale	< 14 or
Systolic blood pressure	< 90 or
Respiratory rate	< 10 or > 29 (< 20 in infant < one year)

YES → Take to a trauma center. Steps 1 and 2 attempt to identify the most seriously injured patients. These patients should be transported preferentially to the highest level of care within the trauma system.

NO → Assess anatomy of injury

2
- All penetrating injuries to head, neck, torso, and extremities proximal to elbow and knee
- Flail chest
- Two or more proximal long-bone fractures
- Crushed, degloved, or mangled extremity
- Amputation proximal to wrist and ankle
- Pelvic fractures
- Open or depressed skull fracture
- Paralysis

YES → Take to a trauma center. Steps 1 and 2 attempt to identify the most seriously injured patients. These patients should be transported preferentially to the highest level of care within the trauma system.

NO → Assess mechanism of injury and evidence of high-energy impact

3
Falls
- Adults: > 20 ft. (one story is equal to 10 ft.)
- Children: > 10 ft. or 2-3 times the height of the child

High-Risk Auto Crash
- Intrusion: > 12 in. occupant site; > 18 in. any site
- Ejection (partial or complete) from automobile
- Death in same passenger compartment
- Vehicle telemetry data consistent with high risk of injury

Auto v. Pedestrian/Bicyclist Thrown, Run Over, or with Significant (> 20 MPH) Impact

Motorcycle Crash > 20 MPH

YES → Transport to closest appropriate trauma center, which depending on the trauma system, need not be the highest level trauma center.

NO → Assess special patient or system considerations

4
Age
- Older Adults: Risk of injury death increases after age 55
- Children: Should be triaged preferentially to pediatric-capable trauma centers

Anticoagulation and Bleeding Disorders

Burns
- Without other trauma mechanism: Triage to burn facility
- With trauma mechanism: Triage to trauma center

Time Sensitive Extremity Injury

End-Stage Renal Disease Requiring Dialysis

Pregnancy > 20 Weeks

EMS Provider Judgment

YES → Contact medical control and consider transport to a trauma center or a specific resource hospital.

NO → Transport according to protocol

When in doubt, transport to a trauma center.

For more information, visit: www.cdc.gov/FieldTriage

U.S. DEPARTMENT OF HEALTH AND HUMAN SERVICES
CENTERS FOR DISEASE CONTROL AND PREVENTION

CDC

Source: Centers for Disease Control and Prevention, CDC

Figure 13-13 Centers for Disease Control and Prevention Field Triage Decision Scheme.

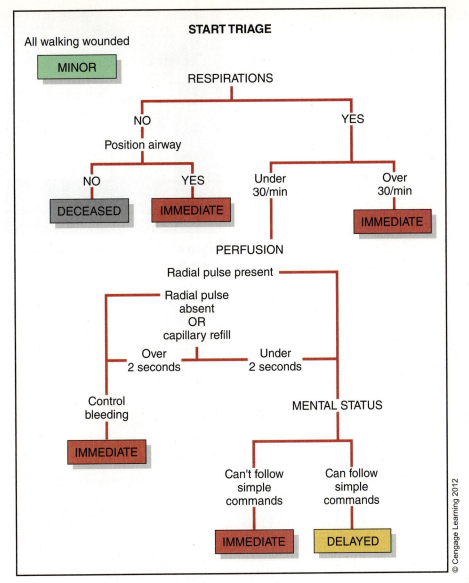

Figure 13-14 START (simple triage and rapid treatment).

Trauma Centers

Using a triage system such as the CDC Field Triage Scheme or START allows the EMR to rapidly triage victims and seek immediate transport to a **trauma center**, an acute care facility that has made special preparations and achieved certain resource and personnel standards to provide care for severely injured patients.

Delivering patients directly to a trauma center rather than to a geographically closer emergency department may be better in the long term for patients with certain injuries or predisposing factors.

Level One Trauma Center

A level one trauma center has the greatest amount of resources and personnel for patient care. These centers provide leadership in patient care, education, and research for trauma, including prevention programs. A severely injured person's risk of death is 25 percent lower at a level one trauma center.[1]

Level Two Trauma Center

A level two facility offers similar resources to a level one facility. A level two trauma center may not offer continuous access to certain subspecialties. A level two facility may also lack sufficient prevention and research activities to acquire a level one designation.[1]

Level Three Trauma Center

A level three center is capable of assessment, resuscitation, and emergency surgery. This kind of center stabilizes injured patients for transfer to a facility with a higher level of care. Transfers are done according to preexisting agreements.[1]

Level Four Trauma Center

A level four center is capable of providing 24-hour physician coverage, resuscitation, and stabilization to injured patients before they are transferred to another facility.[1]

JumpSTART Pediatric MCI Triage®

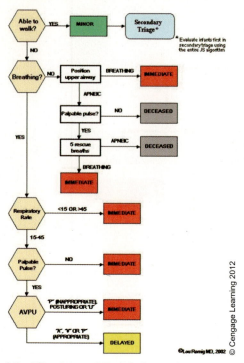

Figure 13-15 JumpSTART (simple triage and rapid treatment) pediatric triage.

Air Transportation

Air transport, where available and when used appropriately, saves time for the most critically injured patients. Many public safety agencies and private companies have helicopters staffed and prepared for immediate deployment to transport critical patients to a medical facility.

Introducing a helicopter to an incident scene creates additional safety concerns. Most regions have protocols to be considered when determining whether a patient should be transported by air. Generally, if you determine during triage that a patient requires rapid treatment and immediate transport to a specialized treatment center, the patient would be a candidate for air transport depending on distance to the trauma center and associated obstacles.

Regional requirements determine which emergency air transportation can be requested and who should request the transportation. EMRs should be familiar with these requirements for their response areas. Table 13-2 lists clinical traumatic conditions that, if suspected to be present in a given patient, might be appropriate indications for air medical transport to a medical facility.

Air Transportation Requests

In general, minimal information needed to request air transport includes:

1. Requesting agency
2. Requester's call-back number
3. Type of accident

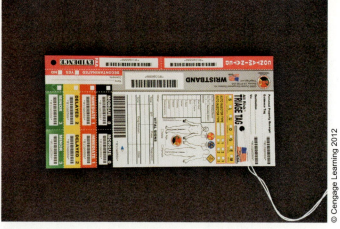

Figure 13-16 Triage tags provide a quick means of communication.

Table 13-2 Trauma Criteria for Potential Air Medical Transport

Trauma
General and mechanism
Unstable vital signs
Significant trauma in young, old, or pregnant patients
Multisystem injuries
Ejection from vehicle
Pedestrian struck by vehicle
Death in the same passenger compartment
Penetrating trauma to the abdomen, pelvis, chest, neck, or head
Crush to the abdomen, chest, or head
Fall from a significant height
Neurologic considerations
Glasgow Coma Scale score <10
Deteriorating mental status
Skull fracture
Spinal cord injury
Thoracic considerations
Major chest wall injury
Pneumothorax or hemothorax
Suspected cardiac injury
Abdominal or pelvic considerations
Significant abdominal pain after blunt trauma
Abdominal wall contusion
Obvious rib fracture below the nipple line
Major pelvic fracture
Orthopedic or extremity considerations
Partial or total ambulation of a limb (exclusive of digits)
Finger or thumb amputation when emergent surgical evaluation is indicated and rapid surface transport is not available
Fracture or dislocation with vascular compromise
Extremity ischemia

© Cengage Learning 2012

(continues)

Table 13-2 (continued)

Open long bone fractures
Two or more long bone fractures
Major burns
>20% body surface area
Involvement of the hands, feet, face, or genitalia
Inhalation injury
Electrical or chemical burns
Burns with associated injuries
Patients with near drowning injuries

© Cengage Learning 2012

4. Patient information
   a. Patient's injuries, including level of consciousness
   b. Patient's weight
5. Incident elevation
6. Incident location and landing zone (LZ) location
7. Incident global positioning satellite (GPS) position
8. LZ landmarks
   a. Highways
   b. Obstructions
9. LZ wind direction
10. Radio frequency being used
11. Call sign of the LZ officer

Landing Zones

An LZ is the area where aircraft land. The ground personnel must find a safe place for the helicopter to land. From a safety stand point, the following LZ guidelines are universal.

1. Landing zone requirements
   a. Landing area of 100 x 100 feet; 150 x 150 feet if emergency personnel are present or 300 x 300 feet if there are spectators
   b. Loose debris removed
   c. Flat: less than a 10 percent grade
   d. Hard surface or grassy area
   e. Free of overhead obstructions
   f. Clearly marked by markers or lights (Figures 13-17 and 13-18)
   g. Secure: no foot or vehicle traffic
2. LZ behavior by ground personnel (Figure 13-19)
   a. Never approach a helicopter until signaled.
   b. Never approach from the rear.
   c. Never go behind the rear elevators on the tail of the aircraft.
   d. Always approach within view of the pilot.
   e. Watch for inclines.
   f. Do not take the patient to the helicopter. The crew will come to you.
   g. Remove or secure pad, sheets, and intravenous (IV) poles on stretchers.
   h. Flight crew directs patient and equipment loading, including operation of doors.
   i. Do not smoke.

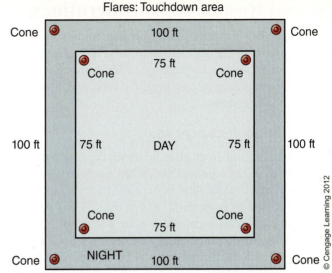

Figure 13-17 The intended touchdown area should be clearly marked with cones, flares, or other secured markers at its four corners.

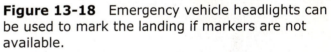
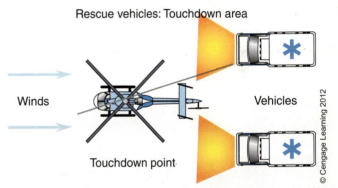

Figure 13-18 Emergency vehicle headlights can be used to mark the landing if markers are not available.

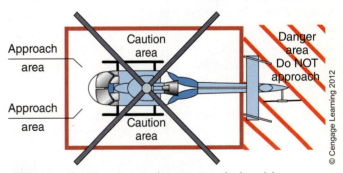

Figure 13-19 Ground personnel should be familiar with the danger zones around a helicopter.

   j. Do not run.
   k. Keep your head and arms down.

Identifying a LZ officer to communicate with the helicopter is recommended and, in some regions, mandatory. This person would be responsible for selecting and preparing the LZ.

Special Response Considerations

At times, EMRs encounter unexpected situations. An EMR must be prepared for responding in rural or remote areas, finding violent scenes, responding during extreme weather conditions, providing extended patient care, and managing various other situations.

Rural Area Responses

Responding in rural areas often increases the length of time necessary to get to a patient and, when necessary, to get a patient to a medical facility. For critical patients, air transportation should be considered early in the incident. Another option for rural responses is to initiate a transport to meet with a higher level, prehospital care professional. In rural transport situations, the patient will be on a gurney for an extended period of time. Try to make the patient as comfortable as possible.

EMRs in rural areas need to be prepared for emergencies involving farm equipment, livestock, silos, and farm chemicals. Farm accidents may include lacerations or limbs caught in belts such as shown in Figure 13-20. Other injuries include puncture wounds or degloving injuries to hands caught within the rollers or cutters of a machine or combine, such as the combine shown in Figure 13-21. Crushing injuries to arms and legs occur when heavy loads shift unexpectedly, such as when a bale of hay falls while being lifted. Injuries from an unshielded power takeoff can easily tear a limb off (Figure 13-22).

The single cause of most deaths on the farm is tractor rollovers. Operators of older tractors without a rollover

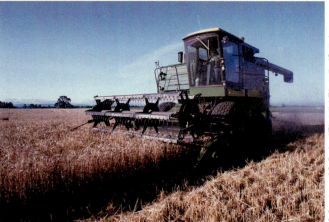

Figure 13-21 Combines can cut an operator's arm.

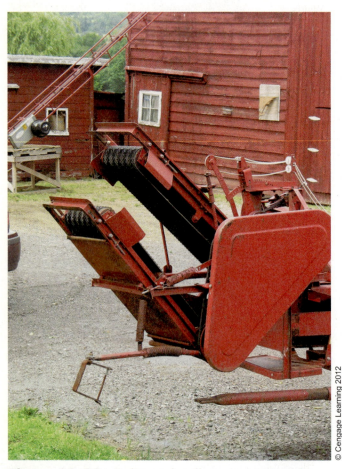

Figure 13-20 Belts and pulleys can entangle and mangle limbs.

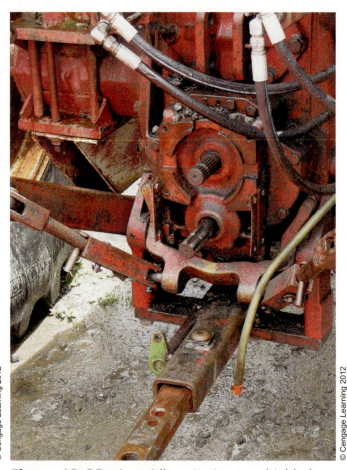

Figure 13-22 A rapidly spinning, unshielded power takeoff can tear off a limb.

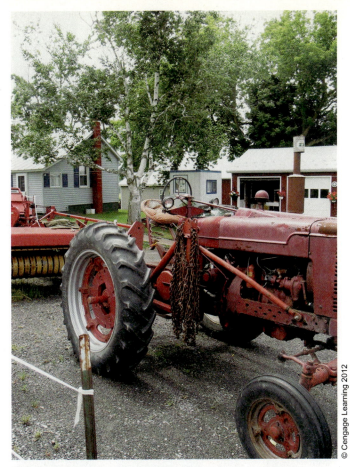

Figure 13-23 Operators of older tractors without rollover protective structures are at risk for being pinned and crushed under the tractor.

protective structure (ROPS) become pinned under the weight of the tractor and are crushed (Figure 13-23).

Search and Rescue

The EMR may respond in a geographical area where terrain makes it difficult to locate and treat patients. Situations may include locating a person lost in the woods or a cornfield as well as locating victims in a collapsed building or after a natural disaster such as a flood, hurricane, or tornado. If a person with a trauma or medical condition is located in a wilderness or other remote area, specialized rescue teams called SAR (search and rescue) and trained dogs may be dispatched. EMRs should not contaminate the area or interfere with search and rescue personnel looking for the lost or injured person.

Violent Scenes

If an incident scene has ongoing violence, stay away from the scene and wait at a location out of sight of the incident location until law enforcement arrives on the scene and renders or determines the scene to be safe. Law enforcement may need to use nonlethal gases to subdue a violent person or crowd. Wear eye protection as well as other PPE after the

Table 13-3 Crime Scene Procedures for Emergency Medical Responders

- Limit the number of responders that enter the scene to only what is needed for patient care and to keep watch on the scene's safety.
- Be prepared for the possibility that the patient may also be the individual who committed the crime. Make sure there are no weapons or potential weapons the patient could suddenly grab.
- Take care to not disturb evidence, such as footprints, broken glass, or any items that look out of place.
- Do not touch anything that is not needed in treating the patient.
- Always wear gloves to avoid leaving your fingerprints at the scene.
- Keep any clothing that is removed from the patient. Additionally, when cutting through clothing, try to avoid cutting through what could be a bullet hole or knife slash.
- Document everything about the scene thoroughly, including who was at the scene upon arrival and any individual items from the scene that were turned over to law enforcement personnel.

scene is deemed safe. If it is a potential crime scene, preserve the scene as much as possible following the procedures listed in Table 13-3.

Suspected Terrorism

Acts of terrorism, or man-made disasters as they are called, are designed to frighten people into one type of concession or another. Acts of terrorism may be either domestic or international. The bombing in Oklahoma City was an act of domestic violence (Figure 13-24). Known all too well, the organized attacks on September 11, 2001, were orchestrated by international terrorists (Figure 13-25). If terrorism is suspected at an incident, the scene should be considered a crime scene, full of evidence and clues that law enforcement will want to collect and examine. During on-scene operations, be careful to preserve the scene by not disturbing evidence. Operations involving terrorism are similar to operations in mass casualty incidence because they are often large-scale operations, requiring several agencies. Safety should be paramount in the EMR's mind. Watch for secondary devices or substances at the scene that can cause injury or death by remembering the acronym of B-NICE, which refers to biological, nuclear, incendiary (flammable), chemical, and explosives.

Confined Space

Confined space is any space that has limited openings for entry or exit and is not designed for occupancy. Examples of confined spaces are listed in Table 13-4. These spaces can be hazardous to workers who may become trapped inside. Many of these spaces have very poor oxygenation and may contain hazardous gases, which can poison a worker or EMR. The National Institute of Occupational Safety and Health (NIOSH) reports that more than 60 percent of fatalities in confined spaces are rescuers. The EMR should never enter any confined space without the proper equipment and training, Figure 13-26.

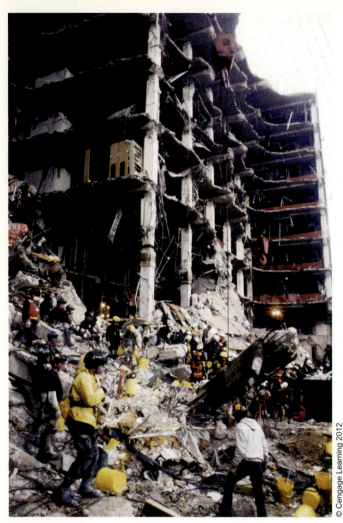

Figure 13-24 Terrorism can be domestic, as in the case of the Oklahoma City bombing.

Table 13-4 Examples of Confined Spaces

Grain bins

Wells

Sewers

Storage

Manholes

Drainage culverts

Natural caves

© Cengage Learning 2012

Extrication

Extrication simply means removing an injured person from an entrapped situation. Patients entrapped may require specialized rescue equipment to be brought to the scene (Figure 13-27). This equipment is primarily provided by the fire department, which has specialized training in this type of rescue. The patient in a vehicle should be protected from flying shards of glass by covering the victim with a heavy tarp or a short backboard, as shown in Figure 13-28.

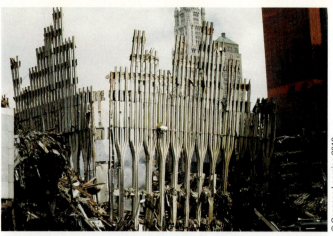

Figure 13-25 Terrorism can be international, as in the September 11, 2001, attacks.

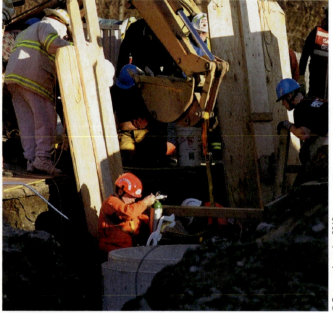

Figure 13-26 Entry into a confined space is limited to specially trained rescue personnel.

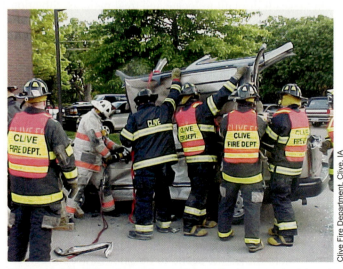

Figure 13-27 A roof can literally be peeled back to allow patient compartment access.

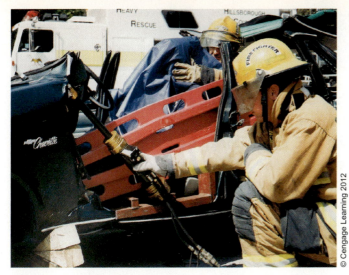

Figure 13-28 The patient should be protected from flying shards of glass by using a heavy tarp or short backboard.

Fire

Firefighting is very difficult and physically demanding work. The excessive demand on firefighters can put them at risk for illness, injury, an even death. Although many EMRs are firefighters, they need to have the proper equipment and training to protect themselves and their fellow firefighters. If a fire scene is prolonged, a concept of emergency incident rehabilitation will be instituted. This rehabilitation system includes intermittent rest and rehydration as well as medical monitoring of the firefighter.

Industrial Safety

Many industrial companies have a trained Emergency Response Team (ERT). These teams are specifically trained to handle the specifics of the industry and environment in which they work. They may be trained as EMRs or have training in basic first aid and CPR. Any EMR responding to a scene in an industrial setting will need to discuss the situation with ERT members before entering the scene.

Extreme Weather Conditions

Weather creates hazards for EMRs and victims. Extreme cold makes performing even the easiest tasks more difficult. Ice and snow conditions slow response times. Extreme heat fatigues EMRs and taxes motorized vehicles and equipment. EMRs must preplan for patient and medical personnel protection from extreme weather conditions. Consider options for safely moving to a sheltered location or for sheltering patients at the scene. If extreme weather displaces victims from their homes, contact a relief agency to assist the victims.

SUMMARY

Safety and the providing prehospital emergency medical care should be an EMR's primary tasks. FADE, a 360-degree perspective, personnel accountability, and ICS techniques are methods for accomplishing these tasks. Using CDC Field Triage Decision Scheme or START, an EMR can determine transport for patients to the correct level of trauma center. Because medical calls are not all the same, EMRs should consider special conditions and potential safety issues that might be involved when responding to a call alone, in rural areas, in violent situations, or in extreme weather conditions. Through continued training, education, and on-scene experience, the professional EMR can be an asset to any medical or trauma incident.

REVIEW QUESTIONS

1. Name the three phases of incident resolution.
2. What does the acronym FADE mean?
3. What does the acronym NIMS mean?
4. To what type of incident does uphill, up wind, and upstream apply?
5. In a HAZMAT response, what zone should the EMR stay in unless specifically trained?
6. What are two triage systems used in the United States?
7. According to ICS, a supervising officer span of control should include how many people?
8. Which level of trauma center can handle the most serious trauma cases?
9. How should you manage a crime scene?
10. With acts of terrorism what secondary devices and chemicals may cause harm to the EMR?

REFERENCE

1. Centers for Disease Control and Prevention: *Field Triage Decision Scheme*. 2009.

APPENDIX A

Emergency Medical Responder Code of Ethics

The Emergency Medical Responder Code of Ethics *is a guide for ethical and professional behavior by Emergency Medical Responders given to you by the authors to use in your own agency.*

Emergency Medical Responders come from diverse agencies, companies, schools, and organizations. As diverse as they are, Emergency Medical Responders are linked together by their responsibilities and desire to protect and preserve the quality of life and reduce the pain and disability of the patients they serve.

Emergency Medical Responders may serve their communities as a career- or volunteer-responder. As volunteers, they leave their primary job duties or homes to respond to various medical and trauma crises. Emergency Medical Responders acknowledge and recognize that they are a vital component of the emergency services profession. They provide the initial safety net for patients until a higher level of responder arrives.

Emergency Medical Responders recognize the importance of continuing education and training and dedicate themselves to continually improving their medical assessment and management of the patients they encounter.

Emergency Medical Responders shall perform their duties without regard to a patient's race, religion, sexual orientation, or creed. While performing their duties and responsibilities, the emergency medical responder shall act selflessly, ethically, and professionally with integrity, and violate no laws.

Emergency Medical Responders shall operate within their prescribed scope of practice and the standard of care in the communities in which they serve, and shall not cause harm to the patients temporarily entrusted in their care.

Emergency Medical Responders shall, to the best of their ability, establish and maintain a safe working environment protecting themselves, their professional associates, their patients, and the public they serve.

The goal of the Emergency Medical Responder, is at all times and to the best of their abilities, shall be to maintain and promote an atmosphere of team cohesiveness, mutual respect, and camaraderie.

To this code of conduct, as an Emergency Medical Responder I shall freely acknowledge and accept as my own.

Chris Miller and Joe Grafft

APPENDIX B

Competency Skill Sheets for the Emergency Medical Responder

Competency skill sheets correlate with the skills introduced in the book and can be used by students to practice skills in the lab. These competencies for the EMR must be approved by the agency's Medical Director.

To access electronic versions of these skill sheets, please visit www.cengagebrain.com. At the CengageBrain home page, search for this book using the search box. On the page illustrating this book, click on the "Access Now" button, and this will direct you to the skill sheets.

Patient Assessment and Management—Medical Competency Skill Sheet

Medical Assessment and Management	YES	NO
Scene size-up/PENMAN		
Scene Safety		
Proper PPE*		
Determines MOI or NOI		
Determines number of patients		
Requests additional help if needed		
Spinal stabilization (if MOI indicates): verbalizes or directs assistant		
Primary Survey and Management		
Verbalizes general impression of the patient		
Determines level of consciousness		
Determines patient's chief complaint		
Assesses airway, breathing, and circulation*		
Verbalizes management: administers oxygen and controls major bleeding if necessary		
Baseline vital signs*		
Secondary Survey or Rapid Survey*		
SAMPLE history		
OPQRST		
Verbalize medical management		
Reassessment*		
Transport decision		
Reassures the patient throughout the procedure		

Critical Criteria

_____ *Did not use or verbalize proper PPE

_____ *Did not properly assess or manage the ABCs

_____ *Did not perform baseline vital signs

_____ *Did not perform a secondary survey or rapid survey

_____ *Did not verbalize reassessment

The above competency skill sheet is based on this text and the NREMT check off sheets – Used with permission.

Patient Assessment and Management—Trauma Competency Skill Sheet

Trauma Assessment and Management	Yes	Yes
Scene size-up/PENMAN		
Scene safety*		
Proper PPE*		
Determines MOI		
Determines number of patients		
Requests additional help if needed		
Spinal stabilization (if MOI indicates)*: verbalize or direct assistant		
Primary Survey and Management		
Verbalizes general impression of the patient		
Determines level of consciousness		
Determines patient's chief complaint		
Assesses airway, breathing, and circulation*		
Verbalizes management: administers oxygen and controls major bleeding if necessary		
Baseline vital signs*		
Secondary Survey or Rapid Survey*		
Head-to-toe assessment		
SAMPLE		
OPQRST		
Verbalizes management of injuries and wounds appropriately		
Reassessment*		
Reassures the patient throughout the procedure		
Transport decision*		

Critical Criteria

_____ *Did not establish scene safety

_____ *Did not use or verbalize proper PPE

_____ *Did not verbalize spinal stabilization

_____ *Did not properly assess or manage the ABCs

_____ *Did not obtain baseline vital signs

_____ *Did not perform a secondary survey or rapid survey

_____ *Did not verbalize reassessment

_____ *Did not indicate a need for rapid transport

The above competency skill sheet is based on this text and the NREMT check off sheets – Used with permission.

Upper Airway Adjuncts—Competency Skill Sheets

Oropharyngeal Airway Insertion

Proper PPE*		
Selects and measures appropriate size OPA*		
Inserts OPA properly*		
NOTE: Patient is gagging		
Removes the OPA		

Critical Criteria

_____ *Did not use or verbalize proper PPE

_____ *Did not select and measure appropriate size airway

_____ *Did not properly insert the OPA

Nasopharyngeal Airway Insertion

Proper PPE*		
Selects and measures appropriate size NPA*		
Verbalizes lubrication of the NPA*		
Fully inserts NPA with bevel toward the septum*		

Critical Criteria

_____ *Did not use or verbalize proper PPE

_____ *Did not select and measure appropriate size NPA

_____ *Did not verbalize lubrication of the NPA

_____ *Did not properly insert the NPA

The above competency skill sheet is based on this text and the NREMT check off sheets – Used with permission.

Suctioning—Competency Skill Sheet

Upper Airway Suction	YES	NO
Proper PPE*		
Turns on device and ensures suction is working properly*		
Inserts catheter into oropharynx without suction*		
Suctions correct amount of time (approximately 15 seconds for adult, child 10 seconds, infant 5 seconds)*		
Explains what to do if catheter becomes plugged		

Critical Criteria

_____ *Did not use or verbalize proper PPE

_____ *Did not prepare suction device or presence of suction

_____ *Used suction while inserting catheter

_____ *Did not suction correct amount of time

The above competency skill sheet is based on this text and the NREMT check off sheets – Used with permission.

Oxygen Tank Assembly—Competency Skill Sheet

Oxygen Tank Assembly	YES	NO
Verbalizes confirmation that the tank is an oxygen tank*		
Secures the oxygen tank*		
Cracks the oxygen tank to clean out the orifice*		
Places a new O ring on the oxygen regulator orifice*		
Places and tightens the regulator properly on the tank*		
Turns the oxygen tank valve (fully to the left and backs off ¼ turn)*		
Verbalizes the pressure of the tank		

Critical Criteria

_____ *Did not determine if this was an oxygen tank

_____ *Did not properly secure the tank

_____ *Did not crack the tank before placing the regulator on the tank

_____ *Did not place a new O ring on regulator orifice

_____ *Did not properly place the regulator on the tank

_____ *Did not open the oxygen tank valve correctly

The above competency skill sheet is based on this text and the NREMT check off sheets – Used with permission.

Ventilation—Competency Skill Sheets

Mouth-to-Mask Ventilation with Oxygen

Mouth to Mask	YES	NO
Proper PPE*		
Opens the airway manually or with airway adjunct		
Establishes and maintains a proper mask to face seal*		
Ventilates the patient to visible chest rise only (adult every 5–6 seconds, pediatric patient every 3–5 seconds)*		
Connects mask to high-flow oxygen*		
Continues ventilation with visible chest rise		

Critical Criteria

____ *Did not use or verbalize proper PPE

____ *Did not have proper mask-to-face seal

____ *Did not ventilate to chest rise only or at proper rate

____ *Did not provide proper liter flow rate

Bag Valve Mask Ventilation with Oxygen

Bag Valve Mask—Apneic Patient		
Proper PPE*		
Places an airway adjunct		
Attaches oxygen tubing to the BVM and while using high-flow oxygen ensures inflation of bag*		
Uses a proper mask-to-face seal with BVM*		
Ventilates the patient to visible chest rise only (adult every 5–6 seconds, pediatric patient every 3–5 seconds)*		

Critical Criteria

____ *Did not use or verbalize proper PPE

____ *Did not have adequate mask-to-face seal

____ *Did not ventilate to chest rise only or at proper rate

____ *Did not provide proper liter flow rate

The above competency skill sheet is based on this text and the NREMT check off sheets – Used with permission.

Supplemental Oxygen
Delivery—Competency Skill Sheets

Nasal Cannula Administration

Nasal Cannula	YES	NO
Proper PPE*		
Attaches the nasal cannula tubing to the assembled oxygen tank		
Adjusts the oxygen regulator to the appropriate liter flow rate (maximum of 6 lpm)*		
Tests the nasal cannula for oxygen flow*		
Applies the nasal cannula properly*		
Verbalizes monitoring the patient for adequate oxygenation		
Reassures the patient during the procedure		

Critical Criteria

_____ *Did not use or verbalize proper PPE

_____ *Did not set the appropriate liter flow rate

_____ *Did not test the nasal cannula for oxygen flow

_____ *Did not properly apply the nasal cannula

Non-Rebreather Mask Administration

Non-Rebreather Mask	YES	NO
Proper PPE*		
Attaches the non-rebreather mask tubing to the assembled oxygen tank		
Adjusts the oxygen regulator to the appropriate liter flow rate (at least 10 lpm)*		
Inflates the non-rebreather bag*		
Applies non-rebreather mask properly*		
Verbalizes monitoring the patient for adequate oxygenation		
Reassures the patient during the procedure		

Critical Criteria

_____ *Did not use or verbalize proper PPE

_____ *Did not set the appropriate liter flow rate

_____ *Did not inflate the non-rebreather bag

_____ *Did not properly apply non-rebreather mask

The above competency skill sheet is based on this text and the NREMT check off sheets – Used with permission.

Bleeding Control and Shock Management—Competency Skill Sheet

Major Bleeding Control and Shock Management	YES	NO
Proper PPE*		
Applies direct pressure with gauze to the wound*		
NOTE: The wound continues to bleed through the dressing. Applies additional dressing and maintains direct pressure*		
NOTE: The wound continues to bleed through the dressing. Places a tourniquet above the site and notes the time placed*		
NOTE: Bleeding is controlled—signs of hypoperfusion.		
Treats the patient for shock* (proper positioning and maintains body heat)		
Verbalizes application of oxygen*		
Verbalizes the need for rapid transport		
Reassures the patient throughout the procedure		

Critical Criteria

_____ *Did not use or verbalize proper PPE

_____ *Did not apply direct pressure

_____ *Did not apply additional dressing and continue direct pressure

_____ *Did not apply a tourniquet or note the time of placement

_____ *Did not treat for shock

_____ *Did not verbalize application of oxygen

The above competency skill sheet is based on this text and the NREMT check off sheets – Used with permission.

Long Bone Fracture Stabilization—Competency Skill Sheet

Lower Leg Fracture Stabilization	YES	NO
Proper PPE*		
Directs assistant to stabilize the lower leg above and below the fracture and adjacent joints*		
Verbalizes exposure of fracture site		
Checks CMS* (shoe and sock removal)		
Places rigid splints along each side of the involved leg		
Properly secures cravats or straps above and below the fracture site first*		
Immobilizes foot in position of function		
Secures the uninvolved leg to the rigid splint*		
Rechecks CMS*		
Reassures the patient during the procedure		

Critical Criteria

_____ *Did not use or verbalize proper PPE

_____ *Did not verbalize stabilization fracture

_____ *Did not check CMS

_____ *Did not secure cravats or straps properly

_____ *Did not secure the uninvolved leg to the rigid splint

_____ *Did not recheck CMS

The above competency skill sheet is based on this text and the NREMT check off sheets – Used with permission.

Immobilization of a Joint Injury—Competency Skill Sheet

Immobilization of a Joint Injury—Knee	YES	NO
Proper PPE*		
Directs assistant to stabilize the affected joint in the position found*		
Verbalizes exposing area of injury		
Check CMS* (shoe and sock removal)		
Places rigid splints along each side of the affected joint		
Properly secures the rigid splints above and below the joint first*		
Recheck CMS*		
Reassures the patient during the procedure		

Critical Criteria

_____ *Did not use or verbalize proper PPE

_____ *Did not direct stabilization

_____ *Did not check CMS

_____ *Did not properly secure the rigid splint

_____ *Did not recheck CMS

The above competency skill sheet is based on this text and the NREMT check off sheets – Used with permission.

Upper Arm Fracture
Stabilization—Competency Skill Sheet

Upper Arm Fracture Stabilization	YES	NO
Proper PPE*		
Directs assistant to stabilize above and below the fracture site and adjacent joints*		
Verbalizes exposure of fracture site		
Check CMS*		
Places a rigid splint under the arm		
Secures the rigid splint above and below the fracture site first*		
Places a roller bandage in the patient's hand in the position of function		
Places a sling and swathe on the fractured arm*		
Rechecks CMS*		
Reassures the patient during the procedure		

Critical Criteria

_____ *Did not use or verbalize proper PPE

_____ *Did not direct stabilization

_____ *Did not check CMS

_____ *Did not properly secure the rigid splint to the arm

_____ *Did not properly place a sling and swathe on the arm

_____ *Did not recheck CMS

The above competency skill sheet is based on this text and the NREMT check off sheets – Used with permission.

Traction Splint of a Closed Femur Fracture—Competency Skill Sheet

Traction Splint of a Closed Femur Fracture	YES	NO
Proper PPE*		
Directs assistant to stabilize above and below the fracture site and adjacent joints*		
Verbalizes exposure of fracture site		
Checks CMS* (shoe and sock removal)		
Directs application of gentle manual traction		
Properly measures and adjusts the traction device*		
Properly places the ankle strap and directs continued gentle traction*		
Places the traction device under the fractured leg and adjusts but does not attach the securing straps		
Secures the ischial strap high in the thigh*		
Attaches the windless to the ring on the ankle hitch		
Applies mechanical traction*		
Applies the straps beginning with above and below the fracture site		
Rechecks CMS*		
Verbalizes securing the body and splint on a long backboard		
Reassures the patient during the procedure		

Critical Criteria

_____ *Did not use or verbalize proper PPE

_____ *Did not direct stabilization

_____ *Did not check CMS

_____ *Did not properly measure the traction device

_____ *Did not properly attach the ankle strap

_____ *Did not secure only the ischial strap before mechanical traction

_____ *Did not recheck CMS

The above competency skill sheet is based on this text and the NREMT check off sheets – Used with permission.

Spinal Immobilization:
Seated Patient—Competency Skill Sheet

Short Board—Seated Patient	Yes	No
Proper PPE*		
Directs assistant to stabilize the neck in neutral alignment*		
Checks for CMS*		
Applies appropriate size cervical collar*		
Positions board and secures straps in correct order: middle, abdominal, top*		
Places pad behind patient's head as needed		
Secures forehead strap then chin strap		
Verbalizes placement of the short board onto a long backboard*		
Rechecks CMS*		
Reassures the patient throughout the procedure		

Critical Criteria

_____ *Did not use or verbalize proper PPE

_____ *Did not properly direct stabilization of the cervical spine

_____ *Did not check for CMS

_____ *Did not properly place cervical collar

_____ *Did not properly secure the patient to the short board

_____ *Did not verbalize placement of the short board on the long board

_____ *Did not recheck CMS

The above competency skill sheet is based on this text and the NREMT check off sheets – Used with permission.

Spinal Immobilization:
Long Board—Competency Skill Sheet

Long Backboard—Supine Patient	YES	NO
Proper PPE*		
Directs assistant to stabilize the neck in neutral alignment*		
Checks for CMS*		
Applies cervical collar correctly*		
Properly positions long backboard		
Directs proper log roll or seven-person lift to the long backboard*		
Directs placement straps properly and in correct order: chest (under the arms), abdominal, upper leg, lower leg*		
Immobilizes patient's head to the device: forehead, then chin strap*		
Rechecks CMS*		
Reassures the patient throughout the procedure		

Critical Criteria

_____ *Did not use or verbalize proper PPE

_____ *Did not direct stabilization the cervical spine

_____ *Did not check CMS

_____ *Did not properly place the cervical collar

_____ *Did not properly place the patient onto the long backboard

_____ *Did not properly place the straps

_____ *Did not recheck CMS

The above competency skill sheet is based on this text and the NREMT check off sheets – Used with permission.

Cardiac Arrest Management:
Adult One or Two Rescuer and Automated External Defibrillator (AED)—Competency Skill Sheet

Cardiac Arrest Management—Adult One or Two Rescuer	YES	NO
Scene safety*		
Proper PPE*		
Directs spinal stabilization if MOI indicates*		
Checks for responsiveness*		
Checks for no breathing or no normal breathing* (5–10 seconds)		
Checks carotid pulse (5–10 seconds)*		
Locates CPR hand position		
Performs 30 compressions and two ventilations for five cycles (<23 seconds per cycle)*		
Additional rescuer arrives with AED and turns it on		
AED pads are attached while the two rescuers continue compressions and ventilations*		
Follows AED prompts of clearing the patient*		
AED delivers shock, and the rescuer immediately begins compressions*		
Continues 30 compressions and two ventilations following the AED prompts		
Transfers care to EMS		

Critical Criteria

_____ *Did not establish scene safety

_____ *Did not use or verbalize proper PPE

_____ *Did not stabilize the cervical spine if MOI indicated

_____ *Did not check for responsiveness and breathing

_____ *Did not check carotid pulse

_____ *Did not perform proper compressions and ventilations

_____ *Did not properly attach the AED to the patient

_____ *Did not continue compressions while attaching the AED

_____ *Did not follow AED prompts

_____ *Did not immediately begin with compressions after the shock

The above competency skill sheet follows the 2010 American Heart Association guidelines and NREMT check off sheets.

APPENDIX C

Patient Care Report (PCR)

The student can use the patient care report to practice documentation in conjunction with scenarios found in the trauma, medical, and environmental emergency chapters.

To access this form, please visit www.cengagebrain.com. At the CengageBrain home page, search for this book using the search box. On the page illustrating this book, click on the "Access Now" button, and this will direct you to the electronic form.

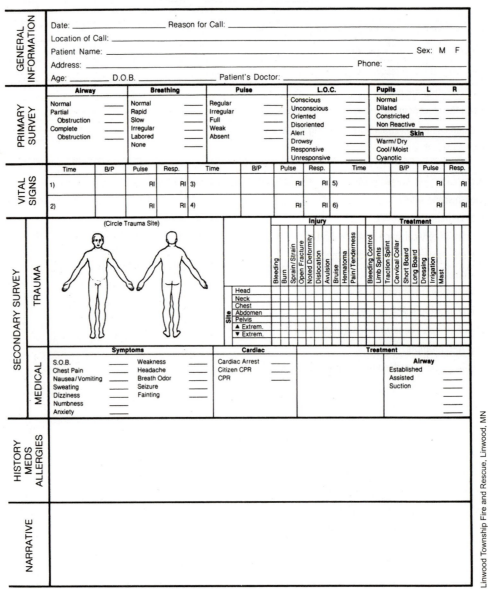

GLOSSARY

Abandonment Occurs in the prehospital setting when an Emergency Medical Responder begins emergency medical treatment of a patient and then leaves that patient, still in need of care, unsupervised.

ABCs Acronym that refers to airway, breathing, and circulation.

Abdominal aortic aneurysm Leak or rupture in the wall of the aorta, the largest artery in the body.

Abdominal cavity Area between the diaphragm and pelvis that contains the organs of digestion and elimination.

Abrasion Superficial scrape of the uppermost layer of skin.

Abuse Intentional physical, emotional, sexual, or economic injury to a dependent person that may lead to serious injury or permanent disability.

Accessory muscles for breathing Muscles not normally involved in breathing.

Active listening Requires the listener to understand, interpret, and evaluate what is heard.

Addiction A strong physiological and psychological dependence on a drug or substance despite negative effects.

Advanced emergency medical technician (AEMT) Emergency Medical Technician who can perform some advanced emergency care, including advanced airway management, intravenous therapy, and administering basic medications.

Advanced life support (ALS) A broad term applied to emergency medical care rendered beyond basic life support.

Agonal breathing Slow breathing at a rate of approximately 3 to 4 breaths/min with shallow, irregular, or gasping breaths.

Airborne pathogens Pathogens suspended in air on water droplets or dust particles.

Airway devices Devices used to maintain an open airway by keeping the tongue from obstructing the back of the mouth.

Allergen A substance that is foreign to the body and can cause an allergic reaction in certain people.

Altered mental status (AMS) A change in level of consciousness, cognition, and behavior from baseline due to a medical or trauma condition.

Alveoli Small air sacs at the end of bronchioles that allow exchange of carbon dioxide and oxygen.

Anaphylactic shock (anaphylaxis) Exaggerated allergic reaction that causes a severe inflammatory response that can be life threatening.

Anatomy The study of the structure of an organism.

Angina pectoris Chest pain or discomfort that results from insufficient oxygenated blood flow to the heart muscle.

Anterior aspect The front of the body.

Apgar score A numerical expression of the condition of a newborn infant, usually determined at 60 seconds after birth, being the sum of points gained on assessment of the color (appearance), heart rate (pulse), reflex irritability (grimace), muscle tone (activity), and respiratory effort (respiration).

Apparatus The transport vehicle for personnel and equipment.

Appendicitis Inflammation or infection of the appendix often characterized by the presence of right lower quadrant pain.

Arteries Blood vessels that lead away from the heart and carry oxygenated blood.

Arterioles Small blood vessels that branch from the arteries.

Aspiration Introduction of vomit, fluid, or other foreign material into the lungs.

Assault A case in which a patient is afraid that he or she may be touched without having given consent.

Asthma A condition consisting of bronchospasm and inflammation of the bronchial tubes in response to a stimuli or combination of stimuli.

Asystole Cardiac arrest; when there is no electrical activity to the heart muscle resulting in no contractions or movement of blood.

Atria Two upper chambers of the heart.

Atrial fibrillation Unorganized electrical impulses in the atria of the heart.

Auscultation Listening to the sounds of the body, usually with a stethoscope.

Automated external defibrillator (AED) A machine that can read the electrocardiogram (ECG); advise the Emergency Medical Responder to shock or defibrillate; and then deliver that shock to the patient.

Autonomic nervous system Collection of nerves that originates in the brainstem and transmits impulses for automatic functioning of organs.

AVPU An acronym to recall the classifications of level of responsiveness: alert, voice, pain, and unresponsive.

Avulsion A wound or flap of body tissue created by a forceful tearing away or separation of tissue from the body.

Axilla Armpit.

Backboarding Providing a hard surface to perform cardiopulmonary resuscitation to transfer a patient who is unable to ambulate or to provide spinal immobilization for a traumatic injury.

Bacterial tracheitis An acute crouplike bacterial infection of the upper airway in children, characterized by coughing and high fever.

Bag valve mask (BVM) Handheld device used to provide positive pressure ventilation to a patient who is not breathing or who is not breathing adequately.

Bandages Strips of cloth used to hold dressings securely in place and provide pressure to control bleeding and protect the wound from further injury.

Baseline vital signs First set of vital signs obtained; used to compare to the following sets.

Battery Unlawfully touching a patient against his or her wishes.

Battle's sign Bruising behind the ears indicating a skull fracture.

Biohazards Short term for biological hazard meaning any biological substance that may be infectious.

Bladder A large muscular sac that holds urine until elimination.

Bloodborne pathogens Pathogens spread by contaminated blood.

Blood pressure (BP) The amount of pressure placed on the walls of blood vessels by the circulatory system.

Blood vessels Complex set of tubes that allows blood to travel around the body.

Bloody show Expulsion of a small amount of bloody mucus from the cervix as the cervix begins to thin and starts to dilate in preparation for childbirth.

Blow-by oxygenation Delivering oxygen by placing oxygen tubing or mask close to the patient's mouth and nose when the patient cannot tolerate a mask.

Body mechanics The proper way to lift, push, or carry that helps prevent physical strain that may cause injury.

Body substance isolation (BSI) Methods of protecting oneself and avoiding direct contact to pathogens from body substances.

Bounding pulse Strong and forceful pulse.

Bowel obstruction Blockage of the flow through the intestine that results in distension, abdominal pain, and vomiting.

Brachial pulse The pulse located in the inner aspect of the arm between the elbow and shoulder.

Bradycardia A slower than normal heart rate.

Bradypnea A slower than normal respiratory rate.

Brainstem The lower part of the brain that extends into the spinal cord and regulates several vital functions.

Braxton Hicks contractions Random contractions, also known as "false labor," that occur in the third trimester that are not associated with cervical effacement or dilation.

Breech presentation The presentation of the buttocks or a limb instead of the fetal head during birth.

Bronchi Large air tubes leading from the trachea to the lungs.

Bronchioles Numerous pathways that branch off the bronchi and terminate in small sacs called alveoli. The alveoli are in direct contact with the lungs and are covered with blood vessels.

Bronchospasm An abnormal contraction of the smooth muscle of the bronchi, resulting in an acute narrowing and obstruction of the airway.

Call data The first component of the patient care report; contains the location of the call, call times, unit number, responding personnel, date, and patient identifying information.

Capillaries The smallest blood vessels that connect arteries to veins.

Capillary refill time (CRT) The time it takes to see the refill of blood (returning to the normal color) in the fingernail or toenail after blanching (pressing to obtain loss of color) and releasing pressure to the area.

Carbon dioxide (CO2) A colorless, odorless gas that is naturally formed in the tissues of the body and eliminated by the lungs; CO_2 is toxic in large amounts but is necessary for life in proper amounts.

Cardiac arrest The heart stops contracting (beating); no electrical impulses seen on an ECG and no pulse felt.

Cardiac muscle A special type of muscle that is able to generate its own electrical impulse.

Cardiogenic shock A hypoperfused state resulting from inadequate cardiac pumping. The heart muscle fails to adequately perfuse the vital organs because of damage to the heart muscle.

Cardiopulmonary resuscitation (CPR) Emergency procedure to provide oxygenated blood flow that consists of external cardiac compressions and pulmonary resuscitation through ventilations.

Carotid pulse The central pulse found in the neck by tipping the head back and sliding your fingers down from the thyroid cartilage to the grove in the neck.

Cartilage A substance, not as firm as bone, that connects and cushion bones in places such as the ribcage, vertebrae, and tip of the nose.

CDC Field Triage Design Scheme A triage system set up by national emergency medical services experts to assist in the proper sorting of patients at a multiple-casualty incident.

Centers for Disease Control and Prevention (CDC) Governmental agency dedicated to disease prevention and control.

Central nervous system Consists of the brain and spinal cord and is involved in the initiation and transmission of sensory and motor messages throughout the body.

Cerebellum Part of the brain located above the brainstem that controls muscular coordination and balance.

Cerebrospinal fluid (CSF) Fluid that serves as a support or cushion for the brain within the skull.

Cerebrovascular accident (CVA) Injury to the brain tissue that occurs as a result of disruption of blood flow to part of the brain; also known as a stroke.

Cerebrum The largest and most highly evolved area of the brain

Cervical immobilization device (CID) A cervical collar device intended to assist in maintaining the cervical spine and head in a neutral inline alignment.

Cervical spine The uppermost section of the spinal column, made up of seven vertebrae in the neck; protects the spinal cord in the neck.

CHART An acronym for chief complaint, history of present illness or injury, assessment, treatment and interventions used, and need for transport.

Chief complaint (CC) The patient's main problem and reason for seeking medical services.

Child abuse Any act, or failure to act, on the part of responsible adults that results in the death, serious physical or emotional harm, sexual abuse or exploitation, or an act or failure to act that presents an imminent risk of serious harm.

Chronic bronchitis Swelling and thickening of the lining of the bronchi and bronchioles and an increase of mucus production causing shortness of breath.

Chronic obstructive pulmonary disease (COPD) A group of lung diseases characterized by chronic airway obstruction and bronchospasms, making it difficult to breathe.

Closed fracture A broken bone in which the ends do not break the skin.

CMS An assessment done on the extremities, usually the hands and feet, that includes circulation, movement, and sensation.

Coccyx The tailbone, or last portion of the spinal column.

Code 3 Emergency response requiring lights and sirens.

Cold zone A designated safe area as established by the hazardous materials response team to assist other responders and provide patient care.

Compensatory mechanism Methods the human body uses to correct distinct deficits that come with illness or injury.

Concussion A mild, closed head injury caused by a blunt force.

Confidentiality Privacy; in the medical system, means ensuring that patient medical information is given only to the patient's health care provider.

Consent Voluntary agreement by a person to allow something to take place.

Contrecoup injury A contusion resulting from a blow on one side of the head with damage to the brain on the opposite side.

Contusion Bruising of tissue usually caused by blunt forces.

Core values Personal beliefs and behaviors that are considered important and necessary among the emergency medical services profession such as integrity, fairness, respect, honesty, courage, and compassion.

Coup-contrecoup Damage to brain tissue at the point of initial impact as well as damage to the side opposite the point of the initial impact.

Cranium The bony skull that encloses the brain.

Cravat A simple cotton triangle bandage folded to approximately two inches in width.

Crepitus Crackling or popping sound heard or felt under the skin or in the joints; the sound of bone ends grinding together.

Critical incident stress debriefing (CISD) A structured conversation between the individual who has experienced a traumatic event and a mental health professional, a peer trained in CISD, or CISD team.

Critical thinking The identification and evaluation of evidence to guide decision making.

Croup Swelling and inflammation of the larynx, the trachea, and (to some extent) the bronchi, usually caused by a viral infection.

Crowning The appearance of the fetal head at the vaginal opening when delivery is imminent.

Culture of emergency medical services The structure and history of an emergency medical services agency.

Data collection Specific health care information collected and documented by the Emergency Medical Responder that is used for consideration of future health care needs and practices.

Deceleration injury Injury that occurs after impact when the forward movement of the body causes the organs to continue moving, causing tearing or rupturing.

Decerebrate posture Abnormal posturing on one or both sides of the body that involves the arms and legs being extended, the toes being pointed downward, and the head and neck arched backward. Muscles are tightened and held rigidly.

Decorticate posture Abnormal posturing on one or both sides of the body that involves rigidity, flexion of the arms, clenched fists, and extended legs. The arms are bent inward toward the body with the wrists and fingers bent and held on the chest.

Degloving avulsion The forceful separation of just the skin from an extremity.

Delirium tremens (DTs) Symptoms associated with the sudden withdrawal of alcohol from an alcohol-dependent person.

Department of Transportation (DOT) The governmental agency responsible for safe transportation on U.S. roadways.

Dependency A physiological and psychological need a person has for a drug.

Depression A mood disorder characterized by persistent sadness and lack of interest in usual life pleasures.

Developmental challenge A challenge that is physical, cognitive, sensory, emotional, or a combination that affects a person's functioning.

Diabetes mellitus A condition in which the pancreas no longer produces enough insulin or cells stop responding to the insulin that is produced, so that glucose in the blood cannot be absorbed into the cells of the body.

Diabetic ketoacidosis (DKA) Seen in diabetics with severe hyperglycemia. A condition when fats are metabolized when glucose cannot be used. Ketones (acids) are produced by the break down of fats. The body attempts to expel the ketones by rapid deep breathing.

Diaphoresis Profuse sweating.

Diaphragm Fibrous structure that inferiorly borders the rib cage and is the main muscle of breathing.

Diastolic blood pressure The pressure of the blood in the vessels at rest between heartbeats when there is no force, represented by the bottom number of the blood pressure reading.

Direct contact Disease transmission via physical contact with an infected medium such as blood, secretions, or contaminated water.

Dislocation A bone slips out of joint and out of alignment.

Distal Directional term used to describe points farther away from the core of the trunk.

Diverticulitis Inflammatory disease caused by impacted diverticula that may lead to an obstructed colon, perforation, and hemorrhage; often associated with left side abdominal pain.

Do not resuscitate (DNR) An order refusing procedures such as CPR if the patient's heart stops or if the patient stops breathing.

DOTS Acronym assessment tool to remind the Emergency Medical Responder to check for deformities, open wounds, tenderness, and swelling during a secondary or rapid survey.

Dressing Sterile, absorbent material placed directly over a wound to control bleeding and protect the open wound from further injury and contamination.

DRGERM An acronym to guide the Emergency Medical Responder in performing a patient assessment by checking for distension, rigidity, guarding, evisceration, rebound tenderness, and pulsating masses.

Drowning Suffocation and death resulting from filling the lungs with water, fluid, or other substances so that gas exchange becomes impossible.

Drug tolerance A decreasing response to repeated constant doses of a drug or the need for increasing doses to maintain a constant response.

Dyspnea Breathlessness or shortness of breath.

Ecchymosis A pooling of blood under the skin, such as a contusion (bruise).

Eclampsia Preeclampsia with seizures.

Ectopic pregnancy Pregnancy in which the fertilized egg implants somewhere outside the uterus, usually in a fallopian tube.

Edema Swelling due to fluid leaving the vessels and entering the body's tissues.

Elastic bandages Bandages that stretch and are self-adhering, secured with tape, or have Velcro or metal fasteners.

Electrocardiogram (ECG or EKG) A recording of the electrical activities of the heart graphically displayed on an oscilloscope or printed on paper.

Emancipated minor A minor who is married, pregnant, in the military, or financially independent and no longer lives with a parent or guardian and is legally responsible for his or her own decisions and consequences of those decisions.

Embolism A thrombus that moves.

Embryo A developing human from the fourth day after fertilization to the end of the eighth week.

Emergency Medical Responder (EMR) A person who has special training in emergency medicine for pre-hospital care. Training includes basic assessment and management, simple airway management, oxygen administration, bleeding control, CPR, and use of an AED.

Emergency Medical Services (EMS) Coordinated network of professionals whose function is to provide a variety of medical services, such as out-of-hospital medical and trauma care and transportation for those in need of emergency care.

Emergency Medical Technician (EMT) Responder, one level above Emergency Medical Responder, who has completed the basic entry level training for prehospital care and trained in expanded airway management and limited medication administration.

Emergency moves Rapid extrication of patients when the risk of harm (fire, flood, unstable vehicle, or gun fire) from the environment outweighs the risk of injury from the move.

Emergency Response Team (ERT) Group trained to handle emergency responses specific to the industry with whom they are employed.

Emesis Vomit.

Emotional intelligence The process of improving our strengths and weaknesses as we navigate our inner conflicts.

Empathy The identification with and understanding of the patient's situation, feelings, and emotions.

Emphysema Disorder in which air flow in the lower airways is restricted, directly affecting the elasticity of lung tissue. Loss of elasticity causes air to become trapped and the alveoli to become distended making it difficult to breathe air out.

Enhanced 9-1-1 9-1-1 system in which the operator receiving the call immediately sees the name and address associated with the telephone number and which fire, police, and rescue agencies serve that address.

Epidural hematoma The collection of blood often from an arterial bleed found outside of the dura mater just under the skull.

Epiglottis A small flap that closes over the trachea when swallowing is initiated, preventing food and fluids from going into the lungs.

Epiglottitis A bacterial infection characterized by a swollen, inflamed epiglottis that can cause upper airway obstruction.

Epilepsy A history of recurrent seizures in a patient.

Epistaxis A nosebleed.

Esophageal varices Dilated veins within the lining of the lower esophagus that may bleed profusely if they rupture.

Ethical behavior Doing what is right based on a set of moral principles and values.

Evisceration Protrusion of abdominal organs through a wound caused by traumatic injury, especially the bowel.

Exhalation The act of expelling air from the lungs.

Exposure control plan Written policies and procedures to prevent or document on-the-job exposure incidents, such as exposure to blood or airborne pathogens.

Expressed consent Act of a competent adult or emancipated minor verbally advising a medical provider to proceed with treatment.

FADE Acronym for incident and patient management, including facts, address facts, decide and act, evaluate.

FAST Four components of the Cincinnati Prehospital Stroke Scale that evaluate a potential stroke patient: Facial droop, arm drift, speech, time.

Fetus A developing human from nine weeks after fertilization until birth.

Figure-of-eight bandage Roller or elastic bandage that turns across itself like a figure-of-eight and holds a dressing on a joint or palm.

Fire-based EMS Emergency medical services provided by fire departments.

First Report of Exposure Form Used by the Emergency Medical Responder to document when, where, and how contact with blood or bodily fluids occurred.

Flail chest A free-floating chest wall segment due to two or more ribs fractured in two or more places.

Flexible splint Any material that can be formed to fit any body angle and then made rigid.

Fomites Inanimate objects such as door knobs, metal surfaces, hand towels, bedding, or equipment in the responding unit that can transmit disease.

Foreign body airway obstruction (FBAO) Any ingested object that is capable of causing airway blockage.

Fowler's position A semi-sitting position in which the person's head and chest are elevated between 45 and 60 degrees.

Frostbite Tissue damage resulting from exposure to freezing and subfreezing temperatures.

Full-thickness burn Involves all layers of skin; the most serious burn.

Gauze dressings Sterile cotton weave material placed over a wound.

Generalized seizure A seizure that involves the entire brain and results in loss of consciousness; also known in the past as a grand mal seizure.

Geriatrics The medical specialty dealing with aging adults 65 years of age and older.

Gestational diabetes mellitus A form of diabetes that occurs only in pregnant women who have no prior history and usually resolves after the birth of the baby.

Glasgow Coma Scale (GCS) A neurological scale used to quantify a patient's level of responsiveness; used to determine the extent of and urgency for transporting a patient with a traumatic brain injury.

Good Samaritan Law A law meant to provide legal protection for certain people who voluntarily administer emergency assistance to an injured or ill person in good faith and with reasonable care.

Hallucinations Thoughts and perceptions that have no basis in reality.

Hallucinogen A substance that induces hallucinations.

Hazardous materials (HAZMAT) A substance (biological or chemical) that has the potential to cause an exposed person illness, injury, or death.

Head-tilt, chin-lift method Maneuver used to open the airway, involving tilting the head back and lifting the jaw up.

Health care directive A legal document establishing the patient's written wishes for medical care in the event the patient becomes incapacitated.

Health Insurance Portability and Accountability Act (HIPAA) A law that governs protection of patient privacy, patient confidentiality, and security of patient health information.

Heart failure A condition in which the heart muscle is not strong enough to pump blood out of the heart as quickly as it enters. The blood backs up into the lungs and causes edema in other areas of the body.

Heat cramps Painful, involuntary muscle spasms caused by dehydration and exposure to heat.

Heat exhaustion A milder form of generalized heat-related illnesses characterized by multiple symptoms and often by dehydration.

Heat stroke A life-threatening form of heat-related illness that involves a rise in body temperature; the patient may exhibit symptoms of seizures, altered mental status, and coma. The body usually ceases to perspire.

Hematoma An accumulation of blood trapped under the skin or within a body compartment.

Hemorrhagic shock Hypoperfusion caused by a significant loss of blood.

Hemorrhagic stroke Stroke that involves a rupture of one of the cerebral vessels in the brain.

Hemostatic dressings Dressings that contain powders or other substances that promote clotting of the blood when applied directly on an open wound.

Hemothorax Accumulations of blood between the lung and chest wall.

High altitude cerebral edema Swelling of the brain as a result of hypoxia at high altitudes.

High efficiency particulate air filter (HEPA) mask A filtration mask intended to remove very small airborne contaminants.

High Fowler's position A position in which the person is sitting upright at 90 degrees.

Hormones Chemical messengers that travel in the bloodstream to tissues or organs.

Hyperglycemia A higher than normal level of glucose.

Hypertension A higher than normal blood pressure.

Hyperthermia Internal body temperature elevated above normal from overall heat gain that is greater than heat loss.

Hyperventilation Overbreathing exhibited by a patient's breathing faster and deeper than normal.

Hypoglycemia A lower than normal level of glucose.

Hypoperfusion Decreased blood flow through an organ; if prolonged, it may result in permanent cellular dysfunction and death.

Hypotension Lower than normal blood pressure.

Hypothermia A condition that occurs when a person's core body temperature falls below 95 degrees Fahrenheit.

Hypovolemic shock A form of shock in which severe blood and fluid loss make the heart unable to supply enough blood to the body.

Hypoxia Deficiency of adequate oxygen in the body.

Immunizations Inoculations that increase a person's resistance to certain infectious diseases by exposing the person to weakened or dead pathogens of a particular disease.

Impaled object A foreign object that penetrates the body and lodges in place.

Implied consent Legal presumption that a patient who is unable to verbally express agreement to treatment would agree to being treated in certain circumstances.

Incident Command System (ICS) A standardized, on-scene, all-hazard incident management concept that was originally designed for emergency scene management by public safety agencies. ICS is based on a flexible, scalable response organization providing a common framework within which people can work together effectively.

Incision Full-thickness wound; a cutting of the skin.

Infectious disease Any disease that can be transmitted from one person to another or from an animal to a person.

Inferior Body part reference meaning below. The head is superior to the chest, and the chin is inferior to the nose.

Informed consent Consent given by a responsive patient after an explanation of the risks and benefits of care or treatment has been given.

Inhalation Breathing in of air or substance through the nose or mouth, past the pharynx into the trachea (windpipe), and then into the lungs as the diaphragm is pulled down by abdominal muscles or the intercostal chest muscles, causing the chest to expand; a transmission route for airborne pathogens.

In loco parentis Someone with the authority to act on the behalf of a minor in the place of a parent.

Inoculation Direct entry of pathogens into the body through a break in the skin such as through open wounds, needle sticks, or animal bites.

Insulin A hormone produced by the pancreas that allows glucose utilization by the body.

Insulin shock Severe hypoglycemia induced by too much insulin administration or too little food intake.

Intracranial pressure (ICP) The pressure within the skull.

Ischemic stroke The injury of tissue in the brain that occurs as a result of a blockage of the vessel that normally supplies that tissue with blood.

Jaw thrust maneuver A method of opening the airway for a potential cervical spinal cord injury.

Jugular venous distension (JVD) Extended jugular veins in the sides of the neck.

JumpSTART triage A triage system that uses the assessment techniques specifically for infants and children.

Ketones Acids created by ineffective metabolism involving the breakdown of fats.

Knowledge-based errors Errors occurring when the Emergency Medical Responder (EMR) does not have the information needed to accomplish the skill. These mistakes occur when the EMR has not had the opportunity to receive the training or has failed to take advantage of new skills that are available.

Kussmaul respirations Deep, labored, almost sighing respirations seen with DKA.

Labor The childbirth process by which the uterus expels the fetus and placenta.

Laceration A type of wound characterized by a full-thickness tear in the skin.

Landing zone (LZ) An area intended for the purpose of landing and taking off in a helicopter.

Lateral Directional term used to describe the side of a structure; areas farther from the midline.

Lateral recumbent Lying on one's side.

Level of consciousness (LOC) The measure of a person's response to stimuli.

Ligaments Connective tissue that connects bone to bone.

Lumbar vertebrae Five vertebrae that make up the lower back and support the weight of the entire upper body.

Manual suction A suctioning unit that is inserted into the oral cavity and suctions secretions as the device is manually squeezed or pumped.

Mechanical suction A suction device that operates on a battery or other power source.

Mechanism of injury or illness (MOI) The event that causes a patient's injury or illness.

Meconium Newborn feces.

Medial A directional term meaning areas closer to the midline or middle of the body.

Medical director A person of highest medical authority who provides direction of on-scene activities, establishes written protocols for emergency medical services providers and grants variances to individual providers that allow them to exceed their standard scope of practice.

Medical oversight Written and verbal instructions for prehospital patient care by the medical director.

Medical patient A patient who verbalizes or appears to have a disease, illness, or reaction.

Meninges Membranes, consisting of three layers, that encase the brain, brainstem, and spinal cord, keeping the cerebrospinal fluid in place.

Midaxillary line Marker that runs from the middle of the axilla to the center of the waist.

Midline The line that runs directly through the center of the body vertically and divides the body into left and right.

Military compresses Dressing and bandage in one package. Has attached "tails" to secure the dressing to the wound.

Miscarriage Spontaneous, unintentional termination of a pregnancy.

Modified Trendelenburg position Position in which a person is lying supine with the legs elevated 12 to 16 inches; also known as shock position.

Motor vehicle collision (MVC) When a vehicle forcefully strikes another vehicle or object. Formerly referred to as a car accident.

Mottling Skin discoloration that is blotchy or patchy in appearance.

Multiple-casualty incident (MCI) An emergency incident with a patient load that overwhelms the immediately available resources of the first emergency medical services responder(s) who arrives on the scene.

Myocardial infarction (MI) Inadequate perfusion of the myocardium (heart muscle) that can cause death or damage to the myocardium. Also known as a heart attack.

Narcotic A drug or chemical agent that blocks pain but also can produce insensibility or stupor.

Nasal cannula A soft, flexible tube with two nasal prongs that can be inserted into the patient's nostrils to deliver oxygen.

Nasopharyngeal airway (NPA) A tube designed to be inserted into the nasal passageway to secure an open airway for a patient by helping to hold the tongue off the back of the throat; also called a nasal airway.

National Highway Traffic Safety Administration (NHTSA) A division of the U.S. Department of Transportation that was established to make national highways safer and sets standards for training in emergency services.

National Incident Management System (NIMS) Derived from the Incident Command System, a structured but flexible framework used nationwide for agencies to respond to disasters, natural or human made, at the local, state, and federal levels of government.

National Registry of Emergency Medical Technicians (NREMT) A certification agency established to standardize minimum training requirements and is the recognized testing agency for emergency medical services professionals and accepted by most states and jurisdictions.

Nature of illness (NOI) The cause or history of an illness or medical emergency; analogous to MOI in trauma.

Near drowning Survival after any amount of time submerged in water.

Necrosis Premature death of living cells or body tissue.

Neglect Failure to provide for the basic needs of a dependent person.

Negligence The failure to provide care in a manner that upholds accepted medical practices and standards of care.

Neonate Newborn infant up to one month of age.

Neurogenic shock Hypoperfused state resulting from injury to the spinal cord and generalized vasodilation.

Neutral inline alignment The natural anatomical position of the head and neck with the eyes looking forward and the chin at a 90-degree angle from the long axis of the body.

9-1-1 system The United States' national emergency number.

Non-adherent dressing Dressing with a special coating that does not allow the dressing to stick to a wound.

Non-emergency moves Moving a patient when there is enough time to plan and execute a patient transfer.

Non-rebreather (NRB) mask An oxygen mask that covers the nose and mouth of the patient and delivers up to 100% oxygen when used at a rate of 10 to 15 liters per minute.

Objective information Data that can be observed and measured.

Obstetrics (OB) A medical specialty involving pregnancy and childbirth.

Occlusive dressings Dressings that do not allow air or secretion penetration.

Occupational Safety and Health Administration (OSHA) A governmental agency created to maintain a safe and healthy work environment.

Open fracture Broken bone in which a bone end at any point has erupted through the skin or an object has penetrated the skin causing a fracture.

Operations The safe application of strategy, tactics, and resources at the site of an emergency incident with the goal of mitigating and resolving the event.

OPQRST An acronym tool to describe a detailed pain assessment. Stands for onset, provocation, quality, region and radiation, severity, and time.

Oropharyngeal airway (oral airway or OPA) A device inserted in the mouth used to maintain a patent airway by keeping the tongue off the back of the throat; also called an oral airway.

Oropharynx Section of the throat that is in the back of the mouth.

Osteoporosis Loss of bone density caused by a progressive loss of calcium, leading to fractures after minimal trauma.

Oxygen (O_2) A colorless, odorless gas required by the body to function normally.

Oxygen regulator A device placed on an oxygen tank that regulates or controls the flow of oxygen to the tubing that leads to the nose of the patient or can be connected to a barrier device to provide positive pressure ventilation.

Oxygen tank A storage vessel for oxygen, which is either held under pressure in gas cylinders or as liquid oxygen and identified by the tank's green color, the national color designated by the U.S. Department of Transportation.

Package To prepare for transport.

Pallor Pale skin color.

Palpate To feel with your hands.

Pancreatitis Inflammation of the pancreas characterized by abdominal pain and often vomiting.

Paradoxical respiration Bilateral movement of a flail chest segment in a direction opposite to that of the rest of the chest wall.

Paramedic The highest level of training for prehospital providers. A paramedic must have advanced life support training in airway management, cardiac monitoring, and administration of medications.

Paraplegia Paralysis of the lower body. Involvement is dependent on the severity and location of spinal cord injury in the thoracic or lumbar area of the spine.

Parasympathetic nervous system A part of the autonomic nervous system that governs the rest-and-repose response; slows body responses and balances against the sympathetic nervous system to maintain a moderation in those responses.

Parietal pain Localized, intense, sharp, constant pain associated with irritation of the peritoneum.

Partial seizure A seizure that affects a limited area of the brain and can be simple to complex.

Partial thickness burn Burn that affects the epidermis and dermal layers of skin.

Patent An unobstructed opening, as in a vessel or passageway.

Pathogens Microscopic organisms such as bacteria, viruses, or parasites that can invade the body and cause disease.

Pathophysiology The study of functional changes associated with or resulting from injury or disease.

Patient advocate A person who makes sure that the care a patient receives is in the patient's best interest.

Patient care report (PCR) A legal written record of the patient's condition and the care that was provided during the patient encounter.

Patient data The second component of the patient care report containing the patient's complaint, medical information, assessment, mechanism of injury or nature of illness, vital signs, and interventions.

Pedal pulse A peripheral pulse located on the top of the foot used to assess for perfusion; also known as the dorsalis pedis pulse.

Pediatric assessment triangle (PAT) A pediatric observational tool for quickly and visually assessing a patient's appearance, work of breathing, and circulation to the skin.

Pediatric Glasgow Coma Scale (PGCS) A scale that is used to quantify a pediatric patient's level of responsiveness.

Pediatrics Branch of medicine that deals with children, the development and care of children, and the nature and treatment of diseases of children.

PENMAN Acronym for personal and personnel safety, environmental hazards, number of victims, mechanism of injury, additional resources needed from your agency, and need for resources outside of your agency.

Peptic ulcer An open sore in the lining of the stomach (gastric ulcer), duodenum (duodenal ulcer), or esophagus (esophageal ulcer).

Perfusion Supply of oxygenated blood to organs or tissues throughout the body.

Peripheral A directional term used to describe points farther away from the core of the body.

Peripheral nervous system Nerves that originate in the spinal cord and transmit messages to and from the body's organs and tissues.

Peripheral pulses Pulses on the extremities, farther away from the core of the body, such as the radial or brachial pulses.

Peristalsis Series of rhythmic contractions that move food from the stomach and through the bowels.

PERRL An acronym to report the results of an eye examination: pupils equal, round, and reactive to light.

Personal accountability report (PAR) Request for all personnel on the scene to verbally or physically check in with the scene supervisor.

Personal health The state of a person's physical, medical, and psychological well-being.

Personal protective equipment (PPE) Specialized clothing or equipment worn by employees for protection against health and safety hazards when caring for all patients.

Physiology Study of the functions and activities of life or living matter.

Placenta Interface between the uterus and the fetus.

Plasma The liquid part of blood.

Pleural space The space between the lung and the chest wall.

Pneumatic splint A splint that conforms to the shape of the injury as it becomes rigid with air by either inflation or vacuum.

Pneumothorax Air in the pleural space potentially causing a collapsed lung.

Pocket mask A barrier device that covers the mouth and nose mask that is used to deliver rescue breaths during a cardiac arrest or respiratory arrest.

Policies Written guidelines informing Emergency Medical Responders of what is expected and what is not allowed.

Position of comfort Position that the patient independently assumes for comfort and for ease of breathing.

Position of function Natural functional position of the hand or foot.

Posterior aspect Directional term referring to a location toward the back.

Posterior tibial pulse Peripheral pulse located below and behind the medial malleolus (the bone that projects at the end of the tibia past the ankle) and is used to assess perfusion.

Postictal phase Phase after seizure activity during which the patient may be confused, sleepy, and exhausted.

Preeclampsia A condition of pregnancy marked by high blood pressure and excess protein in the urine after 20 weeks of pregnancy.

Priapism A prolonged erection of the penis, most often indicative of a spinal cord injury.

Primary survey Systematic assessment of life-threatening conditions including the patient's level of consciousness and ABC's.

Private EMS Emergency medical services in place to handle ambulance services that are both for-profit and not-for-profit operations and may or may not work in conjunction with public services.

Procedures Written, employer-required steps to follow when providing patient care.

Professionalism Behavior, goals, or qualities such as a skilled, caring, confident, and courteous demeanor that characterize a medical professional.

Projectile vomiting Vomiting that is ejected with force.

Prolapsed umbilical cord Presentation of the umbilical cord before the infant, resulting in compression of the cord.

Prone Position when a patient is lying face down.

Protocols Medical guidelines established by an agency's medical director or by a regulatory authority that play an important role in the delivery of emergency medical services.

Proximal A directional term referring to a location closer to the center of the body. The elbow is proximal to the wrist but distal to the shoulder.

Public EMS Emergency medical services provided by a city, county, or other political subdivision that may be funded by a combination of user fees and taxes. These services may be provided as part of a local fire or police department or a third service.

Public safety answering point (PSAP) Local dispatch office staffed with professionals employed to receive 9-1-1 calls from the public and dispatch the required service to the caller as soon as possible.

Pulmonary edema An accumulation of fluid in the lungs.

Pulmonary embolism A blood clot that travels to the lungs and blocks an artery in the lungs.

Pulse The palpable feeling of blood flow through a superficial artery; count of the heartbeat.

Pulse oximeter A device that measures the heart rate and the percentage of oxygen being carried by hemoglobin in the blood.

Puncture wound A wound created by an object that penetrates the skin.

Quadriplegia Paralysis of trunk muscles and muscles of the extremities resulting from a cervical fracture.

Quality assurance (QA) The monitoring and evaluation of all aspects of emergency medical services (EMS) to ensure or improve the quality care the EMS system provides.

Quality improvement (QI) A formal review and analysis of performance and processes within the emergency medical services agency with the goal of reducing medical errors and needless loss of life.

Quality management Ensures not only the quality of the service but also the means by which to achieve the highest quality of service; includes quality assessment and quality improvement.

Raccoon eyes Bruising around the eyes that may indicate a skull fracture.

Radial pulse Pulse found in the wrist.

Rapid survey or secondary survey A secondary survey is a head-to-toe assessment using palpation and visualization. A rapid survey is a secondary survey that is performed as quickly as possible on an unstable or potentially unstable trauma or medical patient.

Rapport A relationship with the patient based on trust in which good communication is possible.

Recovery position Position in which the patient is placed on the side so that secretions may spontaneously drain from the airway; also known as the lateral recumbent position.

Recurrent bandage Roller or elastic bandage used to hold a dressing in place over a large area and consists of turns on top of each other.

Red blood cells (RBCs) Hemoglobin carrying blood cells that deliver oxygen to the tissues.

Referred pain Pain that is felt at a location away from the source.

Rescue breathing The act of assisting respirations in a person who is not breathing or not breathing normally.

Research data The collection of data about emergency medical services calls, including types of illnesses or injuries, date and time of calls, treatment given, and equipment used.

Respiration The act of breathing.

Respiratory compromise Being physically able to inhale and exhale air but not receiving adequate oxygenation with one's own effort.

Respiratory rate (RR) The number of respirations per minute.

Rigid splint Any firm material that can provide support for a limb.

Roller bandage Cotton cloth, usually gauze, rolled into a cylinder for easier control when unwrapping.

Rule-based errors Errors occurring when policies and procedures are not followed.

Rule of nines Formula to determine the percentage of burnt skin.

Sacral vertebrae Five strong vertebrae that close the pelvic ring posteriorly.

Safety and wellness Maintaining physical, emotional, and psychological health on the job.

SAMPLE An acronym to remember important questions to ask for a basic history: signs and symptoms, allergies, medications, past medical history, last oral intake, and events leading up to the incident or illness.

Scope of practice The legal description of the limit of care that an emergency medical services (EMS) provider can give based on the provider's EMS training level and certification.

Search and Rescue (SAR) Organized and disciplined approach to the rescue of the injured, ill, or lost persons.

Secondary cord injury (SCI) A spinal cord injury that is the result of moving a patient with an injury.

Secondary drowning Can take place within 24 to 48 hours of near drowning. Even a small amount of water can collect back into the lungs and cause hypoxia.

Seizure Sudden, abnormal electrical activity in the brain that results in involuntary movements and sometimes loss of consciousness.

Septic shock Hypoperfused state resulting from overwhelming infection and generalized vasodilation.

Sexual assault Physical and psychological trauma to a person of a sexual nature.

Sharps Any items with corners, edges, or projections capable of piercing the skin.

Shock A medical emergency in which organs and tissues of the body are not receiving an adequate flow of blood, resulting in inadequate oxygenation of cells, tissues, and organs.

Short spinal immobilization device (SSID) A short backboard used to temporarily stabilize a patient's spine while transferring him or her to a long backboard.

Skill-based errors Errors occurring because the Emergency Medical Responder failed to follow the correct procedures required to do the skill.

Sling A triangular bandage used to support a fractured arm.

SOAP An acronym for components of documentation: subjective, objective, assessment, and plan.

Social intelligence The state of being intelligent, not just about relationships, but also in them.

Span of control The number of personnel that any position can supervise.

Spinal cord The collection of nerves that run from the brain through the spinal column and branch out as peripheral nerves to the body organs and tissues.

Spinal stabilization Immobilization of the entire spine to prevent further injury and paralysis.

Spiral bandage Roller or elastic bandage that wraps around an extremity, overlapping by half the width of the bandage on each turn.

Sprain An injury to ligaments that is caused by being stretched beyond normal capacity and possibly torn.

Standard anatomical position Facing forward with the legs slightly apart, the feet pointing forward, the arms straight and extended a few inches away from the side, and the palms facing forward.

Standard precautions Methods designed to reduce the risk of transmission of microorganisms from both known and unknown sources of infection.

START Triage system developed to manage victims (simple triage and rapid treatment).

Status epilepticus A potentially life-threatening situation in which the patient has a seizure lasting longer than five minutes or a second seizure occurs after the first without a lucid period between them.

Sternum The bony structure in the center of the chest, also known as the breastbone.

Stimulants Any substance that increases brain activity resulting in alteration of mental, physical, or emotional function.

Stoma Surgically created opening in the body.

Strain An injury to a muscle in which the muscle fibers tear as a result of overstretching.

Straddle injury A soft tissue injury that occurs to the genitals when they are impacted by a fixed object.

Stress management Any method used to control the factors causing stress.

Stroke Disruption of blood flow to part of the brain caused by a blockage or hemorrhage of a blood vessel in the brain.

Subdural hematoma A collection of blood within the subdural space of the skull caused by the tearing of small veins that run between the brain surface and the dura mater.

Subjective information Information offered by a person or patient that is not objectively verifiable.

Substance abuse The use of chemical substances that are not prescribed or are not taken as prescribed.

Substance misuse Taking a substance that was prescribed but not for the purpose intended.

Sucking chest wound An opening in the outside of the chest through which air is moving, creating bubbling or sucking sounds.

Suction catheter A long tube used to remove secretions from the airway.

Sudden infant death syndrome (SIDS) The sudden, unexplained death of an infant in the first year of life.

Sunset clause Requirement that policies and procedures be reviewed every three to five years or as they expire to keep them updated.

Superficial burns Involves the epidermis; a mild sunburn is an example.

Superior A directional term used to refer to a location toward the top of an object. The head is superior to the chest, and the chin is on the inferior part of the head.

Supine Position in which a person is lying face up with the spine to the ground.

Swathe A triangular bandage or cloth folded into a band and used to secure a sling in place.

Sympathetic nervous system A part of the autonomic nervous system that governs the fight-or-flight response.

Synergy When a combination of chemical substances are used causing an intensity of the effect.

Synovial fluid The fluid in a joint that acts as a lubricant.

Systolic blood pressure The amount of force on the vessels when the heart contracts and pushes the blood out of the heart into the system, represented by the top number of the blood pressure reading.

Tachycardia A faster than normal heart rate.

Tachypnea A faster than normal respiratory rate.

Task fixated Being so focused or engaged on an observed object or the accomplishment of a task that awareness of other obstacles or hazards can diminish.

Tendons Connective tissue that attaches muscle to bone.

Tension pneumothorax An increasing collection of air in the pleural space, resulting in collapse of the lung on the affected side and shifting of the heart and other thoracic structures to the uninvolved side.

Third service An emergency medical service not integrated within other agencies such as fire or police, which may serve as the primary or backup responder.

Thoracic cavity The chest cavity; the cavity enclosed within the rib cage where the heart and lungs are located. Also termed the thorax.

Thoracic vertebrae The 12 vertebrae found below the cervical spine and above the lumbar spine; these are attached to the 12 sets of ribs.

Thready pulse Weak and rapid pulse.

360-degree incident assessment An incident size-up technique that reinforces safety by requiring the first and subsequent arriving emergency responders to consider the incident from all angles while looking for safety hazards.

Tonic-clonic seizure Seizure phases in which the patient's muscles relax only to contract again; the jerking phase.

Thrombus Blood clot.

TIC An acronym for tenderness, instability, and crepitus.

Tourniquets A constricting band that stops blood flow to a limb to control major bleeding.

Trachea A cartilaginous tube that is the passageway for air to get from the upper airway to the lungs also known as the windpipe.

Tracheal deviation Positioning of the trachea away from the midline of the neck.

Tracheostomy A surgical opening made in the anterior neck and into the trachea for breathing.

Tracheostomy tube A rigid tube that is inserted into a tracheostomy; also called a trach.

Traction splint A splint that provides a continuous pull along the axis of the bone.

Trauma center An acute care facility that has made special preparations and achieved certain resource and personnel standards to provide care for severely injured patients.

Trauma dressings Large cotton dressings that usually consist of two or more layers of gauze with an absorbent cotton core, large enough to cover major wounds.

Trauma patient A patient who has an injury that may or may not be visible.

Traumatic amputation A body part that is partially or fully pulled away because of trauma.

Traumatic brain injury (TBI) An injury to the brain from a direct cause (penetrating trauma), an indirect cause (blow to the skull), or a secondary cause (hypoxia).

Trending Obtaining multiple sets of vital signs to determine if the patient is improving, staying the same, or getting worse.

Triage A rapid system of distribution of patients into treatment classifications according to their injury severity.

Triangular bandages Triangular pieces of muslin or cotton cloth used to hold dressings on the head or other large areas of the body in place.

Tripod position A position maintained by a person with severe breathing difficulties with the upper body leaning slightly forward, arms straight, and hands supporting the upper body by resting on the legs or a table.

Universal dressings 9- by 36-inch gauze dressing with several layers of absorbent cotton used to control a major bleed.

Universal precautions Method for reducing the risk of transmission of bloodborne pathogens.

Urethra Tube through which urine exits the body.

Vectors Living things such as mosquitoes, flies, fleas, and ticks that can transmit disease.

Veins Vessels that lead to the heart carrying deoxygenated blood.

Ventricles Two lower chambers of the heart. The primary pump chambers.

Ventricular fibrillation (VF) Electrical signals in the ventricles that are disorganized, causing the heart to quiver and be unable to pump an adequate blood for perfusion.

Ventricular tachycardia (VT) Electrical signals to the ventricles that fire too fast and do not allow the heart to fill adequately with blood.

Venuoles Tiny vessels that connect the capillaries and veins.

Vertebrae Individual bones of the spine.

Victim generator A dynamic incident component that continues to produce victims.

Visceral pain Pain that is poorly localized, more general in nature, and originates from an organ.

Vital signs Heart rate, respirations, blood pressure, and temperature.

Vulnerable patient Individuals with disabilities who are susceptible to injury or illness or at risk for abuse because of existing health conditions, impairments, age, or dementia.

White blood cells (WBCs) One of the cells in the blood that fights infection in the body.

Withdrawal symptoms The unpleasant physical and psychological effects experienced by a drug-addicted patient when the drug use is discontinued.

Xiphoid process Narrow cartilage tip at the bottom of the sternum.

Yankauer suction catheter A rigid suction catheter used to remove thick pharyngeal secretions or blood from the mouth.

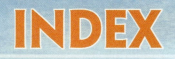

INDEX

Note: f indicates figure, t indicates table, and italicized numbers indicate skill building exercises